Obesity prevention and public health

Obesity prevention and public health

Edited by

David Crawford
Centre for Physical Activity and Nutrition Research
Deakin University, Australia

and

Robert W. Jeffery
Division of Epidemiology and Community Health
School of Public Health
University of Minnesota, USA

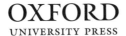

OXFORD
UNIVERSITY PRESS

OXFORD

UNIVERSITY PRESS

Great Clarendon Street, Oxford OX2 6DP

Oxford University Press is a department of the University of Oxford.
It furthers the University's objective of excellence in research, scholarship,
and education by publishing worldwide in

Oxford New York

Auckland Cape Town Dar es Salaam Hong Kong Karachi
Kuala Lumpur Madrid Melbourne Mexico City Nairobi
New Delhi Shanghai Taipei Toronto

With offices in

Argentina Austria Brazil Chile Czech Republic France Greece
Guatemala Hungary Italy Japan South Korea Poland Portugal
Singapore Switzerland Thailand Turkey Ukraine Vietnam

Oxford is a registered trade mark of Oxford University Press
in the UK and in certain other countries

Published in the United States
by Oxford University Press Inc., New York

© Oxford University Press, 2005

A catalogue record for this title is available from the British Library

Library of Congress Cataloging in Publication Data

(Data available)

ISBN 0 19 856600 X   978-019-856600-7
10 9 8 7 6 5 4 3 2 1

Typeset by Cepha Imaging Pvt. Ltd., Bangalore, India

Printed in Great Britain

on acid-free paper by Biddles Ltd, King's Lynn

Acknowledgements

We would like to begin by thanking Oxford University Press for initiating this edited volume. This book is timely and we feel confident it will make an important scholarly contribution to the ongoing debate regarding obesity prevention. We are particularly grateful for the guidance and support provided by Helen Liepman, Tania Pickering, Charlotte Owen, and Kate Martin at OUP.

David Crawford would like to acknowledge all of his colleagues in the Behavioral Epidemiology Program at the Centre for Physical Activity and Nutrition Research, Deakin University. In particular, I would like to recognize Kylie Ball, Karen Campbell, Jo Salmon, Anna Timperio, and Tony Worsley. It is their passion and commitment to research that has inspired me and allowed me to remain focused on obesity research over a prolonged period. Thanks to Bianca Brijnath who provided expert administrative assistance in the final stages of our editing. I would also like to acknowledge the National Health and Medical Research Council and the National Heart Foundation of Australia for their support via a Career Development Award.

Robert Jeffery would like to acknowledge the support and encouragement of numerous colleagues at the University of Minnesota, including especially Sally Miles and Kerrin Brelje for their invaluable administrative and clerical support, Judy Baxter, Carolyn Thorson, Emily Finch and many others who together have been such an effective research team and host of professional colleagues who have been a never-ending source of inspiration and assistance over many years, especially Simone French, Mary Story, Jennifer Linde, Nancy Sherwood, Katie Schmitz, and Lisa Harnack. Financial support for this book has come from the University of Minnesota Obesity Prevention Center, the Minnesota Obesity Center, and the University of Minnesota School of Public Health.

Contents

Contributors ix

Introduction xi

Part 1

1 The epidemiology of obesity: a global perspective 3
  Jacob C. Seidell

2 The role of nutrition and physical activity in the obesity epidemic 21
  Lisa J. Harnack and Kathryn H. Schmitz

3 The role of socio-cultural factors in the obesity epidemic 37
  Kylie Ball and David Crawford

4 Evolving environmental factors in the obesity epidemic 55
  Robert W. Jeffery and Jennifer A. Linde

5 The implications of the nutrition transition for obesity in the developing world 75
  Barry M. Popkin

Part 2

6 Population approaches to promote healthful eating behaviors 101
  Simone A. French

7 Population approaches to increasing physical activity among children and adults 129
  Jo Salmon and Abby C. King

8 Population approaches to obesity prevention 153
  Robert W. Jeffery and Jennifer A. Linde

9 The cost-effectiveness of obesity prevention 165
  Rob Carter and Marj Moodie

Part 3

10 Opportunities to prevent obesity in children within families: an ecological approach 207
  Kirsten Krahnstoever Davison and Karen Campbell

11 Drawing possible lessons for obesity prevention and control from the tobacco control experience 231
Shawna L. Mercer, Laura Kettel Khan, Lawrence W. Green, Abby C. Rosenthal, Rose Nathan, Corinne G. Husten, and William H. Dietz

12 The potential for policy initiatives to address the obesity epidemic: a legal perspective from the United States 265
Ellen J. Fried

13 The potential of food regulation as a policy instrument for obesity prevention in developing countries 285
Mark Lawrence

14 The need for courageous action to prevent obesity 307
Marlene B. Schwarz and Kelly D. Brownell

Index 331

Contributors

Kylie Ball
Centre for Physical Activity and
 Nutrition Research
Deakin University, Melbourne, Australia

Kelly D. Brownell
Department of Psychology
Yale University
New Haven, CT, USA

Karen Campbell
Centre for Physical Activity and
 Nutrition Research
Deakin University
Melbourne, Australia

Rob Carter
Program Evaluation Unit
School of Population Health
University of Melbourne
Melbourne, Australia

David Crawford
Centre for Physical Activity and
 Nutrition Research
Deakin University, Melbourne, Australia

Kirsten Krahnstoever Davison
School of Public Health
University of Albany (SUNY)
Albany, NY, USA

William H. Dietz
Division of Nutrition and
 Physical Activity
National Center for Chronic
 Disease Prevention and
 Health Promotion

Centers for Disease Control and
 Prevention
Atlanta, GA, USA

Simone A. French
Division of Epidemiology and
 Community Health
School of Public Health
University of Minnesota
Minneapolis, MN, USA

Ellen J. Fried
Department of Nutrition, Food Studies,
 and Public Health
New York University
New York, NY, USA

Lawrence W. Green
Department of Epidemiology &
 Biostatistics
University of California at San Franciso
San Francisco, CA, USA

Lisa J. Harnack
Division of Epidemiology and
 Community Health
School of Public Health
University of Minnesota
Minneapolis, MN, USA

Corinne G. Husten
Office on Smoking and Health
National Center for Chronic Disease
 Prevention and Health Promotion
Centers for Disease Control and
 Prevention
Atlanta, GA, USA

Robert W. Jeffery
Division of Epidemiology and
    Community Health
School of Public Health
University of Minnesota
Minneapolis, MN, USA

Laura Kettel Khan
Division of Nutrition and Physical
    Activity
National Center for Chronic Disease
    Prevention and Health Promotion
Centers for Disease Control and
    Prevention
Atlanta, GA, USA

Abby C. King
Stanford Prevention Research Center
Stanford University School of Medicine
Stanford, CA, USA

Mark Lawrence
Centre for Physical Activity and
    Nutrition Research
Deakin University
Melbourne, Australia

Jennifer A. Linde
Division of Epidemiology and
    Community Health
School of Public Health
University of Minnesota
Minneapolis, MN, USA

Shawna L. Mercer
Office of the Chief Science Officer
Centers for Disease Control and
    Prevention
Atlanta, GA, USA

Marj Moodie
Program Evaluation Unit
School of Population Health
University of Melbourne
Melbourne, Australia

Rose Nathan
National Center for Environmental
    Health
Centers for Disease Control and
    Prevention
Atlanta, GA, USA

Barry M. Popkin
Carolina Population Center
University of North Carolina at
    Chapel Hill
Chapel Hill, NC, USA

Abby C. Rosenthal
Office on Smoking and Health
National Center for Chronic Disease
    Prevention and Health Promotion
Centers for Disease Control and
    Prevention
Atlanta, GA, USA

Jo Salmon
Centre for Physical Activity and
    Nutrition Research
Deakin University
Melbourne, Australia

Kathryn H. Schmitz
Division of Epidemiology and
    Community Health
School of Public Health
University of Minnesota
Minneapolis, MN, USA

Marlene B. Schwartz
Department of Psychology
Yale University
New Haven, CT, USA

Jacob C. Seidell
Department for Nutrition and Health
Faculty of Earth and Life Sciences & VU
    University Medical Center
Free University of Amsterdam
Amsterdam, The Netherlands

Introduction

It would be difficult to imagine that there is anyone currently working in health or medical fields who is unaware of the obesity pandemic, its impact on population health, or the debates surrounding its causes and prevention. We enter the 21st century with up to one in four children and adolescents, and more that half of the adults in most developed countries, classified as overweight or obese. Of particular concern is the emerging data clearly showing that the epidemic is not confined to developed countries, with many developing countries and those in transition also affected. There is no disputing that obesity poses a major population health challenge – it is an important contributor to disability and disease, the health costs associated with obesity are substantial, and, as already noted, obesity has reached epidemic proportions in many countries with the incidence continuing to increase in children and adults.

Although recognized clinically for at least the past 50 years as an important condition that increases risk of ill-health in affected individuals, it was only relatively recently, since the release of the World Health Organization's report in 1998, that obesity has become recognized internationally as a serious threat to public health that requires preventive action across whole communities. While now accepted by health authorities as a major population health issue, our understanding of the specific causes of the obesity epidemic is poor, we possess inconsistent and inadequate surveillance systems for obesity and related behaviors, and there has been relatively little population-based research that has focused on the prevention of unhealthy weight gain. The consequence of our overall ignorance is that the ability of public health officials to recommend how and where best to intervene is limited.

The aim of this book is to provide public health professionals (researchers, practitioners, and policy makers) with a scholarly text that provides them with a 'state of the science' overview of the epidemiology of the world-wide obesity epidemic and the case for prevention. It reviews the definitions and trends in obesity world wide; it examines what is known about the causes of the rapid, recent upward trend; and it reviews the existing evidence regarding the effectiveness of intervention strategies in different settings and with different target groups. Expert views are also offered on the potential opportunities for obesity prevention.

This book draws upon the existing literature and expertise with a view to helping set the agenda for future public health action to halt and reverse trends in population obesity. We have brought together some of the most distinguished and experienced scholars on the topic of public health aspects of obesity, in an effort to provide a clear statement about the world-wide growth of obesity as major threat to health, its causes and approaches to stemming its growth, and starting us toward more healthy body weights. The book is intended to be scholarly in the sense of basing its exposition on the best available data and the best available scientific methods. Because the study of the obesity epidemic is so new, however, and because the immediate public health need is so great, we have asked the contributing authors to draw conclusions to the best of their ability on what practical courses of action might best contribute to improvements in the public health problem now. Those recommendations relate to future directions for research, education, demonstration projects, and/or policy debate.

Organization of the book

The book is divided into three parts. Part 1 provides an overview of the context of the problem. Chapter 1 focuses on the epidemiology of obesity. It discusses the assessment and definition of overweight and obesity, and describes the obesity pandemic, drawing upon the latest international prevalence and trend data available for children and adults. The chapter also provides an overview of the health outcomes associated with obesity, and the economic impact of obesity. In Chapter 2, Harnack and Schmitz examine temporal trends in energy intake and energy expenditure, using the US as a case study. They focus particularly on the quality of the available data and discuss its limitations. Chapter 3 provides an overview of socio-cultural influences which impact on obesity, and considers the pathways through which these influences may operate. The authors also speculate about the likely impact of societal trends on future rates and patterns of obesity and the implications for obesity prevention. Chapter 4 presents a thought-provoking review of available data on environmental factors that may have contributed to trends in population body weight over the past 30 years. In addition to traditional epidemiological data on energy intake and expenditure, the authors take a novel approach by drawing upon a variety of other information from the public and private sectors. The implications of the nutrition transition for obesity in the developing world are discussed by Popkin in Chapter 5.

Part 2 focuses on the existing evidence regarding strategies to promote healthful eating, increase physical activity, and prevent population obesity. As well as reviewing intervention research across key settings and in different population groups, Part 2 includes an exploration of the economics of obesity prevention. In Chapter 6, French presents an overview of the state of the science of population-based interventions to promote healthful food choices. In doing so she identifies the most promising strategies to promote population-wide healthful food choices and dietary intake. Chapter 7 provides an overview of the latest evidence for population approaches to increasing physical activity in children, adolescents, and young, mid-life, and older adults, and discusses emerging issues and future directions for physical activity promotion. In Chapter 8, Jeffery and Linde review the limited available empirical work that has attempted to address obesity treatment and/or prevention in entire populations. In the final chapter in Part 2, Carter and Moodie present an analysis of the economics of obesity prevention, focusing particularly on the evidence of the cost-effectiveness of interventions and how the economic credentials for obesity prevention might be further developed.

Part 3 explores a range of novel approaches to tackle the obesity pandemic in the developed and developing world. In Chapter 10, Davison and Campbell consider the opportunities to prevent childhood obesity within families. They examine the context of parenting and the relationship between parenting and obesity-risk behaviors and suggest ways that parents might foster healthful behaviors among children, and how practitioners and policy makers can support parents' efforts. In Chapter 11, Mercer and her colleagues draw lessons from the successes of the tobacco control experience for the organization of more successful efforts to reduce and prevent obesity. The potential of legal approaches to combat obesity is addressed in Chapter 12 by Fried. In that chapter she uses the US as a case study to describe regulatory and legislative issues, and the role of litigation as a public health tool. Chapter 13 approaches the topic of obesity prevention in developing countries by exploring opportunities to work within existing rules and procedures of international trade agreements to construct the case for using food regulation as a policy instrument. In the final chapter, Schwartz and Brownell mount a strong case for the need for courageous action to prevent a further increase in population obesity. They focus particularly on the need for a shared vision and on the role of the food industry, and conclude by proposing a series of target actions to reverse current trends.

Part 1

Chapter 1

The epidemiology of obesity: a global perspective

Jacob C. Seidell

Introduction

Over the last two to three decades, overnutrition and obesity have been transformed from relatively minor public health issues that primarily affect the most affluent societies to a major threat to public health that is being increasingly seen throughout the world. The plight of the most affected populations, like the US, has been well publicized. However, less recognized has been increases in population obesity elsewhere in the world that are now increasingly being monitored. In this chapter we focus on the prevalence of overweight and obesity, as indicated by the body mass index, in a variety of populations world wide. The emphasis is on recent surveys and time-trends and data have been selected that are based on representative population surveys with measured weight and height. Most attention is devoted to the affluent countries with established market economies (North America, Europe, Australia, New Zealand, and Japan) because the data quality and time span covered by it are reasonably comparable. Data on time-trends in the developing world and in countries undergoing an economic transition are given in Chapter 5 and elsewhere (1). The intent of this chapter is to convey a balanced sense of the temporal trends being experience overall in societies around the world and their variability.

Classification of obesity and fat distribution

The epidemiology of obesity has for many years been difficult to study because many countries had their own specific criteria for the classification of different degrees of overweight. Gradually, during the 1990s, however, the body mass index (BMI = weight/height^2) became a universally accepted measure of the degree of overweight and now identical cut-off points are recommended. This most recent classification of overweight in adults by the World Health Organization (WHO) is given in Table 1.1. In many community studies in affluent societies, this scheme has been simplified and cut-off points of 25 and 30 kg/m^2 are used for descriptive purposes. Both the prevalence of very low BMI (<18.5 kg/m^2) and very high BMI (40 kg/m^2 or higher) are usually low, in the order of 1 to 2 per cent or less.

Table 1.1 Classification of overweight in adults by the World Health Organization (2)

Classification	BMI (kg/m²)	Associated health risks
Underweight	< 18.5	Low (but risk of other clinical problems increased)
Normal range	18.5–24.9	Average
Overweight	25.0 or higher	
Preobese	25.0–29.9	Increased
Obese class I	30.0–34.9	Moderately increased
Obese class II	35.0–39.9	Severely increased
Obese class III	40 or higher	Very severely increased

A recent WHO expert consultation (3) addressed the debate about interpretation of recommended body mass index (BMI) cut-off points for determining overweight and obesity in Asian populations, and considered whether population-specific cut-off points for BMI are necessary. They reviewed scientific evidence that suggests that Asian populations have different associations between BMI, percentage of body fat, and health risks than do European populations. The consultation concluded that the proportion of Asian people with a high risk of Type 2 diabetes and cardiovascular disease is substantial at BMIs lower than the existing WHO cut-off point for overweight ($\geq 25\,kg/m^2$). However, available data do not necessarily indicate a clear BMI cut-off point for all Asians for overweight or obesity. The cut-off point for observed risk varies from $22\,kg/m^2$ to $25\,kg/m^2$ in different Asian populations; for high risk it varies from $26\,kg/m^2$ to $31\,kg/m^2$. No attempt was made, therefore, to redefine cut-off points for each population separately. The consultation also agreed that the WHO BMI cut-off points should be retained as international classifications. The consultation identified further potential public health action points (23.0, 27.5, 32.5, and $37.5\,kg/m^2$) along the continuum of BMI, and proposed methods by which countries could make decisions about the definitions of increased risk for their population (Figure 1.1).

Much research over the last decade has suggested that, for an accurate classification of overweight and obesity with respect to the health risks, one needs to factor in abdominal fat distribution. Traditionally, this has been indicated by a relatively high waist-to-hip circumference ratio. Recently, it has been proposed that the waist circumference alone may be a better and simpler measure of the health risks associated with abdominal fatness (4). In 1998, the US National Institutes of Health (National Heart, Lung, and Blood Institute) adopted the BMI classification and combined this with waist cut-off points (5). In this classification, the combination of overweight (BMI between 25 and $30\,kg/m^2$) and moderate obesity (BMI between 30 and $35\,kg/m^2$) with a large waist circumference ($\geq 102\,cm$ in men or $\geq 88\,cm$ in women) is proposed to carry additional risk (5).

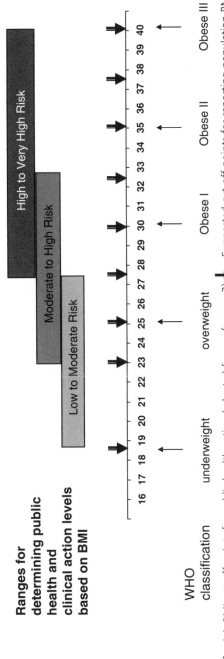

Fig. 1.1 BMI cut-off points for public health action (adapted from reference 2). ▶ = Suggested cut-off points for reporting population BMI distribution and specific action levels for populations and individuals.

Obesity prevalence and trends in adults

North America

In the US, there are two important sources of data on the prevalence of obesity. One is the Behavioral Risk Factor Surveillance System (BRFSS) which is based on an annual survey by telephone in random representative samples of the population in the US (6). Figure 1.2 shows the time-trends of the prevalence of obesity in adult men and women (two lower lines). The other set of data comes from the National Health and Nutrition Examination Survey (NHANES) which is also based on random representative samples of the US population but here weight and heights are measured in people attending a health examination (7). Figure 1.2 shows that the estimates of the prevalence of obesity are considerably higher in the latter study and that in women a higher prevalence of obesity is seen compared to men, which was not found in the BRFSS.

Although the slopes of the time-trends are similar in both studies, this illustrates how difficult it is to assess the true prevalence of obesity. Because of likely under-reporting of weight with increasing obesity, and the lower non-response rate in NHANES, it can be assumed that the data of NHANES give a more valid estimate of the true prevalence compared to those based on the self-reported weights and heights in the telephone survey. However, there also may be other methodological differences that account, at least partly, for the large differences in the estimates of the prevalence of obesity. These methodological issues regard sampling design, response rate (including selective response), and selection based on telephone ownership (many people may have unlisted numbers, cell-phones or no phone and this may lead to bias).

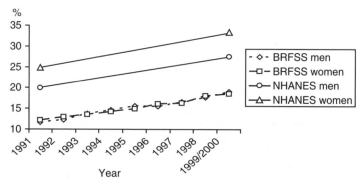

Fig. 1.2 Time-trends of the prevalence of obesity (BMI ≥ 30 kg/m²) in the United States based on the annual behavioral risk factor surveillance system (BRFSS; self-reported height and weight). The NHANES III (National Health and Nutrition Examination Survey III) was conducted between 1988 and 1994 (depicted here as the midpoint of the survey in 1991) and continuously after 1999, in a nationally representative sample based on measured weight and height.

Table 1.2 Sex-specific prevalence data of obesity (BMI $\geq$ 30 kg/m^2) and sex ratio by ethnicity in men and women aged 20–74 in the US; data from the NHANES III, 1988–1994 (Flegal KM *et al.* (8))

Race – ethnic group	Men %	Women %	Sex ratio (women/men)
Non-Hispanic white	20.0	22.4	1.12
Non-Hispanic black	21.3	37.4	1.76
Mexican-American	23.1	34.2	1.48

There are important ethnic differences in the prevalence of obesity in the US, particularly in women (Table 1.2). The female: male prevalence ratio is highest among non-Hispanic blacks (ratio about 1.8), lower in Mexican-Americans (ratio about 1.5) and lowest in non-Hispanic whites (ratio about 1.1). It is important to note that shifts in the distribution of body mass index have significant implications for the increase in severe obesity. Figure 1.3 shows that a doubling in obesity (BMI > 30 kg/m^2) is accompanied by a five to six-fold increase in severe obesity. These different rates of increases in the prevalence of obesity of different degrees of severity have quite different implications for health care and management (8).

The prevalence of obesity in Canada in much lower than in the neighboring US. Canada has also experienced an increase in the prevalence of overweight and obesity,

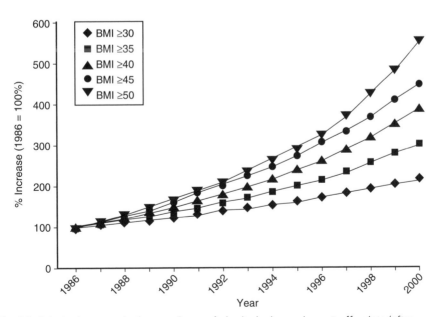

Fig. 1.3 Relative increases in the prevalence of obesity by increasing cut-off points (after reference 8).

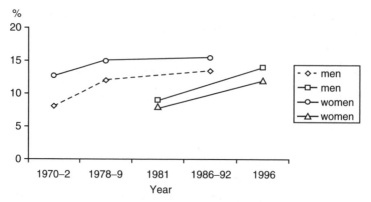

Fig. 1.4 Time-trends in the prevalence of obesity (BMI ≥ 30 kg/m²) in Canadian men and women (after references 9 and 10).

particularly in men (Figure 1.4). One publication documented the increase in the prevalence between 1970 and 1992 (9). A more recent study described an increase in the prevalence of obesity from 9 per cent in 1981 to 14 per cent in 1996 in men (10). In women the corresponding figures were 8 per cent in 1981 and 12 per cent in 1996. Both time-trend studies used data on measured height and weight in nationally representative samples. Like the data for the US, the curves generated from these two studies do not correspond well. In the earlier study, the prevalence was higher in women than in men, and in the later study this situation was reversed. However, it seems reasonable to assume that about a decade ago the prevalence of obesity among adults in Canada was somewhere between 12 and 15 per cent. The prevalence of obesity varies between different population groups. As in the US, the highest prevalence is observed in indigenous populations (11). These groups are also among the least privileged and often live under economically disadvantaged conditions.

Europe

In Europe, only the UK can provide us with truly nationally representative annual estimates of the prevalence of obesity based on measured height and weight. Figure 1.5 shows the long-term trends in the UK (12). These data suggest that in just under a quarter of a century (1980–2002) the prevalence of obesity has increased four-fold.

In most other European countries the existing estimates of obesity prevalence and trends are either based on national interview surveys with self-reported height and weight, or on regional or local studies. In order to make a comparison between countries, it is necessary to compare population-based data on measured height and weight in which identical protocols for measurement were applied and which were collected in the same period. The most comprehensive data on the prevalence of obesity in Europe are provided by the WHO MONICA study (13). The majority of these data were collected between 1983 and 1986, with a third survey performed approximately

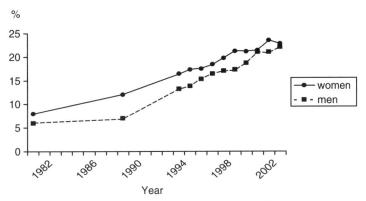

Fig. 1.5 Time-trends in the prevalence of obesity (BMI ≥ 30 kg/m²) in the UK (after reference 12).

10 years later. However, it is important to note that the populations included in the MONICA study are not necessarily representative of the countries in which they were located.

Tables 1.3 and 1.4 show the increases in the prevalence of obesity in men and women aged 35–64 years in several centers participating in the MONICA study (13). It is clear that there has been a rapid increase in the prevalence of obesity in most centers from countries in the European Union, particularly in men. The prevalence of obesity in men and women in European countries in the EU region (Table 1.3) is similar, with a female: male prevalence ratio of 1.07 (range 0.56–1.29). In central and eastern European countries (Table 1.4) the prevalence is generally much higher in women than in men (average female: male prevalence ratio 2.03; range: 1.27–2.87).

In centers from countries in Central and Eastern Europe it appears that the prevalence of obesity in women has stabilized or even slightly decreased, although the prevalence still remains among the highest in Europe. A study by Molarius *et al.* (13) showed that the social class differences in the prevalence of obesity are increasing with time. The available data suggest that obesity is increasingly becoming a lower class problem in Europe. Similarly, data from the Netherlands (14) illustrate the striking inverse association between educational level and the prevalence of obesity (Figure 1.6). Time-trends of the prevalence of overweight and obesity are shown in Figure 1.7. These data are based on self-reported weight and height and it has been shown (unpublished data) that the prevalence of obesity is underestimated by about 3 to 4 percentage points.

Reasonably accurate data (although not recent) based on measured height and weights have been obtained in eastern Finland (Figure 1.8) and Germany (Figure 1.9). In Eastern Finland, there has been a steady high prevalence of obesity in women and a rapid increase in men (15). In Germany, data from before and after the reunification of East and West Germany show that in men there has been an increase in obesity on both

Table 1.3 Prevalence of obesity (age standardized % with BMI ≥ 30 kg/m²) in centers in EU countries plus Switzerland and Iceland participating in the first round of the MONICA study (May 1979 to February 1989) and the third round (June 1989 to November 1996)

Country (Center)	Men		Women		Sex ratio 3rd round women/men
	1st round	3rd round	1st round	3rd round	
Belgium (Ghent)	9	10	11	11	1.10
Denmark (Glostrup)	11	13	10	12	0.92
Finland (north Karelia)	17	22	23	24	1.09
Finland (Kuopio)	18	24	20	25	1.04
Finland (Turku/Loimaa)	19	22	17	19	0.86
France (Toulouse)	9	13	11	10	0.77
France (Lille)	13	17	17	22	1.29
Germany (Augsburg, urban)	18	18	15	21	1.17
Germany (Augsburg, rural)	20	24	22	23	0.96
Iceland (Iceland)	12	17	14	18	1.06
Italy (area Brianza)	11	14	15	18	1.29
Italy (Friuli)	15	17	18	19	1.12
Spain (Catalonia)	10	16	23	25	1.56
Sweden (North)	11	14	14	14	1.00
Switzerland (Vaud/Fribourg)	12	16	12	9	0.56
Switzerland (Ticino)	19	13	14	16	1.23
United Kingdom (Belfast)	11	13	14	16	1.23
United Kingdom (Glasgow)	11	23	16	23	1.00
Mean	13.7	17.0	16.4	18.8	1.07

*Men and Women combined

sides of the former wall. In women from the former East Germany, there has been some increase in obesity whereas in the western part there was an increase (16). The overall prevalence in Germany was over 20 per cent in 1998. Table 1.5 shows the high prevalence of obesity in the Baltic states and in some republics in Eastern Europe (17).

Another systematic examination of the prevalence of obesity across Europe comes from the *European Prospective Investigation into Nutrition and Cancer (EPIC)* (18) which showed that in men and women aged 50 to 64 years the prevalence of obesity varied from 8 to 40 per cent in men and 5 to 53 per cent in women, with high prevalence (over 25 per cent) in the centers from Spain, Greece, and Italy. In women, the lowest prevalence was seen in France, but this estimate was based on a rather unrepresentative sample of the populations (teachers).

Table 1.4 Prevalence of obesity (age standardized % with BMI ≥ 30kg/m^2) of centers in countries in Central and Eastern Europe participating in the first round of the MONICA study (May 1979 to February 1989) and the third round (June 1989 to November 1996)

Country (Center)	Men		Women		Sex ratio 3rd round women/men
	1st round	3rd round	1st round	3rd round	
Poland (Warsaw)	18	22	26	28	1.27
Poland (Tarnobrzeg)	13	15	32	37	2.47
Russia (Moscow)	14	8	33	21	2.63
Russia (Novosibirsk)	13	15	43	43	2.87
Czech Republic (rural CZE)	22	22	32	29	1.32
Yugoslavia (Novi Sad)	18	17	30	27	1.59
Mean	16.3	16.5	32.7	30.8	2.03

Many counties have quite extensive data on obesity prevalence from health interview surveys. It is unclear whether a comparison between countries can be made based on this kind of information. There has no systematic research into degree of selective participation and under-reporting in these kinds of surveys. However, some countries do have sufficiently detailed information to allow regional comparisons to be made. An example is Spain (19) where it was shown that the prevalence of obesity based on self-reported data increased from 7.8 per cent in 1987 to 12.8 per cent in 2001 (obesity was a slightly more common in women compared to men). The data from 2001 also

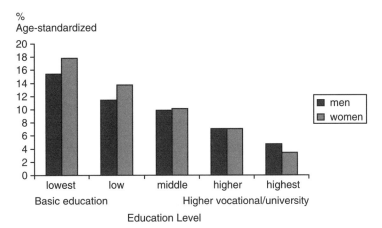

Fig. 1.6 Age-standardized prevalence of obesity (BMI ≥ 30 kg/m^2) in the Netherlands by level of education.

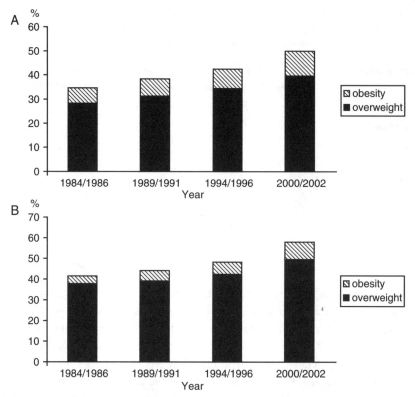

Fig. 1.7 Age-standardized prevalence of overweight (BMI between 25 and 30 kg/m^2) and obesity (BMI ≥ 30 kg/m^2) in the Netherlands: (a) men; (b) women.

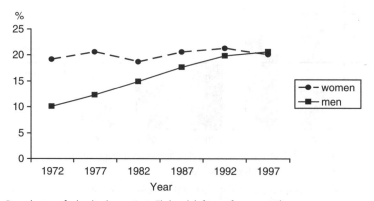

Fig. 1.8 Prevalence of obesity in eastern Finland (after reference 15).

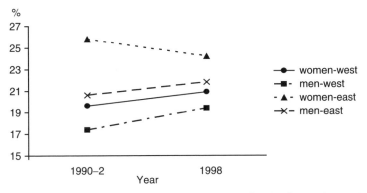

Fig. 1.9 Prevalence of obesity in Germany pre- and postreunification (east = former Deutsche Democratische Republik; west = Bundes Republik Deutschland; after reference 16).

showed that the prevalence of obesity ranged from 7.5 per cent in the province of Navarra in the north to 16.9 per cent in Andalucia in the south. The authors did not provide an explanation for the regional difference but similar geographical variation has been reported in Italy where obesity seems to be more common in the southern regions than in the northern regions (particularly in women). In Italy this seems to be linked to the relatively poorer economic circumstances in the south.

The Eastern Mediterranean

Generally, there is a lack of good representative data (e.g. national surveys) from this region. Table 1.6 shows the prevalence of overweight and obesity in Northern Africa and the Middle East (20). The available data show that the prevalence of obesity is higher in women than in men (particularly in the Middle East and the Gulf States).

Table 1.5 Overweight (BMI 25–29.9 kg/m^2) and obesity (BMI $\geq$ 30 kg/m^2) levels in the Baltic States (adapted from Pomerleau et al. (17))

Country	Year of survey	Sample size	% Overweight		% Obese	
			Men	Women	Men	Women
Estonia	1997	1154	32.0	23.9	9.9	6.0
Latvia	1997	2292	41.0	33.0	9.5	17.4
Lithuania	1997	2096	41.9	32.7	11.4	18.3
Lithuania[a]	2000	2195	45.6	31.6	16.9	23.4
Kazakstan	1995	3538	–	21.8	–	16.7
Uzbekistan	1996	4077	–	16.3	–	5.4

[a]Finbalt study based on self-reported height and weight (Janina Petkeviciene personal communication).

Table 1.6 Overweight (BMI 25–29.9 kg/m²) and obesity (BMI 30 ≥ kg/m²) levels in women aged 15–49 years in North Africa and the Middle East (adapted from Doak (20))

Country	Year of survey	Sample size	% Overweight		% Obese	
			Men	Women	Men	Women
Bahrain	1991/1992	290	16.0	31.3	26.3	29.4
Kuwait	1993/1994	3435	35.2	32.3	32.3	40.6
Saudi Arabia	1996	13177	29.0	27.0	16.0	24.0
Jordan	1994/1996	2836	–	–	32.7	59.8
Morocco	1984/1985	41921	18.7*		5.2*	
Morocco	1992	2850	–	22.3	–	10.5
Morocco	1998/1999	17320	28.0	33.0	5.7	18.3
Tunisia	1997	2760	23.3	28.2	6.7	22.7
Egypt	1995/1996	6769	–	31.7	–	20.1
Turkey	1993	2401	–	31.7	–	18.6

*Men and women combined

Australia, New Zealand, Oceania, and Japan

Trend data on the prevalence of overweight and obesity are available for Australia (21). The AusDiab study showed that the prevalence of obesity in 1999/2000 was 19.3 per cent in men and 22.2 per cent in women. This was 2.5 times higher than in 1980. The prevalence in young adult men aged 25–34 years is particularly high (17.4 per cent; see Figure 1.10). In New Zealand obesity prevalence was 11 per cent in 1989 and in 1997 this had risen to 17 per cent (14.7 per cent in men and 19.3 per cent in women) (22).

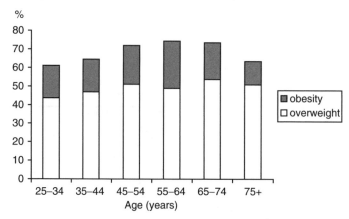

Fig. 1.10 Prevalence of overweight (BMI between 25 and 30 kg/m²) and obesity (BMI ≥ 30 kg/m²) in Australian males, 1999–2000 (after reference 21).

There is data that indicate some of the Pacific island populations have extremely high rates of obesity. The prevalence of obesity in Nauru in 1987, for example, was reported to be around 65 per cent in men and 70 per cent in women (23). Similar high rates have been observed in urban areas of Papua New Guinea (36 per cent in men and 54 per cent in women) whereas the prevalence in the highlands was not higher than about 5 per cent in men and women. Urban Samoans, in 1991, had a prevalence of 58 per cent in men and 77 per cent in women, and in rural areas obesity prevalence was high as well (42 per cent in men and 59 per cent in women).

In Japan, the prevalence of obesity over the past 20 years has increased in men from 0.8 per cent in 1976/1980 to 2.0 per cent in 1991/1995. In women there has been no change over this period (25). However, the International Diabetes Institute has proposed that the international classification of obesity should be adapted for Asian countries (24). They indicated that overweight should be classified as BMI above 23 and obesity as a BMI of 25 or higher. If such a classification were applied, then the prevalence of obesity (BMI ≥ 25) in Japan would be substantially higher (20 per cent rather than 2 per cent) (25).

Childhood obesity

Over the last few decades, it has been difficult to compare estimates of the prevalence of overweight and obesity in children between different time-points and in different populations. This is because definitions of overweight and obesity were based on populations and time-specific BMI-for age specific percentiles (e.g. 85th percentile for overweight and 95th percentile for obesity). An additional problem was that these reference points did not match adult criteria. Thus, someone aged 18 could be classified differently according to centile criteria and by adult BMI cut-off points. In 1999, an expert committee of the International Obesity Task Force (IOTF) used data from six different populations to develop centile curves that passed though the points of 25kg/m^2 and 20kg/m^2 at age 18. These tables are now increasingly used for epidemiological purposes and they allow comparisons across time and populations (26), although they have not been sufficiently validated for clinical use.

In a recent report to the World Health Organization, Lobstein and others (27) have estimated that the worldwide prevalence of obesity in children aged 5 to 17 years is about 10 per cent (of which 2–3 per cent are obese). The Americas had a combined overweight and obesity prevalence of about 30 to 35 per cent, Europe about 20 per cent, the Near and Middle East about 15 per cent, the Asian Pacific region about 5 per cent, and in Sub-Saharan Africa about 1 per cent. As in adults, there are doubts as to whether the same BMI cut-off points can be applied to different ethnic groups and there have been suggestions to lower cut-off points for Asians to match adult criteria.

In most countries, there has been documentation of a rapid increase in the prevalence of obesity among children. Lobstein *et al.* have shown sharp increases

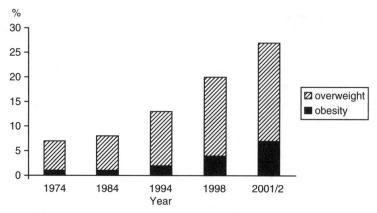

Fig. 1.11 The prevalence of overweight and obesity (using the classification of the International Obesity Task Force) in 7 to 11-year-old children in England in the period 1974–2002 (source: Health Survey for England).

between 1980 and 2000 for Australia, Brazil, Canada, China, Spain, the UK, and the US based on classification of overweight according to the IOTF BMI-for-age cut-off points (27). In the US, the NHANES III shows that the current prevalence of over-weight is slightly over 20 per cent in 6 to 8 year olds (18 per cent in boys and 23 per cent in girls) and about 30 per cent in 12 to 14-year-old children (29 per cent in boys; 31 per cent in girls) (28). In Canada, the prevalence of obesity had increased from about 12 per cent in 1981 to about 30 per cent in 1996 (10). Figure 1.11 shows the almost four-fold increase in the prevalence of overweight in the UK in the past quarter century. According to Lobstein and Frelut (29), the prevalence of obesity in 7 to 10-year-old children in Europe is somewhat lower in Northern Europe (e.g. Netherlands: 12 per cent, Denmark: 15 per cent, Germany: 16 per cent, Sweden: 18 per cent, Belgium: 18 per cent, France: 19 per cent, UK: 20 per cent, Switzerland: 22 per cent) compared to countries in the South (e.g. Italy: 36 per cent; Malta: 25 per cent, Spain: 34 per cent, Crete: 33 per cent, Greece: 31 per cent). It is clear from the available data that, as in adults, overweight and obesity are common and becoming increasingly common in populations throughout the world.

Health consequences of obesity

Obesity is associated with increased risk of ill health and carries with it significant eco-nomic costs to society. Table 1.7 shows estimates of the increased risk of disease associ-ated with obesity based on an extensive literature review by the UK National Audit Office (30). The table has some curious omissions, since some diseases are absent from the list despite a well-documented relationship with obesity (e.g. breast cancer in post-menopausal women and endometrial cancer in all women). Nonetheless, the National

Table 1.7 Estimated increased risk for the obese of developing associated diseases taken from international studies (adapted from (30))

Disease	Relative risk in women	Relative risk in men	Estimated sickness absence due to obesity in UK (days/year)
Type 2 diabetes	12.7	5.2	5 960 000
Hypertension	4.2	2.6	5 160 000
Myocardial infarction	3.2	1.5	1 230 000
Angina pectoris	1.8	1.8	2 390 000
Osteoarthritis	1.4	1.9	950 000
Stroke	1.3	1.3	440 000
Gout	?	?	530 000
Gall bladder disease	1.8	1.8	20 000 (gallstones)
Cancer of the colon	2.7	3.0	970 000 (all cancers)
Ovarian cancer	1.7	–	
Total			17 650 000

Audit Office has estimated that, based on claims for certified incapacity benefit supplied by the Department for Social Security, almost 18 million days of sickness absence can be attributed to obesity (Table 1.7). This is likely to be an underestimate because it excludes both self-certified and uncertified sickness absence, and takes no account of sickness due to diseases for which the proportion of cases attributable to obesity cannot be quantified (e.g. low back pain).

Visscher and Seidell have recently reviewed the evidence for the association between obesity and other diseases (31). Apart from the well-documented diseases associated with the metabolic syndrome (hypertension, dyslipidemia, insulin resistance, abdominal obesity) leading to an increased risk of Type 2 diabetes mellitus and cardiovascular disease, there is also increasing evidence that obesity is related to diseases that partly reflect the mechanical stress on the body by increased fatness (e.g. shortness of breath, sleep apnea, low back pain). In addition to these disabling chronic conditions, obesity also contributes to psychological and social burdens such as social stigma, low self-esteem, reduced mobility, and a generally poorer quality of life. Obesity seems to particularly affect the physical dimension of the quality of life scales and less the emotional and social domains (except for clinical samples).

The magnitude of the obesity epidemic has prompted researchers in many countries to capture obesity-associated economic costs by using cost of illness (COI) methodology (32). These include estimates of resources costs (diseases-specific health-care-related costs) as well as loss of healthy years and productivity losses. Roux and Donaldson have summarized the COI estimates for obesity (32). There are difficulties in making cross-country comparisons, due to the variability of included comorbidities and different

BMI cut-off criteria. US estimates seem to be the highest with obesity accounting for about 7 per cent of the total health care budget (32). Other countries have estimated that obesity accounts for 2 to 3.5 per cent of the health care budget.

Conclusions

The prevalence of obesity is increasing at an alarming rate in many parts of the world. In populations living in the west and north of Europe, Australia, Canada, and the US the prevalence of obesity is high in men and women, as well as in children. Based on the existing prevalence and trend data, and the epidemiological evidence linking obesity with a range of physical and psychosocial health conditions, it is reasonable to describe obesity as a public health crisis that severely impairs the health and quality of life of people and adds considerably to national health-care budgets. Action is urgently required to reverse current trends.

References

1. Seidell JC, Rissanen A (2004). Global prevalence of obesity and time trends. In: Bray GA, Bouchard C, eds. *Handbook of obesity. Etiology and pathophysiology,* 2nd edn, pp. 103–7. Dekker Inc, New York.
2. World Health Organization (2000). *Obesity: preventing and managing the global epidemic.* WHO Technical Report Series, No. 894.WHO, Geneva.
3. Barba C, Cavalli-Sforza T, Cutter J, *et al.* (2004). Appropriate body-mass index for Asian populations and its implications for policy and intervention strategies. *Lancet* **363**, 157–63.
4. Lean MEJ, Han TS, Seidell JC (1998). Impairment of health and quality of life in men and women with a large waist. *Lancet* **351**, 853–6.
5. NIH (1998). Clinical guidelines on the identification, evaluation, and treatment of overweight and obesity in adults. The Evidence Report. National Institutes of Health. *Obes Res* **6**, 51S–209S.
6. Mokdad AH, Ford ES, Bowman BA, *et al.* (2001). Prevalence of obesity, diabetes, and obesity-related health risk factors. *JAMA* **289**, 76–9.
7. Flegal KM, Carrol MD, Ogden CL, Johnson CL (2002). Prevalence and trends in obesity among US adults, 1999–2000. *JAMA* **288**, 1723–7.
8. Sturm R (2003). Increases in clinically severe obesity in the United States, 1986–2000. *Arch Intern Med* **163**, 2146–8.
9. Torrance GM, Hooper MD, Reeder BA (2002). Trends in overweight and obesity among adults in Canada (1970–1992): evidence from national surveys using measured height and weight. *Int J Obesity* **26**, 797–804.
10. Tremblay MS, Katzmarzyk PT, Willms JD (2002). Temporal trends in overweight and obesity in Canada 1981–1996. *Int J Obesity* **26**, 538–43.
11. Kuhnlein HV, Receveur O, Soneida R, Egeland GM (2004). Arctic indigenous peoples experience the nutrition transition with changing dietary patterns and obesity. *J Nutr* **134**, 1447–53.
12. *Health Survey for England.* Available from http://www.publications.doh.gov.uk/stats/trends1.htm. Accessed 15 March 2004.
13. Molarius A, Seidell JC, Sans S, Tuomilehto J, Kuulasmaa K (2000). Educational level and relative body weight and changes in their associations over ten years – an international perspective from the WHO MONICA project. *Am J Public Health* **90**, 1260–8.

14. Visscher TLS, Kromhout D, Seidell JC (2002). Long-term and recent time trends in the prevalence of obesity among Dutch men and women. *Int J Obesity* **26**, 1218–24.

15. Lahti-Koski M, Jousilahti P, Pietinen P (2001). Secular trends in body mass index by birth cohort in eastern Finland from 1972 to 1997. *Int J Obes Relat Metab Disord* **25**, 727–34.

16. Bergmann KE, Mensink GB (1999). Anthropometric data and obesity (in German). *Gesundheitswesen* **61**, S115–20.

17. Pomerleau J, Pudule I, Grinberga D, *et al.* (2000). Patterns of body weight in the Baltic republics. *Public Health Nutr* **3**, 3–10.

18. Haftenberger M, Lahmann P, Panico S, *et al.* (2002). Overweight, obesity, and body fat distribution in individuals aged 50- to 64-year-old participants in the European Prospective Investigation into Cancer and Nutrition (EPIC). *Public Health Nutr* **5**, 1147–62.

19. Martinez JA, Moreno B, Martinez-Gonzales MA (2004). Prevalence of obesity in Spain. *Obes Rev* **5**, 171–2.

20. Doak CM, Popkin BM (2001). The emerging problem of obesity in developing countries. In: Semba RD, Bloem MW, eds. *Nutrition and health in developing countries*, pp. 447–64. Humana Press, Totowa, NJ.

21. Cameron AJ, Welborn TA, Zimmet PZ, *et al.* (2003). Overweight and obesity in Australia: the 1999–2000 Australian Diabetes, Obesity and Lifestyle Study (AusDiab). *Med J Aust* **178**, 427–32.

22. Wilson BD, Wilson NC, Russel DG (2001). Obesity and body fat distribution in the New Zealand population. *NZ Med J* **114**, 127–30.

23. Hodge AM, Dowse GL, Toelupe P, Collins VR, Imo T, Zimmet PZ (1994). Dramatic increase in the prevalence of obesity in Western Samoa over the 13 year period 1978–1991. *Int J Obesity* **18**, 419–28.

24. Examination Committee of Criteria for "obesity disease" in Japan (2002). *Circ J* **66**, 987–92.

25. Yoshiike N, Seino F, Tajima S, *et al.* (2002). Twenty-year changes in the prevalence of overweight in Japanese adults: the National Nutrition Survey 1976–1995. *Obes Rev* **3**, 183–90.

26. Cole TJ, Bellizzi MC, Flegal KM, Dietz WH (2000). Establishing a standard definition for child overweight and obesity worldwide: international survey. *BMJ* **320**, 1240–3.

27. Lobstein T, Baur L, Uauy R (2004). Obesity in children and young people: a crisis in public health. *Obes Rev* **5**(suppl 1), 4–85.

28. Flegal KM, Ogden CL, Wei R, Kuczmarski RL, Johnson CL (2001). Prevalence of overweight in US children: comparison of US growth charts from the Centers for Disease Control and Prevention with other reference values for body mass index. *Am J Clin Nutr* **73**, 1086–93.

29. Lobstein T, Frelut ML (2003). Prevalence of overweight children in Europe. *Obes Rev* **4**, 195–200.

30. National Audit Office (2001). *Tackling Obesity in England*. Report by the comptroller and auditor general HC 220 Session 2000–2001.

31. Visscher TLS, Seidell JC (2001). The public health impact of obesity. *Ann Rev Public Health* **22**, 355–75.

32. Roux L, Donaldson C (2004). Economics and obesity: costing the problem or evaluating solutions? *Obes Rev* **12**, 173–9.

Chapter 2

The role of nutrition and physical activity in the obesity epidemic

Lisa J. Harnack and Kathryn H. Schmitz

Introduction

In order to develop effective public health strategies for the prevention of obesity it is critical to understand both the proximal and distal factors contributing to the rising rates of obesity. Proximally, body fatness is a function of the balance of energy intake and energy expenditure. If energy intake exceeds energy expenditure, the excess energy is stored as body fat. If energy expenditure is lower than energy intake the unexpended energy is stored as adipose tissue. Consequently, the proximal cause of the rising prevalence of obesity is a growing imbalance between energy intake and energy expenditure that may be attributable to an increase in total energy intake and/or a downward shift in total energy expenditure. Distal causes of the obesity epidemic include changes in behavioral and environmental factors that may spur energy intake or depress energy expenditure.

There has been considerable scientific debate over the relative importance of diet vs. physical activity in relation to the epidemic of obesity. While interesting from a scientific perspective, this debate may be less helpful in terms of determining the focus of public health efforts to prevent obesity. The paucity of surveillance data and methodological limitations of the measurements used have resulted in scant data and conflicting findings on trends in energy intake and energy expenditure.

In this chapter, information on temporal trends in energy intake and energy expenditure in the US are reviewed, with the quality and limitations of available data discussed as part of this review. The focus will be on trends in the US because of the availability of surveillance data and the complications of differences in obesity trends across countries. The surveillance issues that have arisen in this country may serve as a valuable example for other countries regarding the pitfalls of tracking risk factors for obesity. Further, because the US has experienced a steady and steep increase in the prevalence of obesity over the past 25 years it serves as good case study for attempts to understand the relative contributions of diet and physical activity to the development of obesity.

Trends in energy intake

Information available for assessing trends in energy intake in the US include dietary intake information collected as part of national and local surveys and food disappearance data for the US food supply. Overall, although results are not entirely consistent across data sources, findings suggest that energy intake in the US has risen in tandem with rising rates of obesity.

Survey findings

National surveys that allow for examining trends in energy intake in the US include the National Health and Nutrition Examination Surveys (NHANES) conducted by the Department of Health and Human Services (DHHS) and the Nationwide Food Consumption Survey (NFCS) and Continuing Survey of Food Intakes of Individuals (CSFII) conducted by the United States Department of Agriculture (USDA). Four NHANES surveys have included assessments of dietary intake: NHANES I from 1971–1974; NHANES II from 1976–1980; NHANES III from 1988–1994; and NHANES 1999–2000. As depicted in Figure 2.1, among both adult males and females a statistically significant increase in average energy intake occurred between 1971 and 2000, with most of the increase occurring between 1976–1980 and 1988–1994 (1).

A rise in energy intake across the USDA surveys was also found (Figure 2.2) with average energy intake increasing from 1795 kcal/day in 1989–1991 to 1985 kcal/day in 1994–1996, although average energy intake was similar between the 1977–1978 and 1989–1991 surveys (2). It is interesting to note that although results suggest energy intake in the US population has shifted upward, the patterns of the increases seen are not entirely consistent with the steep and steady increase in obesity seen in the US between the mid to late 1970s and 1999–2000 (Figure 2.3) (3).

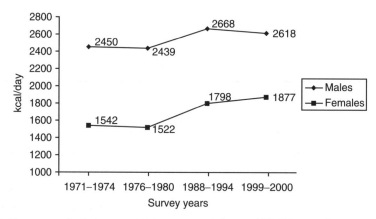

Fig. 2.1 Mean age-adjusted energy intake among adults aged 20–74 years, by sex (National Health Nutrition Examination Surveys (NHANES), US, 1971–2000).

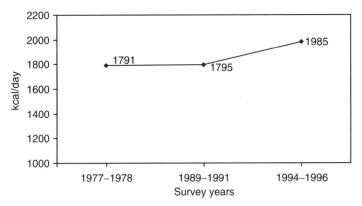

Fig. 2.2 Mean age-adjusted energy intake among those aged ≥ 2 years (Nationwide Food Consumption Survey (NFCS) and Continuing Survey of Food Intakes of Individuals (CSFII), US, 1977–1996).

In contrast to findings from the NHANES and USDA surveys, two surveys of specific populations in the US, the Minnesota Heart Survey and the Bogalusa Heart Study, have found little evidence of an increase in energy intake. The Minnesota Heart Survey is an ongoing observational epidemiologic study to assess trends in risk factors for cardio-vascular disease. The survey has been conducted every 5 years since 1980 with cross-sectional random samples of adults in the Minneapolis St Paul, MN metropolitan area. Results from this survey indicate no significant change in average energy intake between 1980–1982 and 1995–1997 among males. Among females average energy intake increased significantly between these years, although the increase occurred pre-dominately between 1990–1992 and 1995–97 with average energy intake increasing from 1683 to 1822 kcal/day between these years (4). In the Bogalusa Heart Study, children attending the fifth grade in the Bogalusa, Los Angeles school system were

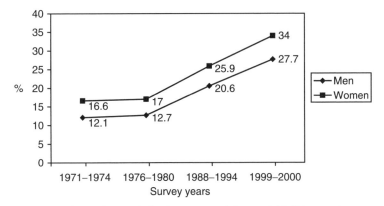

Fig. 2.3 Age-adjusted prevalence of obesity among adults aged 20–74 years, by sex (National Health Nutrition Examination Surveys (NHANES), US, 1971–2000).

recruited for participation in seven cross-sectional surveys from 1973 to 1994 with dietary intake information collected from a subset of participants as part of each survey. No significant change in average energy intake was found across the surveys (5).

There are several possible explanations for these conflicting survey finding on trends in energy intake. Trends in energy intake found in each of the national surveys could be artifacts of inherent methodological shortcomings. For each of the surveys the methods used to collect dietary information and derive nutrient estimates varied between some of the survey periods. For example with NHANES beginning in 1988, dietary recalls were collected for weekend days as well as weekdays (previously they were collected for weekdays only). Because energy intake has been found to be higher on weekend days compared with weekdays (6) an increase in average estimated energy intake between the survey periods would be expected due to this change in data collection procedure. Also, beginning in 1988 the dietary recall interview format was changed and questions were added that might have resulted in the collection of more complete dietary intake data (1). In contrast to the national surveys, the dietary intake assessment methods used in the Minnesota Heart Survey and the Bogalusa Heart Study remained consistent, which provides support for the dietary intake results from these studies.

It is important to note that both the national and local surveys relied on self-reported dietary information (dietary recalls and/or food records), which presents an opportunity for bias in the results. Underreporting of dietary intake is a well-documented shortcoming of self-reported dietary intake information (7), and it has been speculated that the magnitude of underreporting of intake may be growing over time (8, 9). Indeed, it is well known that underreporting of intake is greater among overweight compared with non-overweight individuals (10–14). Hence, the magnitude of underreporting of intake in surveys is likely increasing along with prevalence of obesity. Also, larger sized food portions tend to be underestimated (15–17), which may contribute to growing underestimation of intake with the increasing availability (18) and consumption (19) of larger sized food products.

Food disappearance data

In consideration of the limitations of surveillance data it is important to consider alternative sources of information about trends in food and nutrient intake, namely food disappearance data. For the purpose of agricultural planning and evaluation of food security, in most countries the amount of food available in the food supply is tracked and reported on an annual basis. In the US, food availability data is collected and reported as part of the US Food Supply Series, which provides measures of per capita availability of several hundred food commodities and per capita per day nutrient availability estimates (20). As shown in Figure 2.4, a sizeable increase in average per capita availability of energy has occurred between 1970 and 1999, with the pattern of the increase congruent with trends obesity.

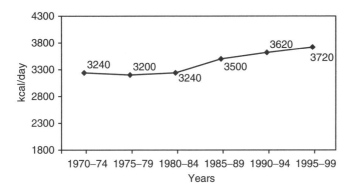

Fig. 2.4 Average annual per capita availability of energy in the food supply (Food Supply Series, US, 1970–1999).

Strengths of the Food Supply Series data include its reliance on objective measures of food availability and the consistent manner in which the data has been collected and analyzed over time. The primary limitation of the data relates to its representation of food availability rather than consumption. Because food that is wasted or that spoils during the marketing process or in the home (e.g. food that is thrown away or fed to pets) is not subtracted in calculating food available for consumption, estimates of per capita availability are usually overestimates of actual consumption. Thus, food-disappearance data are not useful for estimating absolute intake. The data may be useful as an indicator of trends in consumption over time, however, assuming that food spoilage and waste remains constant. The USDA Economic Research Service has developed a method for adjusting food supply data for spoilage, plate waste, and cooking and other losses in the home and marketing system (21), and has applied these adjustments to food supply series data collected since 1970. Trends in per capita energy availability adjusted for spoilage and wastage are similar to trends seen with unadjusted estimates (22).

Although food disappearance data is generally considered inferior to dietary intake information collected from individuals because it represents food and nutrient availability vs. consumption, given the limitations of self-report dietary intake information delineated earlier it may serve as a valuable adjunct. Indeed, in contrast to surveillance data, trends in energy availability from the Food Supply Series data correspond remarkably well with trends in the prevalence of obesity.

Trends in energy expenditure

The total amount of energy an individual expends on a daily basis is a function of the amount of energy required to maintain basic bodily functions (resting energy expenditure), digest food eaten (thermic effect of food), maintain posture and spontaneous activity, and support voluntary bodily movement (physical activity).

Ideally, trends in each of these components of energy expenditure should be considered in evaluating the extent to which trends in energy expenditure may contribute to rising rates of obesity. Unfortunately, surveillance data on trends in energy expenditure in the US are sparse and mostly limited to assessing only one domain of voluntary energy expenditure—leisure time physical activity. Nonetheless, available data is reviewed herein.

Involuntary activity

Involuntary activity comprises the largest proportion of total energy expenditure. More specifically, resting energy expenditure (REE) accounts for about 60 to 70 per cent (23) and the thermic effect of food approximately 10 per cent (24) of total daily energy expenditure, respectively. Surveillance data is lacking regarding trends in these components of energy expenditure. It could be speculated that REE has risen in accord with rising body weights as it has long been known that REE is a linear function of body size, with the widely used Harris–Benedict equation for estimating resting energy expenditure based on this premise (25). On the other hand, it could also be speculated that REE has declined per unit of body weight as body weights have risen, because fat-free mass (FFM) is much more metabolically active than fat mass (FM) and adult weight gain is largely fat gain. The correlation of REE with FFM is high, between 0.70 and 0.80 (26). It could be hypothesized that some portion of the increase in the prevalence of obesity that occurs with aging results from the decline in REE from atrophy of muscle tissue resultant to sedentary lifestyles. However, there is ongoing debate in the scientific literature as to the contribution of a low REE to weight gain. Studies of Pima Indians showed low REE to be associated with subsequent weight gain (27). By contrast, follow-up of men from the Baltimore Longitudinal Study on Aging and of non-obese women from Italy showed no association of REE and subsequent weight gain (28, 29). If there is a contribution of low REE to weight gain, it is likely smaller than day-to-day variability and measurement error for REE, which makes it extremely difficulty to measure. The amount of decrease in REE that can be expected per 1 kg loss of FFM is approximately 21 kcal per day (30).

A variety of factors influence the amount of energy expended in digesting food (thermic effect of food) including: meal size and composition; palatability of the food; time of the meals; and perhaps fitness level (31). Thus, it is possible that the amount of energy expended digesting food has shifted in response to changes in the eating patterns and physical activity habits of Americans. For example both surveillance and food disappearance data indicate the macronutrient distribution of the American diet has shifted over the last several decades, with the percent of energy from fat declining while the percent of energy from carbohydrate has increased (1, 2, 4, 5, 20). Because the thermic effect of carbohydrate is greater than that of fat (32), one might surmise thermic energy expenditure has risen. However, there have been shifts in some of the factors just listed that could potentially reduce the amount of energy expended digesting food. As a result, it is difficult to project the direction and magnitude of any temporal changes in thermal energy expenditure in the US. Further, thermic effect of food accounts for a small proportion of total daily energy expenditure. Therefore, any contribution of changes in the thermic effect of food to the rise in obesity prevalence is likely to be small.

Energy expended in physical activity

Reflecting its voluntary nature, physical activity is the most variable component of total daily energy expenditure. It comprises 20 to 30 per cent of total energy expenditure in sedentary adults and the proportion is notably higher among active individuals (31). Leisure time pursuits such as running, bicycling, dancing, and playing sports are one domain of physical activity. Other domains include occupation, transportation, self-care, volunteer work, non-exercise leisure time activities, and domestic-related activities. Although each of these domains may have a significant influence on energy expended in physical activity and consequently total daily energy expenditure, until recently leisure time physical activity has been the focal point for research on energy expenditure in relation to obesity and public health efforts aimed at obesity treatment and prevention. Consistent with this focus, surveillance data on trends in physical activity have centered almost exclusively on quantifying engagement in leisure time physical activities.

Leisure time pursuits

Leisure time pursuits include activities that are energy intense (e.g. running, bicycling, swimming) as well as activities that require minimal exertion (e.g. television viewing, reading, socializing). Two national surveys have consistently measured engagement in energy intense leisure time physical activities. The National Health Interview Survey (NHIS) provides data on physical activity from 1985, 1990–1991, and 1997–2000. During each survey period engagement in moderate, vigorous, and no activity were assessed via self-report. Results from NHIS indicate overall changes in leisure time physical activity level were minimal between 1985 and 2000, although in some demographic subgroups a decline in the proportion reporting no engagement in moderate or vigorous activity was evident (33, 34). As part of the Behavioral Risk Factor Surveillance Survey (BRFSS), a random-digit-dialed telephone survey of US adults, data on leisure time physical activity were collected in 11 surveys conducted between 1988 and 2002. BRFSS results indicate a decrease in leisure time physical inactivity between 1988 and 2002, with most of the decline occurring after 1996 (Figure 2.5) (35).

A variety of methodological shortcomings of the NHIS and BRFSS surveys could explain why findings on trends in leisure time physical activity run counter to changes that would be expected given trends in obesity. First and foremost, both surveys rely on self-report measures of leisure time physical activity. Self-report instruments are subject to both recall and social desirability bias. Also, both surveys rely on brief physical

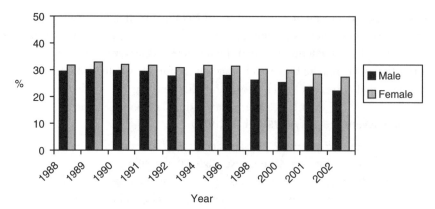

Fig. 2.5 Prevalence of no leisure time physical activity, by sex (Behavioral Risk Factor Surveillance System (BRFSS), 35 states and the District of Columbia, 1988–2002).

activity assessment questions for which reliability and validity have not been established. For example as a measure of physical inactivity in the BRFSS, participants were asked just one question "During the past month, other than your regular job, did you participate in any physical activities or exercise such as running, callisthenics, golf, gardening, or walking for exercise?"

In consideration of the limitations of national surveillance data on trends in leisure time physical activities, it is worth considering findings from two other studies; the Americans' Use of Time Study (36) and the National Human Activity Pattern Survey (37). Both surveys assess how Americans spend their time. The Americans' Use of Time Study has been conducted several times and so it also provides data on how use of time has changed over time.

For the National Human Activity Pattern Survey (NHAPS), 4185 women and 3330 men, age 18 or older, reported detail of how they spent their time over a 24-hour period. The sample was weighted to be representative of US adults in the contiguous 48 states. Time spent in each activity was multiplied by an intensity score based on multiples of REE (METs) to produce a rank for each activity as to contribution to total daily energy expenditure for US adults. Results from the NHAPS study indicate that moderate to vigorous leisure time physical activity contributed only 5 percent to total daily energy expenditure, compared to 8.6 percent for watching TV, 5.8 percent for activities performed while sitting quietly, 3.8 percent for talking or visiting in person or on the phone, 2.2 percent for attending social events, and 2.1 percent for shopping for non-food items (37). Though there are no trends from this study, the results indicate that the US adult population spends more of its leisure time in sedentary than active pursuits.

As part of the Americans' Use of Time Study three national time-diary surveys were conducted. In 1965, 1244 adult respondents kept a single-day diary of activities. A second survey was conducted in 1975, in which 2406 adult respondents kept diaries for a single day. A third survey conducted in 1985 included 5358 adult respondents. The open-ended responses on the time diaries collected at each time period were coded using a coding scheme that first divides activities into non-free time activities and free time activities. Non-free time activities are further subdivided into paid work, family care, and personal care. Free time activities were further subdivided under the general categories of adult education, organizational activities, social life, recreation, and communication.

Results from the Americans' Use of Time Study suggest that counter to Americans' perception that they are increasingly time pressured (36), the amount of time available for leisure time pursuits has increased. In 1985, free time averaged almost 40 hours a week for all people aged 18–64, compared with less than 35 hours a week in 1965. Increases in free time were seen for both sexes and across age categories, although the amount of gain differed somewhat by these demographic factors. The proportion of free time in 1985 allocated to specific activities for adults aged 18–64 is illustrated in Figure 2.6. Activities that tend to be sedentary or require minimal physical exertion accounted for most of the available free time, with three sedentary activities (television, socializing, and home communication) accounting for over two-thirds of all free time. Leisure time pursuits which may require greater physical exertion (sports/exercise and hobbies) were found to account for less than 10 percent of all free time (36).

With respect to trends in how leisure time is used, data from the Americans' Use of Time Study indicate time spent participating in sports and exercise activities more

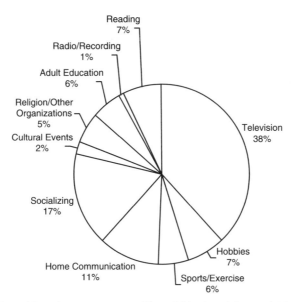

Fig. 2.6 Proportion of free time spent on specific activities by adults aged 18–64 years (Americans' Use of Time Study, 1985).

Table 2.1 Average number of hours per week of free time spent on specific activities for those aged 18–64 years (Americans' Use of Time Project, 1965–1985)

Activity	1965	1975	1985	1985 minus 1965
Adult education	1.8	2.3	2.2	+ 0.4
Cultural events	1.2	0.6	0.9	+ 0.3
Hobbies	2.2	2.8	2.8	+ 0.6
Home communication	3.6	3.4	4.4	+ 0.8
Socializing	8.2	7.1	6.7	− 1.5
Radio/recording	0.6	0.7	0.4	− 0.2
Reading	3.6	3.1	2.8	− 0.8
Sports/exercise	1.0	1.6	2.2	+ 1.2
Religion/other organizations	2.2	2.4	2.1	− 0.1
Television	10.4	14.9	15.0	+ 4.6

than doubled between the mid-1960s and mid-1980s, from an average of 1.0 hours per week in 1965 to 2.2 hours per week in 1985 (Table 2.1). This doubling of participation was found for both sexes and across age and employment groups.

Interestingly though, the greatest absolute increase was seen for television viewing. Free time spent watching television increased from an average of 10.4 hours per week in 1965 to 15.1 hours per week in 1985, an increase of 4.6 hours per week. This increase was found for both sexes and across income, education, race, age, and employment categories, although the magnitude of the increase varied somewhat across these demographic groups (36). It is possible that television viewing displaces other sedentary free time activities producing little change overall in time spent in sedentary leisure time activities. Data from the study provide some support for this hypothesis as free time spent reading, listening to the radio/recordings, involved in religious and other organizations, and socializing decreased between 1965 and 1985. On the other hand, the possibility that television viewing has replaced more active pursuits is supported by the observation that the aggregate decrease in time spent on these activities (2.6 hours per week) is less than the increase in the amount of time spent watching television (4.6 hours per week). Results from the NHAPS survey indicate even higher television viewing in 1992 to 1994, with an estimate of 25.2 hours weekly (37).

Occupation-related physical activities

It has been hypothesized that an increasing proportion of Americans are employed in more sedentary occupations, thus reducing physical activity levels. Moreover, it has been speculated that the physical demands of many occupations have changed over time due to mechanization of job-related tasks (38). Indeed, the proportion of the workforce employed in various industries has undergone notable changes over the past several decades as indicated by data compiled by the US Census Bureau (39, 40). The proportion of the workforce employed in several industries that tend to require more laborious activity (manufacturing and agriculture) have declined significantly since 1970. For example, in 1970, 26.4 per cent of the workforce was employed in manufacturing compared with 14.3 per cent in 2000. Alternatively, several industries that contain occupations that tend to be sedentary (business and repair services, entertainment and recreation, finance, and professional services) have undergone large increases in employment. For example, in 1970, 16.4 per cent of the workforce was employed in professional and related services, compared with 21.3 per cent in 1990. Limited data is available to examine possible changes in the physical demands within occupations. US Census Bureau data indicate that, in 1998, 49.8 per cent of workers used computers at work, an increase from 45.8 per cent in 1993 (39). Earlier data for computer use at work is not available.

Transportation-related physical activities

The means by which Americans commute have changed over the past several decades with use of generally less physically demanding modes of transportation increasing (Table 2.2) (40, 41). Most notably, an increasing proportion of Americans are driving to work. In 1970, 77.7 per cent of the working population commuted via car, truck, or van compared with 87.9 per cent in 2000. Concomitantly, a decreasing proportion of Americans are using public transportation or walking to work.

Decreases in walking or bicycling for transportation may relate to an increase in the proportion of the population residing in the suburbs as well as decreasing population densities in a large number of US metropolitan areas, particularly those outside the southwest (42). Census data indicate that the share of housing units within metropolitan areas but outside city centers, the commonest approximation for measuring suburbs, increased from 19 per cent in 1940 to 44 per cent in 1990 and 61 per cent in 2000 (39). This could influence walking and bicycling behaviors because suburbs are commonly less pedestrian friendly than more dense, urban residential areas. Indeed, an analysis of

Table 2.2 Proportion of workers aged ≥ 16 years using various means of transportation to work (US Bureau of the Census, United States, 1970–2000)

Means of transportation to work	1970 (%)	1980 (%)	1990 (%)	2000 (%)
Car, truck, van	77.7	84.1	86.5	87.9
Public transportation	8.9	6.4	5.3	4.7
Bicycle	N/A	0.5	0.4	0.4
Walked only	7.4	5.6	3.9	2.9
Worked at home	3.5	2.3	3.0	3.3

N/A: not available

NHANES data indicates that the amount of walking is associated with a proxy measure of urban form (age of home) (43). Those who lived in older homes (presumably in more urban neighborhoods that are more walkable) were significantly more likely to walk one or more miles 20 times per month or more than those who lived in newer homes (presumably in suburban, less walkable neighborhoods). These authors were careful to note that the purpose of the walking was not specified in the NHANES survey, but the question on walking was separate from the questions on leisure time physical activities. A recent review concluded that walking to get somewhere (as opposed to walking for leisure time physical activity) is consistently greater in areas with greater residents per unit of space and greater mix of land use compared to less dense residential only developments (44).

It is clear from available data that time spent commuting has increased, leading to more time spent each day in a relatively sedentary activity. According to US Census data, mean travel time to work for those working outside the home has increased from 21.7 minutes in 1980 to 25.5 minutes in 2000 (40, 45). Further evidence that time spent driving/riding in a car may have contributed to the current obesity epidemic comes the NHAPS study (37) which reported that, after sleeping, the single largest contributor to total daily energy expenditure in US adults was driving/riding in a car (10.9 per cent of total daily energy expenditure), simply because US adults spend so much time driving (11.8 hours per week, on average).

Domestic-related physical activities

Although it may seem obvious that improvements in technology over the past several decades have reduced the amount of energy expended in domestic related activities, data is lacking to document this and to quantify the magnitude of any decline that has occurred. Examples of labor-saving devices that have become commonplace in households over the past 50 years include microwave ovens, dishwasher machines, electric garage door openers, blow dryers, motorized push and riding lawn mowers, electric (power) car windows, and television remote controls. Labor saving devices continue to enter the market place and include products such as remote control window blinds, keyless remote control car entry systems, and automated home light switches.

Although labor-saving devices for use in the home may reduce the amount of energy expended completing domestic tasks, it is important to consider that many of the devices also save time. Indeed, the Americans' Use of Time Study found that time spent on domestic activities such as cleaning, cooking, and lawn care has declined (36). If saved time is spent on alternate activities that are energy intense (e.g. running, bicycling, walking) the net effect on total energy expenditure may be neutral or positive. Conversely, if the time saved is spent on sedentary activities, such as television viewing or computer use, the net effect may be a reduction in total energy expenditure. As discussed earlier, results from the Americans' Use of Time Study indicate that gains in free time that occurred between 1960 and 1985 were, in part, spent engaging in additional sports and exercise activities, but the majority of added free time was allocated to television viewing (36). These findings suggest that most of the time potentially saved due to labor-saving domestic devices may be spent in a sedentary activity.

Interestingly, the NHAPS study (37) reported that household activities account for 20.1 per cent and 33.3 per cent of total daily expenditure in men and women, respectively. Therefore, despite declines, household activities still account for a significant portion of daily energy expenditure, more than work, television viewing, or other leisure time pursuits.

Summary and conclusions

Although survey results are not entirely consistent in indicating an increase in energy intake in the US population, Food Supply Series data do suggest energy intake has risen in concert with rising rates of obesity. The objective nature of the Food Supply Series data, combined with the consistent approach used in calculating food availability over time, lends support to findings from this data source. Surveillance of energy intake needs to be improved so that energy intake trends may be monitored with greater confidence. Suggestions for improving surveillance of diet include the need to quantify the effect of methodological changes on intake estimates so that the implications of these changes on intake estimates are known. In addition, accuracy of reporting of dietary intake should be assessed on an ongoing basis so that changes in accuracy or the magnitude of bias in reporting may be detected and considered when interpreting survey findings.

Data support a decline in energy expenditure from transportation and an increase in television viewing, with limited changes in leisure time physical activity. Unfortunately, there is inadequate surveillance data of other activity domains to determine whether they have changed over time. The finding that 20 to 30 per cent of our energy expenditure comes from domestic activities (37) indicates that if there have been any declines in energy expenditure from meal preparation or household chores, these changes could have contributed to a population decline in energy expenditure. Overall, the paucity of data on trends in energy expenditure and the shortcomings of available data limit the certainty regarding the specific domains of energy expenditure that have contributed to the obesity epidemic in the US. Surveillance of trends in energy expenditure should be expanded to include objective measures of activity (such as accelerometry) and 24-hour diaries to address these limitations. The NHANES protocol now includes accelerometry for child and adults participants (46), and these data will assist in further understanding trends in energy expenditure in the US.

Reviews of trends in energy intake and expenditure in other countries (47–51) indicate that, similar to the US, available data is scant and subject to methodological limitations. With respect to energy expenditure, surveillance has been conducted in a limited number of countries, with little data available from developing countries (47).

Among those countries that have tracked trends in physical activity, most have assessed only leisure-time physical activity. Trends observed appear to vary by country. For example surveillance data collected as part of the Australian National Physical Activity Survey (1997–1999) suggest the prevalence of engagement in moderate or vigorous activity has decreased markedly in Australia, while data from the National Health Survey for England (1994–1999) suggests a small increase in high levels of physical activity in England (47). With respect to energy intake, trends also appear to vary by country. For example in an analysis of Food Balance Sheets for Greece, a 26.6 per cent increase in per capita availability of calories was found between 1961 and 1986 (52). Likewise, cross-sectional surveys conducted in Russia between 1992 and 2000 suggest an increase in energy intake in that country (53). In contrast, surveillance data for Spain suggests total energy intake has remained stable in that country (48). The diverse trends in energy intake and expenditure observed across countries may reflect real global differences in the relative contribution of diet and physical activity to rising obesity rates. Conversely, it is possible that the differences observed are the result of the use of varied measurement methods across surveillance systems in conjunction with differing surveillance periods.

In summary, available data suggest increased energy intake and decreased energy expenditure are jointly responsible for the rising rates of obesity in the US. Consequently, public health approaches to obesity prevention must address both of these components of the energy balance equation.

References

1. Wright J, Kennedy Stephenson J, Wang C, McDowell M, Johnson C (2004). Trends in intake of energy and macronutrients – United States, 1971–2000. *MMWR* **53**, 80–2.
2. Nielsen S, Siega Riz A, Popkin B (2002). Trends in energy intake in U.S. between 1977 and 1996: Similar shifts seen across age groups. *Obes Res* **10**, 370–8.
3. Flegal K, Carroll M, Ogden C, Johnson C (2002). Prevalence and trends in obesity among US adults, 1999–2000. *JAMA* **288**, 1723–7.
4. Arnett D, McGovern P, Jacobs D, *et al.* (2002). Fifteen-year trends in cardiovascular risk factors (1980–82 through 1995–97): The Minnesota Heart Survey. *Am J Epidemiol* **156**, 929–35.
5. Nicklas T, Elkasabany A, Srinivasan R, Berenson G (2001). Trends in nutrient intake of 10-year old children over two decades (1973–1994). *Am J Epidemiol* **153**, 969–77.
6. Beaton GH, Milner J, Corey P, *et al.* (1979). A. Sources of variation in 24-hour dietary recall data: implications for nutrition study design and interpretation. *Am J Clin Nutr* **32**, 2546–9.
7. Willett W (1998). *Nutritional epidemiology*. Oxford University Press, New York.
8. Harnack L, Jeffery R, Boutelle K (2000). Temporal trends in energy intake in the United States: an ecologic perspective. *Am J Clin Nutr* **71**, 1478–84.
9. Heitmann B, Lissner L, Osler M (2000). Do we eat less fat, or just report so? *Int J Obes* **24**, 435–42.
10. Johnson R, Soultanakis R, Matthews D (1998). Literacy and body fatness are associated with underreporting of energy intake in US low-income women using the multiple-pass 24-hour recall: A doubly labeled water study. *J Am Diet Assoc* **98**, 1136–40.

11. Bandini L, Schoeller D, Cyr H, Dietz W (1990). Validity of reported energy intake in obese and nonobese adolescents. *Am J Clin Nutr* **52**, 421–5.

12. Fischer J, Johnson R, Lindquist C, Birch L, Goran M (2000). Influence of body composition on the accuracy of reported energy intake in children. *Obes Res* **8**, 597–603.

13. Briefel R, Sempos C, McDoweel M, Chien S, Alaimo K (1997). Dietary methods research in the third National Health and Nutrition Examination Survey: underreporting of energy intake. *Am J Clin Nutr* **65**, 1203S–9S.

14. Pryer JA, Vrijheid M, Nichols R, Kiggins M, Elliott P (1997). Who are the 'low energy reporters' in the Dietary and Nutritional Survey of British adults. *Int J Epidemiol* **26**, 146–54.

15. Harnack L, Steffen L, Arnett D, Gao S, Luepker R (2004). Accuracy of estimation of large food portions. *J Am Diet Assoc* **104**, 804–6.

16. Faggiano F, Vineis P, Cravanzola D, *et al.* (1992). Validation of a method for the estimation of food portion size. *Epidemiol* **3**, 379–82.

17. Chambers E, McGuire B, Godwin S, McDowell M, Vecchio F (2000). Quantifying portion sizes for selected snack foods and beverages in 24-hour dietary recalls. *Nutr Res* **3**, 515–20.

18. Young L, Nestle M (2003). Expanding portion sizes in the US marketplace: Implications for nutrition counseling. *J Am Diet Assoc* **103**, 231–4.

19. Nielsen S, Popkin B (2003). Patterns and trends in food portion sizes, 1977–1998. *JAMA* **289**, 450–3.

20. Putnam J, Allshouse J (1997). *Food consumption, prices and expenditures, 1970–95, 939*. United States Department of Agriculture, Economic Research Service, Food and Consumer Economics Division, Washington, DC.

21. Kantor L (1998). *A dietary assessment of the U.S. food supply: comparing per capita consumption with food guide pyramid serving recommendations, ARS-772*. USDA, ERS, Washington D.C.

22. Putnam J (1999). U.S. food supply providing more food and calories. *Food Review* **22**, 2–12.

23. Ravussin E, Lillioja S, Anderson T, Christin L, Bogardus C (1986). Determinants of 24-hour energy expenditure in man: Methods and results using a respiratory chamber. *J Clinical Investigation* **78**, 1568–78.

24. Weinsier R, Hunter G, Heini A, Goran MI, Sell SM (1998). The etiology of obesity: relative contribution of metabolic factors, diet and physical activity. *Am J Med* **105**, 145–50.

25. Harris K, Benedict F (1919). *A biometric study of basal metabolism in man*. Carnegie Institute, Washington, DC.

26. Luke A, Rotimi C, Adeyemo A, *et al.* (2000). Comparability of resting energy expenditure in Nigerians and US Blacks. *Obes Res* **8**, 351–9.

27. Ravussin E, Lillioja W, Knowler S, *et al.* (1988). Reduced rate of energy expenditure as a risk factor for body-weight gain. *N Engl J Med* **318**, 467–72.

28. Seidell J, Muller D, Sorkin J, Andres R (1992). Fasting respiratory exchange ratio and resting metabolic rate as predictors of weight gain: The Baltimore Longitudinal Study on Aging. *Int J Obes* **22**, 601–3.

29. Marra M, Scalfi L, Covino A, Esposito-Del Puente A, Contaldo F (1998). Fasting respiratory quotient as a predictor of weight change in non-obese women. *Int J Obes* **22**, 601–3.

30. Weinsier R, Schutz Y, Bracco D (1992). Reexamination of the relationship of resting metabolic rate to fat-free mass and to the metabolically active components of fat-free mass in humans. *Am J Clin Nutr* **55**, 790–4.

31. Tataranni P, Ravussin E (2002). Energy metabolism and obesity. In: Wadden T, Stunkard A (eds), *Handbook of obesity treatment*. Guilford Press, New York.

32. de Jong L, Bray G (1997). The thermic effect of food and obesity: a critical review. *Obes Res* 5, 622–31.

33. United States Department of Health and Human Services (1996). *Physical Activity and Health: A Report of the Surgeon General. Centers for Disease Control and Prevention,* National Center for Chronic Disease Prevention and Health Promotion, Atlanta, GA.

34. United States Department of Health and Human Services. *Data 2010: the Healthy People 2010 database.* Available at: http://wonder.cdc.gov/data2010/. Accessed July 15, 2004.

35. Ham S, Yore M, Futon J, Kohl H (2004). Prevalence of no leisure-time physical activity – 35 States and the District of Columbia, 1988–2002. *MMWR* 53, 82–6.

36. Robinson JP, Godbey G (1997). *Time for life.* Pennsylvania State University Press, University Park, PA.

37. Dong L, Block G, Mandel S (2004). Activities contributing to total energy expenditure in the United States: Results from the NHAPS study. *Int J Behav Nutr Physical Activity* 1, 4–14.

38. Hill J, Peters J (1998). Environmental contributions to the obesity epidemic. *Science* 280, 1371–4.

39. US Bureau of the Census (1999). *Statistical Abstract of the United States, the National Data Book.* Washington DC.

40. US Bureau of the Census. *United States Census 2000.* Available at http://www.census.gov. Accessed July 15, 2004.

41. US Bureau of the Census. *Private vehicle occupancy for the United States: 1990, 1980 and 1970 Census.* Available at: http://www.census.gov/population/socdemo/journey/mode6790.txt. Accessed July 6, 2004.

42. Pendall R, Fulton W, Harrison A (2000). *Losing ground the sprawl? Density trends in metropolitan America.* Fair Growth Conference. Fannie Mae Foundation, Atlanta, GA.

43. Berrigan D, Troiano R (2002). The association between urban form and physical activity in US adults. *Am J Prev Med* 23, 74–9.

44. Saelens B, Sallis J, Frank L (2003). Environmental correlates of walking and cycling: findings from the transportation, urban design, and planning literatures. *Ann Behav Med* 25, 80–91.

45. US Bureau of the Census. *Travel time to work for the United States: 1990 and 1980 census.* Available at: http://www.census.gov/population/socdemo/journey/ustime.txt. Accessed July 6, 2004.

46. National Center for Health Statistics. *National health and nutrition examination survey. Survey questionnaires, examination components and laboratory components 2001–2002.* Available at: http://www.cdc.gov/nchs/about/major/nhanes/questexam01_02.htm. Accessed August 3, 2004.

47. International Agency for Research on Cancer, WHO (2002). Weight control and physical activity. *IACR Handbooks of Cancer Prevention. Volume 6.* IARC Press, Lyon.

48. Gutierrez-Fisac J, Regidor E, Lopez-Garcia E, Banegas-Banegas J, Rodriguez-Artalego F (2003). The obesity epidemic and related factors: The case of Spain. *Cad Saude Publica* 19, 101–10.

49. Seidell J (1999). Obesity: a growing problem. *Acta Paediatrica* 88, 46–50.

50. Livingstone M (2001). Childhood obesity in Europe: a growing concern. *Public Health Nutr* 4, 109–16.

51. Kemper H, Stasse-Wolthuis M, Bosman W (2004). The prevention and treatment of overweight and obesity. Summary of the advisory report by the Health Council of the Netherlands. *Neth J Med* 62, 10–17.

52. Zilidis C (1993). Trends in nutrition in Greece: Use of international data to monitor national developments. *Public Health* 107, 271–6.

53. Baturin J, Popkin B (2003). Obesity, diet, and poverty: trends in the Russian transition to market economy. *Eur J Clin Nutr* 57, 1295–302.

Chapter 3

The role of socio-cultural factors in the obesity epidemic

Kylie Ball and David Crawford

Introduction

Obesity is socio-culturally distributed; that is the prevalence of obesity is known to vary according to socio-cultural factors, including socio-economic position, social roles and circumstance, and cultural factors. Further, these socio-cultural patterns are complex and specific to sex, age, and sometimes racial groups, as well as type of society, with patterns of relationships observed in developed countries sometimes reversed in developing countries. As described in Chapter 4, there is little doubt of the importance of the changing physical environment to the increases in obesity observed over the past several decades. However, far less attention has been paid to investigating the potential contribution of socio-cultural factors and to changes in the socio-cultural environment over time to the current obesity pandemic. The mechanisms through which socio-cultural factors may influence body weight and risk for obesity are also not well understood.

In discussing socio-cultural influences we refer to systems of social relations (roles and relationships that define class, gender, ethnicity, and other social factors) and the meanings attached to these (1). For the purposes of this chapter, we focus on the impact of social, economic, and value systems on individuals' obesity-related behaviors (particularly, certain eating patterns and physical inactivity). In particular, we examine socio-cultural categories (socio-economic status, ethnicity, marital/family roles) for which evidence exists that rates of obesity are differentially distributed. We have not focused on the role of physical environmental factors, which is covered in Chapter 4, and we have largely restricted our focus to developed countries, from where the majority of the evidence for socio-cultural influences on obesity is derived. Issues relating to influences on obesity in developing countries are covered in detail in Chapter 5.

This chapter provides an overview of the impact of socio-cultural influences on obesity in developed countries, and considers the potential pathways through which these influences may operate. The chapter concludes by speculating about the potential impact of societal trends on future rates and patterns of obesity in developed countries.

Associations of socio-cultural factors with obesity

It has been suggested that "social factors must be considered as among the most important, if not the most important, influence on the prevalence of obesity" (2, 3). While socio-cultural forces driving obesity have often been mentioned rhetorically in the literature and in official reports on obesity as an important determinant (4–6), the definition and range of socio-cultural influences that may be important influences on obesity are typically not well elucidated. A range of potential socio-cultural factors have been investigated in relation to obesity risk. These can be classified into three broad groups: social roles and relationships; ethnicity and cultural factors; and socio-economic status.

Social roles and relationships

Much of the research on social roles and relationships and obesity has focused on marital status. Research dating back to the 1950s suggests links between body weight/obesity risk and marital status (7, 8), marital progression (including studies showing a tendency for spouses' weight to "synchronize" over years of marriage: see Sobal (9) for a review), marital problems (10), and marital termination (11–17, 9, 18, 19). Research findings, however, are inconsistent, particularly among cross-sectional studies, with some suggesting that married and previously married men and women weigh more than never-married individuals (18); others suggesting gender-specific associations such that ever-married men weigh more than never-married men, whereas ever-married women weigh less than never-married women (12); and other studies finding no relationships (20, 21). Longitudinally, evidence is more consistent, suggesting that marriage predicts weight gain in both men and women, whereas marital termination (through divorce or widowhood) predicts weight loss (14–16, 19).

While studies of social roles and obesity have primarily focused on marital status, it is possible that other social roles and relationships are also important. For example limited data suggest associations of weight gain and obesity with work roles (for instance those involving high work demands and job strain (22, 23)) and with a caregiving role (24). Motherhood has also been linked to greater weight gain (25), only some of which is likely to be attributable to weight gained during pregnancy (26). Other research findings that attest to the influence of social relationships on body weight includes evidence of familial clustering of obesity, beyond that expected by shared genes alone (27), and findings that social support predicts greater weight loss in treatment populations (28).

Ethnicity and cultural factors

Cultural influences on body weight have often been inferred through investigations comparing obesity rates among individuals of different ethnic backgrounds living in the same country. For example, in the US, where much of the research on ethnicity and obesity has been conducted, rates of overweight and obesity are reportedly higher among African-American populations than either Caucasian or Hispanic populations, which in turn demonstrate higher rates than Asian populations (29, 30). One limitation of such studies is that it is very difficult to determine whether differential rates of obesity are attributable to biological or socio-cultural factors. Differences in the prevalence of obesity among neighboring countries, such as the Netherlands, Germany, and England (see Chapter 1), may also be suggestive of cultural influences on body weight. Other evidence comes from "acculturation" studies of differences or changes in body weights of individuals migrating to different countries (31–34). Lauderdale and Rathouz (32), for instance, reported that among Asian Americans born outside the US, the longer the duration in the US, the higher the risk for overweight. Similar findings were reported in a study examining length of time spent in Australia by women having immigrated from a variety of countries (31).

The origins of such racial and ethnic variations in obesity rates are not well-understood. While biological factors may contribute to ethnic group differences in obesity rates, the evidence from acculturation studies particularly suggests that environmental, as well as psycho-social and cultural variables (e.g. values ascribed to a large body size) are also likely to be important determinants of the differential rates of obesity across ethnic groups. These determinants are discussed in further detail below.

Socio-economic status

Much of the existing research on socio-cultural influences on obesity has focused on socio-economic status (SES). Typically, this work has investigated links between SES (assessed using a range of indicators including income, education, and occupation) and relative body weight or risk of obesity. In the seminal review of the literature in 1989, Sobal and Stunkard (35) examined 144 studies that investigated associations of SES with obesity. That review concluded that, in developed societies, SES was consistently inversely associated with obesity among women, but inconsistently related among men and children. The earliest studies of these associations demonstrated the strength of these relationships among women: obesity was six times more prevalent among women of lower SES than those of higher SES (36, 37). In developing societies, Sobal and Stunkard's (35) review showed that SES was strongly directly associated with obesity for men, women, and children. The majority of studies included in that review were cross-sectional, however, and therefore could not provide insight into the longer term relationships between SES and obesity risk.

More recently, we have reviewed evidence from 34 longitudinal studies of SES and weight change over time among adults in developed societies (38). While not unequivocal, our review showed inverse associations between SES and weight gain among white women, and slightly less consistently, among white men in developed societies (no consistent relationships were found for black men or women). Similarly, a review of longitudinal studies of childhood SES and subsequent obesity in adulthood showed a strikingly consistent inverse relationship between SES in childhood and obesity in adulthood (39). These findings rule out the possibility that SES–weight associations are solely attributable to "social mobility" (i.e. obesity leading to low SES), since the majority of studies included in both reviews used baseline measures of SES and examined subsequent weight change.

Other researchers (see (40)) have called for further studies disaggregating SES into components in order to give greater insight into associations of specific aspects of SES that may be more strongly predictive of obesity. In the review described above (38), we attempted to identify those components of SES that were the most important predictors of obesity. This demonstrated that occupation was most consistently related to obesity, education somewhat less consistently related, and income was relatively inconsistently related. While this finding may reflect varying measurement issues (e.g. survey questions on income tend to be fairly poorly answered), it may also suggest different etiological pathways by which SES may act on weight change and obesity. These pathways are discussed below in more detail.

Pathways linking socio-cultural factors with obesity

The mechanisms by which socio-cultural factors (including social roles and relationships, ethnic background, and SES) are associated with obesity are not well-understood. As described earlier, studies examining socio-cultural factors and obesity have found associations in different directions or of different magnitudes across different populations or population subgroups (for instance SES–obesity relationships in developed vs. developing countries, or black vs. white populations). Such findings suggest that it is not social relationships, ethnicity, or socio-economic position *per se* that influences obesity risk, but potentially the meanings attached to obesity in these different societies or groups that are important. It is likely that multiple such "meanings" are important, and that multiple mechanisms underpin socio-cultural influences on obesity. Sobal and Stunkard (35) and Stunkard (40) have suggested a number of potential mechanisms by which SES may influence obesity (for instance through heredity, social mobility, or SES differences in eating patterns, dieting/restraint, or physical activity) but these, and other factors potentially linking other socio-cultural factors to obesity, have not been widely tested empirically. Furthermore, socio-cultural influences may operate in different directions or with varying strength to influence obesity across different populations or subgroups.

Behavioral risk factors for obesity

In speculating about the pathways linking socio-cultural factors and obesity, it seems logical to begin by considering what is known about the development of obesity. As discussed in Chapter 2, obesity results from an energy imbalance, where energy intake exceeds expenditure. While there is no doubt that genetic factors make some contribution, this imbalance is largely a result of behavioral factors relating to certain eating behaviors and physical inactivity. These behaviors serve as the interface between broader social and environmental variables and our personal biology (41).

Currently we have a poor understanding of the specific behaviors important in the etiology of obesity. Even the relative importance of energy intake (i.e. eating behaviors) vs. energy expenditure (i.e. physical activity behaviors) is contentious. It is likely that a multitude of specific behavioral factors contribute to this energy imbalance through increasing overall energy intake and promoting low levels of energy expenditure. Limited evidence implicates behaviors such as fast food consumption, skipping breakfast, low intakes of fruits and vegetables, meat eating, and TV viewing as risk factors for the development of obesity (e.g. 25, 42–45). However, much further research on the eating, physical activity, and sedentary behaviors that are important in relation to risk of weight gain and obesity is required.

Acknowledging that good evidence regarding the role of specific behavioral risk factors in the development of obesity is lacking, it is likely that both dietary patterns and physical inactivity are key contributors to the etiology of obesity. It seems reasonable, then, to hypothesize that socio-cultural variations in obesity risk are largely attributable to socio-cultural variations in these determinant behaviors. Although it is possible that the associations between socio-cultural factors may operate in the reverse direction (i.e. through downward social mobility resulting from obesity), as discussed earlier, evidence from acculturation studies and longitudinal studies of SES suggest that this is unlikely to be the sole explanation. The following section provides an overview of evidence demonstrating socio-cultural variations in diet and physical activity consistent with the above hypothesis.

Socio-cultural variations in obesity-related behaviors

There is a substantial body of research showing that both eating patterns and leisure-time physical activity are differentially distributed across socio-cultural groups. Compared with those of low SES, individuals of high SES tend to follow a diet that is more in line with dietary guidelines (46–50). For example, compared to high SES individuals, those of lower SES are more likely to eat diets that are high in fat and to consume fast food more frequently, and fruit and vegetables less frequently (51–55). Persons of low SES are also less likely than those of high SES to participate in organized sport and leisure-time physical activity (56–58). These associations seem to hold across a range of different indicators of SES.

Variations in obesity-related behaviors by other socio-cultural factors have also been documented. For instance, consumption of vegetables has been reported to be lower among adults who are single, divorced/separated, widowed or living alone compared to those living with a spouse (59, 60). Eating patterns of women with young children are also more closely aligned with dietary recommendations than those of other women (48). Although marital status is inconsistently associated with physical activity, motherhood has been linked with lower levels of activity (61, 62). Lower levels of physical activity have also been reported to be more common among racial and ethnic minorities (including African-Americans and Mexican-Americans) than among Caucasians (62, 63), and these differences do not seem to be wholly attributable to variations in SES (63). There is also some evidence that non-whites have diets that are less closely aligned with recommendations for health (64).

Despite evidence of socio-cultural variations in diet and physical activity, it is noteworthy that only a limited number of studies have attempted to quantitatively test the hypothesis that socio-cultural variations in obesity are explained by socio-cultural variations in the determinant behaviors. Three such studies focused on the role of behavioral factors (including dietary patterns, dieting behavior, leisure-time physical activity, and television viewing) in explaining SES gradients in obesity among adolescent females (65), a working population (66), and a general population sample of men and women (67). In general, these studies showed that some, but not all, of the SES gradients in obesity could be explained by SES variations in the behavioral factors examined. In each of these studies, part of the variance in obesity remained unexplained by the mediating behaviors. It is possible, however, that this unexplained variance is at least partly attributable to imprecise measurement, since behaviors such as physical activity and diet are notoriously difficult to assess accurately. These studies used self-report measures of activity and eating, the validity of which may have been affected by socially desirable response bias, which may vary by weight status.

Why are diet and physical activity behaviors socio-culturally distributed?

If we accept that at least some of the socio-cultural variations in obesity are attributable to socio-cultural variations in obesity-related behaviors, we might then question why these behaviors are themselves socio-culturally distributed? Despite a large body of literature on the influences on eating and physical activity behaviors generally, there has been much less research that directly investigates the extent to which the determinants of eating and physical activity vary by socio-cultural factors, and if so, whether socio-cultural differentials in these determinants might contribute to explaining socio-cultural variations in diet and physical activity behaviors, or in obesity risk.

With regards to SES, there is evidence that greater nutrition knowledge is related to better diet (68), and that higher SES is associated with better knowledge (69–71), and hence we might infer that knowledge mediates the relationship between SES and diet. There is also good evidence of SES variations in: body weight dissatisfaction and weight control attempts (66); values and beliefs about diet and health (72); confidence in cooking skills (73); and discretionary income for food/recreation. However, we might also consider whether socio-economic variations in factors such as enjoyment of physical activity, food taste preferences, stress or depression, access to and uptake of new knowledge/information (e.g. through media/"diffusion of innovation"), discretionary time or energy levels, or social norms relating to diet play a role in increasing obesity risk among persons of low SES through their influence on obesity-related behaviors.

Alternatively, if we consider social roles, there is evidence that social support for healthy behavior from partner, family, or work colleagues (74, 75) is a key influence on health behaviors. Behavioral modeling, psychosocial characteristics of workplaces or opportunities for eating or activity in workplaces, sense of responsibility for diets of others (e.g. partner, family), or discretionary time and energy for physical activity or food shopping, preparation, and cooking are other factors associated with social roles that may influence diet and physical activity behaviors and therefore obesity risk. Factors associated with employee roles specifically (including employment status and grade, occupational conditions, workloads, and job demands) have been associated with food choice (76).

Finally, how might cultural values translate into behavior? There is good evidence of ethnic and cultural differences in: attitudes about ideal body weight and social pressure for thinness (77); definitions of what constitutes healthy eating (78); levels of body weight dissatisfaction and dieting behavior (79, 31, 80); and eating beliefs, customs, and practices (e.g. "fattening" practices for young women in Pacific Island communities (81)). Evidence of cultural differences in attitudes to food, for instance, was demonstrated in a study by Rozin *et al.* (82) exploring the role of food among adults and college students in Flemish Belgium, France, the US, and Japan. That study demonstrated substantial between-country differences in the importance of food, with Americans most likely to associate food with health rather than pleasure, and the French being the most food-pleasure oriented and the least food-health oriented.

Cultural differences regarding the role of women in society may be another important explanation of cultural variations in obesity among women. It is likely that the accepted role of women in traditional Muslim societies may make them less likely to be physically active and thus more susceptible to obesity than men, whereas women's roles in Asian countries may make them less so. On the other hand, the high value placed on education and academic pursuits in some Asian cultures (e.g. Singapore) may mean that many of these children spend a large amount of their free time being tutored, leaving little free time for sport or active play, and this may have contributed to recent rises in childhood obesity observed in some Asian cultures (83). Religious beliefs and ceremonies (e.g. feasting and fasting), and attitudes and beliefs relating to the role of food in social settings, the role of physical activity, and the importance of appearance may also be significant in translating cultural values into weight-related behaviors.

Cultural variations in values may also be important in explaining differences in obesity prevalence. For example in cultures where there are greater concerns about the environment (i.e. environmentalism), people may be more likely to make transportation choices that result in them being more physically active. For example active transport (walking and bicycling) is much more common in The Netherlands than in the UK, where it is more common that in the US. Cultural values reflecting greater consumerism in many Western societies (84) may result in increased purchasing of ready-made meals and convenience meals, which are often of larger portion sizes and higher in energy than foods made in the home. Other cultural values widely considered as increasingly characteristic of Western societies include individualism and secularism (84). Such values may also impact on the dietary patterns and physical activity habits, and hence the risk of obesity in these societies, although the nature and extent of their influence is unknown.

A key challenge in attempting to explore culturally-bound influences and their impact on obesity risk is the complexity inherent in attempting to measure factors such as cultural values and beliefs. Future attempts to understand these influences will require creative methodologies, such as scans of media articles to derive quantitative (count) and qualitative (content/context) indicators of important concepts, that may help explain cultural expectations regarding weight and weight-related behaviors.

Proposed model of socio-cultural influences on obesity

In order to better understand the pathways by which socio-cultural factors influence obesity risk, we argue that further insight into the mediators of socio-cultural influences on diet and physical activity behaviors, such as those suggested above, are required. Several other commentators have also proposed hypothetical models to facilitate understanding of the influences on obesity (e.g. International Obesity Taskforce (85), Sobal (86)). Recently, for example, an expert working group convened to consider options for obesity prevention concluded that there were a small number of overarching social and cultural variables that were likely to be important in influencing obesity-related behaviors, including social roles, relationships and socio-economic status, and ethnic identities (87). However, that expert group noted that the research base identifying specific important socio-cultural influences on obesity is extremely limited. Perhaps for this reason, previous conceptual models have not tended to discuss in detail the specific pathways through which different socio-cultural influences might operate.

Current theoretical models used to explain diet and physical activity behaviors, such as ecological models, posit that a range of factors at the level of the individual, social, and physical environments should be considered when attempting to understand the influences on health behaviors. Taking this into account, Figure 3.1 presents a conceptual model of the way in which we might consider the factors that may contribute to explaining socio-cultural variations in diet and physical activity, and ultimately obesity risk. We propose this model as a general conceptual framework to guide thinking regarding socio-cultural influences on obesity, rather than a comprehensive model of all possible pathways between socio-cultural factors and obesity. Data on many of the variables hypothesized in the model currently do not exist and hence the empirical testing of such a model remains a task for future research.

It should be noted that not all of the pathways suggested in the proposed conceptual model will operate for all socio-cultural determinants. Not only is there a lack of empirical

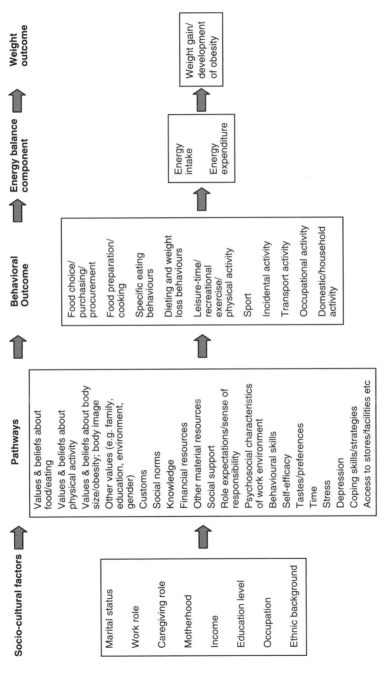

Fig. 3.1 Conceptual model of pathways linking selected socio-cultural factors with obesity.

data to specify which socio-cultural factors are important, as discussed earlier, there is also little evidence of the most important behavioral outcomes for obesity (e.g. the dietary patterns leading to greatest risk of obesity; or the contribution of leisure time vs. transport vs. occupational physical activity to weight gain). However, the model proposes a number of plausible links between socio-cultural factors, dietary and physical activity behaviors, and obesity. For instance, researchers may hypothesize a pathway by which a new parenting role leads to less available time and increased psychological stress, which in turn lead to lower levels of leisure-time physical activity and eventually to weight gain; or a pathway by which low income leads to fewer financial resources available for purchasing fresh fruits and vegetables, which leads to a diet higher in energy density, and eventually to obesity.

Pathways between socio-cultural factors and different behavioral factors may also vary. For instance, whereas knowledge of nutrition and health has been demonstrated to predict healthy eating, knowledge of the health benefits of physical activity has consistently shown no association with physical activity behavior (62). As well as considering the multiple plausible pathways by which socio-cultural factors might lead to increased obesity risk, it should be noted that the relative importance of pathways such as those suggested in Figure 3.1 may vary across population groups (e.g. men vs. women; children vs. adults; Caucasian vs. African-American persons) and societies (e.g. developed vs. developing). The moderating role of such factors as sex, age, race, and societal stage of development should also be considered in any study of socio-cultural influences on obesity.

Socio-cultural change and the obesity epidemic

If socio-cultural factors are indeed an important influence on obesity risk and therefore in the genesis of the obesity pandemic, as we and others have proposed, we would expect that the marked increases in the prevalence of obesity observed over the past 30 years in Europe, Scandinavia, North America, Australasia, and other developed countries would coincide with significant changes in socio-cultural factors in these countries. What evidence, then, is there that developed countries have experienced shifts over the past several decades in the kinds of socio-cultural factors that have been proposed here to be important (i.e. changes in social roles and relationships, the ethnic and cultural composition of societies, and in socio-economic factors)?

There have been significant changes in household composition and family structure since the early 1970s that are likely to have had an important impact on social roles and relationships, and thus on obesity risk. In the UK, for example, the number of "traditional families", defined as a couple with dependent children, has declined from one-third of households in 1971 to only one-quarter in 2001. During this period the proportion of lone parent households doubled (88). The number of marriages decreased by 20 per cent between 1971 and 1994, while the divorce rate doubled during this period (89). Over the past 30 years there has been a marked increase in the proportion of single person households, with an increasing trend for younger people, particularly men, to live alone (88). According to the Office of National Statistics, the decline in marriage that has been observed, the increases in the age at which people first marry, and the rise in separations and divorces means that by 2021 one in seven households in the UK will contain men under the age of 65 living alone.

Another socio-cultural change that is likely to affect our social roles relates to participation in the labor market. Again taking the UK as an example, between 1984 and 2002 there was a decrease in the proportion of adult men in the workforce but an increase in the proportion of women who were working (88). Patterns of employment have also changed over the past two decades, with major declines in the manufacturing sector and increases in the financial and business services sectors, which accounted for approximately one in five jobs in 2002. It is also noteworthy that in the UK, one in four men and just over one in ten women worked more than 50 hours/week in 2002 (88). These observations regarding the UK serve to highlight that socio-cultural factors likely to be important in obesity risk have changed over the last several decades. Importantly, the trends described for the UK in working status, employment type, household composition, and family structure are common to many developed countries.

The ethnic and cultural mix in many developed countries has also changed markedly during the period of the obesity epidemic. In Australia, for example, there have been major changes in the patterns of migration over the past 50 years. According to data from the Australian Bureau of Statistics (90), the cultural mix of migrants has diversified significantly since the 1950s. At that time, most immigrants were from Europe, particularly Germany, the UK, and Italy. Toward the end of the 1960s, there were an increasing number of immigrants from Southern Europe, particularly Yugoslavia and Greece. The pattern of migration changed again during the late 1970s and 1980s, with immigrants increasingly likely to have been born in the Asia-Pacific region, such as New Zealand, Vietnam, and the Philippines. The consequence of these changing patterns of migrations is that Australia is now a multiethnic society of people with a diversity of cultural values and practices. Again, it is important to recognize that Australia's experience of changing patterns of migration, and thus the ethnic composition of its population over the past several decades, is by no means unique in the developed world.

Income inequalities in countries including the US, UK, and other European countries have also widened in recent decades (see (91)). This is thought to be attributable to substantial economic shifts in these countries, such that demand for less skilled workers is reduced. This has resulted in a growing economic divide between those most and least disadvantaged. The impact that such a divide might have on trends in obesity rates in populations is uncertain. Plausibly, however, the increased economic disadvantage of the poor relative to their higher income peers might serve as a barrier to obesity-protective behaviors such as consumption of a diet high in fresh fruits and vegetables, or access to certain physical activity facilities (e.g. gyms, sports), and this may serve to further exacerbate existing socio-economic inequalities in obesity rates.

Clearly there have been significant changes in social roles and relationships, socio-economic inequalities and the ethnic and cultural mix within developed societies during the period of the obesity epidemic, and, as discussed earlier, there is evidence that socio-cultural factors such as these are associated with obesity. It is important to recognize that the kinds of societal changes that have occurred over the last 30 years are likely to continue into the future. These changing patterns of household structure, family composition, employment, migration, and socio-economic inequalities within developed societies will have an important impact on future trends in population obesity and implications for its prevention.

Conclusions

There is a growing body of evidence from the sociological, anthropological, psychological, nutritional, health, and medical research literatures that has examined associations of socio-cultural variables with eating, physical activity, and obesity. We have not attempted to summarize that research exhaustively or systematically; rather we have sought to provide an overview of the evidence related to selected socio-cultural factors and obesity, to review the limited evidence investigating pathways linking socio-cultural factors to obesity, and to provide a suggested conceptual framework to understand the mechanisms by which socio-cultural factors might operate to influence obesity.

Much remains to be learnt about the impact of socio-cultural factors on obesity risk, and how these influences operate. Further research is required to elucidate the range of socio-cultural factors that might impact on obesity. For example future work should disaggregate SES into specific components such as education, occupation, and income, to provide further insight into the specific aspects of SES that are most important. While the majority of studies in this area have focused on SES, this is far from the only important socio-cultural influence on obesity, and additional research is required to examine the nature of associations of social roles/relationships, social institutions, and cultural factors. Ideally, future studies should incorporate multiple socio-cultural factors, in order to investigate their independent and interacting effects. Identifying the extent of socio-cultural influences and how they affect different groups within society (e.g. by sex, age, race) will also be important. Studies of the pathways by which socio-cultural factors influence obesity are particularly required.

While the specific means by which socio-cultural factors operate to influence obesity remains unclear, there seems little doubt that socio-cultural factors do play an important role in influencing eating, physical activity, and sedentary behaviors, and thus risk of obesity. It will therefore be important for those concerned with the development and implementation of strategies aimed at reversing the current epidemic to consider the role of socio-cultural factors in the etiology of obesity and the implications of future socio-cultural change for trends in obesity.

References

1. **Hays S** (1994). Structure and agency and the sticky problem of culture. *Sociol Theory* **12**, 57–72.

2. **Stunkard AJ** (1975). From explanation to action in psychosomatic medicine: the case of obesity. *Psychosom Med* **37**, 195–236.

3. **Stunkard AJ** (1980).The social environment and the control of obesity. In: Stunkard AJ, ed. *Obesity*, pp. 438–62. W.B. Saunders, Philadelphia.

4. Australian National Obesity Taskforce (2003). *Healthy weight 2008: Australia's future.* Available from http://www.healthyactive.gov.au/docs/healthy_weight08.pdf. Accessed 26 October 2003.

5. **Swinburn BA, Caterson I, Seidell JC, James WP** (2004). Diet, nutrition and the prevention of excess weight gain and obesity. *Public Health Nutr* **7**, 123–46.

6. **Nestle M, Jacobson MF** (2000). Halting the obesity epidemic: a public health policy approach. *Public Health Rep* **115**, 1–13.

7. **Shurtleff D** (1956). Mortality among the married. *J Am Geriatr Soc* **4**, 654–66.

8. **Noppa H, Hallstrom T** (1981). Weight gain in adulthood in relation to socioeconomic factors, mental illness and personality traits: a prospective study of middle-aged women. *J Psychosom Res* **25**, 83–9.

9. **Sobal J** (1984). Marriage, obesity and dieting. *Marriage and Fam Rev* **7**, 115–39.

10. **Craddock D** (1975). Psychological and personality factors associated with successful weight reduction: a 10-year follow-up of 134 personal cases. In: Howeard A, ed. *Recent advances in obesity research*, pp. 220–3. Technomic, Westport, CT.

11. **Chen E, Cobb S** (1960). Family structure in relation to health and disease: a review of the literature. *J Chron Dis* **12**, 544–67.

12. **French SA, Jeffery RW, Forster JL, McGovern PG, Kelder SH, Baxter J** (1994). Predictors of weight change over two years among a population of working adults: the Healthy Worker Project. *Int J Obes Relat Metab Disord* **18**, 145–54.

13. **Jeffery R, Rick AM** (2002). Cross-sectional and longitudinal associations between body mass index and marriage-related factors. *Obes Res* **10**, 809–15.

14. **Kahn HS, Williamson DF** (1990). The contributions of income, education and changing marital status to weight change among US men. *Int J Obesity* **14**, 1057–68.

15. **Umberson D** (1992). Gender, marital status and the social control of health behavior. *Soc Sci Med* **34**, 907–17.

16. **Rissanen AM, Heliovaara M, Knekt P, Reunanen A, Aromaa A** (1991). Determinants of weight gain and overweight in adult Finns. *Eur J Clin Nutr* **45**, 419–30.

17. **Rauschenbach B, Sobal J, Frongillo EA** (1995). The influence of change in marital status on weight change over one year. *Obes Res* **3**, 319–27.

18. **Sobal J, Rauschenbach B, Frongillo EA** (1992). Marital status, fatness and obesity. *Soc Sci Med* **35**, 915–23.

19. **Sobal J, Rauschenbach B, Frongillo EA** (2003). Marital status changes and body weight changes: a US longitudinal analysis. *Soc Sci Med* **56**, 1543–55.

20. **Kittel F, Rustin RM, Dramaix M, DeBacker G, Kornitzer M** (1978). Psycho-socio-biological correlates of moderate overweight in an industrial population. *J Psychosom Res* **2**, 145–58

21. **Register CA, Williams DR** (1990). Wage effects of obesity among young workers. *Soc Sci Q* **71**, 131–41.

22. **Hellerstedt W, Jeffery R** (1997). The association of job strain and health behaviours in men and women. *Int J Epidemiol* **26**, 575–83.

23. **Wamala S, Wolk A, Orth-Gomer K** (1997). Determinants of obesity in relation to socioeconomic status among middle-aged Swedish women. *Prev Med* **26**, 734–44.

24. **Vitaliano PP, Russo J, Scanlan JM, Greeno CG** (1996). Weight changes in caregivers of Alzheimer's care recipients: psychobehavioral predictors. *Psychol Aging* **11**, 155–63.

25. **Ball K, Brown W, Crawford D** (2002). Who does not gain weight? Prevalence and predictors of weight maintenance in young women. *Int J Obes* **26**, 1570–8.

26. **Harris HE, Ellison GT, Clement S** (1999). Do the psychosocial and behavioral changes that accompany motherhood influence the impact of pregnancy on long-term weight gain? *J Psychosom Obstet Gynaecol* **20**, 65–79.

27. **Katzmarzyk PT, Perusse L, Rao DC, Bouchard C** (2000). Familial risk of overweight and obesity in the Canadian population using the WHO/NIH criteria. *Obes Res* **8**, 194–7.

28. **Jeffery RW, Drewnoski A, Epstein LH,** *et al.* (2000). Long-term maintenance of weight loss: current status. *Health Psychol* **19**, 5–16.

29. **Matthews KA, Abrams B, Crawford S,** *et al.* (2001). Body mass index in mid-life women: relative influence of menopause, hormone use, and ethnicity. *Int J Obesity* **25**, 863–73.

30. **Gordon-Larsen P, Adair LS, Popkin BM** (2002). Ethnic differences in physical activity and inactivity patterns and overweight status. *Obes Res* **10**, 141–9.

31. **Ball K, Kenardy J** (2002). Body weight, body image, and eating behaviours: relationships with ethnicity and acculturation in a community sample of young Australian women. *Eating Behaviors* **3**, 205–16.

32. **Lauderdale DS, Rathouz PJ** (2000). Body mass index in a US national sample of Asian Americans: effects of nativity, years since immigration and socioeconomic status. *Int J Obes Relat Metab Disord* **24**, 1188–94.

33. **Popkin BM, Udry JR** (1998). Adolescent obesity increases significantly in second and third generation U.S. immigrants: the National Longitudinal Study of Adolescent Health. *J Nutr* **128**, 701–6.

34. **Sundquist J, Winkleby M** (2000). Country of birth, acculturation status and abdominal obesity in a national sample of Mexican-American women and men. *Int J Epidem* **29**, 470–7.

35. **Sobal J, Stunkard AJ** (1989). Socioeconomic status and obesity: a review of the literature. *Psychol Bull* **105**, 260–75.

36. **Goldblatt PB, Moore ME, Stunkard AJ** (1965). Social factors in obesity. *JAMA* **192**, 1039–44.

37. **Moore ME, Stunkard AJ, Srole L** (1962). Obesity, social class, and mental illness. *J Am Med Assoc* **181**, 962–6.

38. **Ball K, Crawford D** (2005). Socioeconomic status and weight change in adults: a review. *Soc Sci Med,* **60,** 1987–2010.

39. **Parsons TJ, Power C, Logan S, Summerbell CD** (1999). Childhood predictors of adult obesity: a systematic review. *Int J Obes Relat Metab Disord* **23** (Suppl 8), S1–S107.

40. **Stunkard AJ** (1996). Socioeconomic status and obesity. *Ciba Found Symposium* **201**, 174–82.

41. **Crawford D, Ball K** (2003). Behavioural determinants of the obesity epidemic. *Asia-Pacific J Clin Nutr* **11** (Supp l), S718–S721.

42. **Quatromoni PA, Copenhafer DL, D'Agostino RB, Millen BE** (2002). Dietary patterns predict the development of overweight in women: The Framingham Nutrition Studies. *JAMA* **102**, 1239–46.

43. **Spencer EA, Appleby PN, Davey GK, Key TJ** (2003). Diet and body mass index in 38,000 EPIC-Oxford meat-eaters, fish-eaters, vegetarians and vegans. *Int J Obes Relat Metab Disord* **27**, 728–34.

44. **Gortmaker SL, Must A, Sobol AM, Peterson K, Colditz GA, Dietz WH.** (1996). Television viewing as a cause of increasing obesity among children in the United States, 1986–1990. *Arch Pediatr Adolesc Med* **150**, 356–62.

45. **Ma Y, Bertone ER, Stanek EJ 3rd,** *et al.* (2003). Association between eating patterns and obesity in a free-living US adult population. *Am J Epidemiol* **158**, 85–92.

46. **Steele P, Dobson A, Alexander H, Russell A** (1991). Who eats what? A comparison of dietary patterns among men and women in different occupational groups. *Aust J Public Health* **15**, 286–94.

47. **Milligan R, Burke V, Beilin L, Dunbar D** (1998). Influence of gender and socio-economic status on dietary patterns and nutrient intakes in 18 year old Australians. *Aust NZ J Public Health* **22**, 485–93.

48. **Roos E, Lahelma E, Virtanen M, Prattala R, Pietinen P** (1998). Gender, socioeconomic status and family status as determinants of food and behaviour. *Soc Sci Med* **46**, 1519–29.

49. **Pryer J, Nichols R, Elliott P, Thakrar B, Brunner E, Marmot M** (2001). Dietary patterns among a national random sample of British adults. *J Epidemiol Comm Health* **55**, 29–37.

50. **Martikainen PT, Brunner E, Marmot M** (2003). Socioeconomic differences in dietary patterns among middle-aged men and women. *Soc Sci Med* **56**, 1397–410.

51. **Smith A, Baghurst K** (1993). Dietary vitamin and mineral intake and social status. *Aust J Nutr Diet* **50**, 163–71.

52. **Davey Smith G, Brunner E** (1997). Socioeconomic differentials in health: the role of nutrition. *Proceed Nutr Soc* **6**, 75–90.

53. **Giskes K, Turrell G, Patterson C, Newman B** (2002). Socio-economic differences in fruit and vegetable consumption among Australian adolescents and adults. *Public Health Nutr* **5**, 663–9.

54. **Mishra G, Ball K, Arbuckle J, Crawford D** (2002). Dietary patterns of Australian adults and their association with socioeconomic status: results from the 1995 National Nutrition Survey. *Europ J Clini Nutr* **56**, 687–93.

55. **French SA, Story M, Neumark-Sztainer D, Fulkerson JA, Hannan P** (2001). Fast food restaurant use among adolescents: associations with nutrient intake, food choices and behavioral and psychosocial variables. *Int J Obes Relat Metab Disord* **25**, 1823–33.

56. **Britton JA, Gammon MD, Kelsey JL,** *et al.* (2000). Characteristics associated with recent recreational exercise among women 20 to 44 years of age. *Women's Health* **31**, 81–96.

57. **Crespo CJ, Ainsworth BE, Keteyian SJ, Heath GW, Smit E** (1999). Prevalence of physical inactivity and its relation to social class in U.S. adults: results from the Third National Health and Nutrition Examination Survey, 1988–1994. *Med Sci Sports Exer* **31**, 1821–7.

58. **Kuh DJ, Cooper CJ** (1992). Physical activity at 36 years: patterns and childhood predictors in a longitudinal study. *J Epidemiol Comm Health* **46**, 114–9.

59. **Billson H, Pryer JA, Nichols R** (1999). Variation in fruit and vegetable consumption among adults in Britain. An analysis from the dietary and nutritional survey of British adults. *Europ J Clini Nutr* **53**, 946–52.

60. **Shahar D, Schultz R, Shahar A, Wing R** (2001). The effect of widowhood on weight change, dietary intake, and eating behavior in the elderly population. *J Aging Health* **13**, 186–99.

61. **Sallis J, Owen N** (1999). *Physical activity and behavioral medicine.* Sage Publications, London.

62. **Trost SG, Owen N, Bauman AE, Sallis JF, Brown W** (2002). Correlates of adults' participation in physical activity: review and update. *Med Sci Sports Exerc* **34**, 1996–2001.

63. **Crespo CJ, Smit E, Andersen RE, Carter-Pokras O, Ainsworth BE** (2000). Race/ethnicity, social class and their relation to physical inactivity during leisure time: results from the third National Health and Nutrition Examination Survey, 1988–1994. *Am J Prev Med* **18**, 46–53.

64. **Patterson BH, Harlan LC, Block G, Kahle L** (1995). Food choices of whites, blacks, and Hispanics: data from the 1987 National Health Interview Survey. *Nutr Cancer* **23**, 105–19.

65. McMurray RG, Harrell JS, Deng S, Bradley CB, Cox LM, Bangdiwala SI (2000). The influence of physical activity, socioeconomic status, and ethnicity on the weight status of adolescents. *Obes Res* **8**, 130–9.

66. Jeffery RW, French SA, Forster JL, Spry VM (1991). Socioeconomic status differences in health behaviours related to obesity: The Healthy Worker Project. *Int J Obes* **15**, 689–96.

67. Ball K, Mishra M, Crawford D (2003). Social factors and obesity: an investigation of the role of health behaviours. *Int J Obes* **27**, 394–403.

68. Wardle J, Parmenter K, Waller J (2000). Nutrition knowledge and food intake. *Appetite* **34**, 269–75.

69. Crawford D, Baghurst KI (1990). Diet and health – a national survey of beliefs, behaviours and barriers to change in the community. *Aust J Nutr Diet* **47**, 97–104.

70. Buttriss JL (1997). Food and nutrition: attitudes, beliefs, and knowledge in the United Kingdom. *Am J Clin Nutr* **65** (Supp 6), S1985–S1995.

71. Parmenter K, Waller J, Wardle J (2000). Demographic variation in nutrition knowledge in England. *Health Edu Res* **15**, 163–74.

72. Hupkens C, Knibbe R, Drop M (2000). Social class differences in food consumption: the explanatory value of permissiveness and health and cost considerations. *Europ J Public Health* **10**, 108–13.

73. Lawrence J, Thompson R, Margetts B (2001). Food choice and socio-economic variables in relation to young women's confidence in cooking specific foods. *Proceed Nutr Soc London* **60**, 77A.

74. Kelsey K, Earp JA, Kirkley B (1997). Is social support beneficial for dietary change? A review of the literature. *Family Comm Health* **20**, 70–82.

75. Sorenson G, Stoddard A, Macario E (1998). Social support and readiness to make dietary changes. *Health Edu Behav* **25**, 586–98.

76. Devine CM, Connors MM, Sobal J, Bisogni CA (2003). Sandwiching it in: spillover of work onto food choices and family roles in low- and moderate-income urban households. *Soc Sci Med* **56**, 617–30.

77. Powell AD, Kahn AS (1995). Racial differences in women's desires to be thin. *Int J Eat Disord* **17**, 91–5.

78. Margetts BM, Martinez JA, Saba A, Holm L, Kearney M, Moles A (1997). Definitions of 'healthy' eating: a pan-EU survey of consumer attitudes to food, nutrition and health. *Eur J Clin Nutr* **51** (Suppl 2), S23–9.

79. Altabe M (1998). Ethnicity and body image: quantitative and qualitative analysis. *Int J Eat Disord* **23**, 153–9.

80. Gluck ME, Geliebter A (2002). Racial/ethnic differences in body image and eating behaviors. *Eat Behav* **3**, 143–51.

81. Pollock NJ (1995). Cultural elaborations of obesity – fattening practices in Pacific societies. *Asia Pacific J Clin Nutr* **4**, 357–60.

82. Rozin P, Rischler C, Imada S, Sarubin A, Wrzesniewski A (1999). Attitudes to food and the role of food in life in the U.S.A., Japan, Flemish Belgium and France: possible implications for the diet–health debate. *Appetite* **33**, 163–80.

83. Florention RF (2002). Summary of the symposium – forging effective strategies for prevention and management of overweight and obesity in Asia. *Asia Pacific J Clin Nutr* **11**, S670–5.

84. Eckersley R (2001). Culture, health and well-being. In: Eckersley R, Dixon J, Douglas B, eds. *The social origins of health and well-being.* Cambridge University Press, Cambridge.

85. International Obesity Taskforce. Available at http://www.iotf.org. Accessed 27 October 2004.

86. Sobal J (1991). Obesity and socioeconomic status: a framework for examining relationships between physical and social variables. *Med Anthr* **13**, 231–47.

87. **Booth SL, Sallis JF, Ritenbaugh C, *et al.*** (2001). Environmental and societal factors affect food choice and physical activity: rationale, influences, and leverage points. *Nutr Rev* **59**, S21–39.

88. **Summerfield C, Babb P, eds** (2003). *Social trends. National Statistics No. 33*, 2003 Edition. The Stationery Office, London.

89. **European Communities, World Health Organization** (1997). *Highlights on health in the United Kingdom.* Available from www.euro.who.int/document/e62043.pdf, Accessed 27 October 2004.

90. **Australian Bureau of Statistics** (2001). *Australian social trends 2001. Population – population growth: coming to Australia.* Available from www.abs.gov.au/Ausstats/abs@.nsf/ 94713ad445ff1425ca25682000192af2/d650a8e2782a347aca256bcd00825564!OpenDocument). Accessed 27 October 2004.

91. **Blank RM** (1995). Changes in inequality and unemployment over the 1980s: comparative cross-national responses. *J Pop Eco* **8**, 1–21.

Chapter 4

Evolving environmental factors in the obesity epidemic

Robert W. Jeffery and Jennifer A. Linde

Introduction

In the last 20 to 30 years, much of the world has experienced a remarkable increase in the prevalence of obesity. Obesity rates have long varied significantly between and within populations, primarily along dimensions of relative population affluence and demographics. However, starting in about 1980, steady increases have been observed in many populations around the world that have made overweight and obesity a serious threat to world health. The seriousness of the phenomenon is underscored by the situation in the US, where average body mass index (BMI) has increased nearly 15 per cent since 1980 and the prevalence of clinical obesity has more than doubled (1). Obesity rates are not uniformly distributed in the US, being concentrated especially in lower income populations and some ethnic minority groups. The upward trend in body weights has been virtually universal, however. It is seen in adults of all ages, including the elderly. It is also seen in children of all ages. It is seen in every social class and every ethnic population. Similar increases have been seen in many populations around the world, including not only those in the upper tiers of economic affluence but also in many developing countries (see Chapter 5).

The causes of the world-wide epidemic of obesity are simple at one level (i.e. the balance between energy intake and expenditure is changing). The specific timing of the behaviors driving the epidemic and its pervasive world-wide character are mysterious (2). The international obesity epidemic was not predicted in advance. It was not recognized until years after it had begun, and its causes are not clearly known. Given the short timeframe in which the changes in world body weight have occurred, it is almost certainly the case that the causes are environmental and behavioral rather than biological. However, the historical data available on potentially causative factors are not good enough to make a compelling case for any specific causal agents. Changes in body weight are certainly being caused by changes in behaviors; increases in energy intake, decreases in physical activity, or both. There is little consensus yet, however, on the relative importance of eating vs. physical activity and even less consensus on what factors could have contributed to such widespread and pervasive changes in these behaviors. The present chapter presents a systematic review of available data on environmental factors that may have contributed to recent trends in population body weight. The review will focus especially on the US population, where data on environmental change and body weight are more complete than in most populations. Emerging data from elsewhere in the world, however, is also very instructive.

Efforts to identify associations between environment and body weight are relatively new. Thus, the data search used for this chapter was intentionally very broad. In addition to examining peer-reviewed scientific literature, a variety of other data sources were also explored, including those from both public and private sources. The review was also intentionally broad in the types of data examined. It includes descriptive data on temporal trends in eating and exercise behavior, and in environmental factors that have occurred in temporal coincidence with recent increases in body weight. It also examines cross-sectional and longitudinal studies of associations between particular environmental exposures and body weight. Peer-reviewed scientific papers were identified by computerized database searches such as Medline and PsycINFO. Governmental data sources were identified through searches of Internet sites of specific government agencies and through databases such as FirstGov. Business and industry data were identified through searches in the ABI/Inform Global, Business and Industry and LEXIS/NEXIS databases, and a search of Internet sites of professional trade organizations and independent companies. Business and industry sources included corporate reports, trade journals, and market research reports.

Because the search for potentially relevant data on environmental factors was so broad, a few caveats should be kept in mind about the limitations of such a strategy. First, because there is no comprehensive index of data sources on environmental trends, the search is almost certainly incomplete. Second, the accuracy of the data in the sources identified is almost certainly variable and may not have the same degree of inaccuracy consistently over time. Third, and perhaps most difficult, the volume of data available in some of the databases identified is so large as to preclude a comprehensive presentation. Therefore, editorial judgment had to be exercised in selecting which pieces of data to report in the chapter.

A final introductory comment is a reminder that the data forming the bulk of this chapter are, for the most part, observational and often ecological. Such data does not lend itself especially well to definitive causal inference and should be judged with epidemiologic principles of causal inference in mind. Observational associations are most likely to be causally related if the associations are strong, consistent across populations and measurement methods, include evidence of temporality to establish that putative causes precede effects, and that hypothesized causal sequences are plausible with respect to what is known about biological mechanisms related to obesity.

Diet versus exercise as a cause of obesity

Obesity, from a biological perspective, is an energy balance problem. When energy intake exceeds energy expenditure, extra energy is stored as body fat. Obesity is typically defined as body weight that exceeds optimal weight for height by about 30 per cent. For the vast majority of people, 30 per cent excess weight represents a cumulative energy imbalance between intake and expenditure that is quite large. For a man of average height, for example, 30 per cent excess body weight represents about 150 000 kcal of energy storage as fat, enough to provide basic energy needs for 2–3 months. Although "obesity" so defined represents a cumulative energy store that is obviously very large, it should be remembered that it does not represent an especially large excess when viewed from the perspective of how obesity typically develops, which is slowly over a period of many years. A daily error in energy balance of 100 kcal would be capable of producing a net increase in energy store of this magnitude in less than 5 years. To produce obesity in a person over a 20-year time span, which is a very common course, requires a daily error of only 25 kcal.

In considering the likely contributions of eating vs. physical activity to obesity, the numbers presented above indicate that it is clearly plausible that either activity or diet could have a major influence on changing body weights. It is believed, however, on both biological and behavioral grounds, that energy intake (i.e. eating) is a more logical candidate for causing changes in weight. The biological underpinnings of this argument are as follows. First, accounting for the cumulative increase in average population body weight of 15 per cent seen in the US in the last 20 years requires an increase in intake or decrease in expenditure of 15 per cent. Because 100 per cent of energy intake comes from food, this could be accomplished by increasing daily energy intake by 15 per cent. For a typical adult requiring 2000 kcal of energy intake per day for energy balance, the change would be 300 calories per day. A 300 calorie per day increase in food intake seems conceptually very plausible. Many food items that have this much energy might plausibly be added to one's diet (e.g. one large soft drink or a chocolate candy bar).

The plausibility of changing energy expenditure by 300 calories is more challenging than the argument for diet. There are two important reasons. First, most of the energy required in humans is not modifiable, that is energy required to maintain temperature homeostasis and basic maintenance functions are pretty constant (3). By most estimates, the proportion of energy expenditure in humans that is occupied by non-modifiable activities is 60–80 per cent. The remaining 20–40 per cent goes to intentional physical activity. Using 20–40 per cent of energy expenditure as the range seen in most human populations, the amount of energy available for modification to produce weight gain is between 400 and 800 calories a day. Thus, changing energy balance to produce a 15 per cent shift relative to intake would require somewhere between a 40 and 75 per cent change in volitional physical activity. We believe that a reduction of this magnitude is not very plausible. In populations such as the US, that were already relatively sedentary at the beginning of the obesity epidemic, a 40 per cent reduction in physical activity would be difficult. A reduction of 300 calories of energy expenditure could be achieved by decreasing the amount of walking by approximately 3 miles a day, for example. However, few would suggest that the average American was walking much more than 3 miles a day before 1980, so average walking time would have to be reduced to near zero. It has been suggested that modern lifestyle conveniences such as cell phones, power lawn mowers, TV remote controls, and other labor-saving devices have made it possible for people to spend significantly less time on their feet during everyday activities (4, 5). This is undoubtedly true. Nevertheless, achieving a reduction in energy expenditure of 300 calories by changing from standing to sitting would require a 3 to 5 hour per day change in relative activity, sitting vs. standing, which also seems to stretch credibility.

In sum, these authors believe that the biology of energy balance in humans combined with a consideration of the magnitude of the behavior change necessary to produce large changes in energy intake vs. large changes in energy expenditure, makes it likely, in the absence of data to the contrary, that changes in food intake probably have played a major role in population changes in body weight. It has, to be sure, been argued that at high enough levels of energy expenditure, people spontaneously regulate their body weight much better than they do at lower rates of expenditure (3). This certainly may be true. However, the observation of sharp increases in body weights in populations at nowhere near these proposed activity threshold levels, suggest that factors other than changes in physical activity are driving changes in body weight in those groups.

Trends in weight-related behavior

International food supply data, from the World Health Organization, suggest cause for alarm with regard to trends in global dietary intake patterns. Over-nutrition, rather than under-nutrition, is now a concern, even in developing nations (6, 7). Reports from the Food and Agriculture Organization of the United Nations indicate that total availability of energy in kcal per capita per day has increased steadily in all nations in the period spanning the mid-1960s to the late 1990s, by approximately 450 kcal per capita per day in developed countries and by over 600 kcal per capita per day in developing countries (7). Food supply data indicate that many developing countries are showing patterns of reductions in intake of dietary fiber and complex carbohydrates, increased intake of fats and saturated fats (particularly from animal sources), and increased intake of sugars, that characterize the "nutrition transition" to a diet that resembles that of developed nations (7, 8) (see Chapter 5). As populations transition to diets that are higher in fats and sugar, and lower in fiber and complex carbohydrates, we would expect obesity rates to increase accordingly world wide.

One of the difficulties in pinpointing specific environmental causes of the obesity epidemic or apportioning relative emphases on diet vs. activity is that reliable data on temporal trends in energy intake and expenditure are not as easily documented as temporal trends in body weight. The primary source of data on trends in population energy intake in the US comes from the US Department of Agriculture (USDA) surveys of individual dietary intake from representative population samples (9). Over much of the time period spanned by the obesity epidemic, estimates of total energy intake per capita have not shown much change in these surveys. For example data from the USDA's Nationwide Food Consumption Surveys (NFCS 1965 and NFCS 1977) and Continuing Survey of Food Intake in Individuals (CSFII 1991 and NSFII 1996) indicated a significant drop in per capita food energy intake between 1965 and 1980, no change between 1980 and 1990, and an increase back to 1965 levels between 1990 and 1995 (10). The latest surveys have shown additional increases in intake (11). However, the fact remains that individual level data on diet have shown essentially no change in energy intake during a period when the average body weight increased substantially.

If correct, the dietary survey data outlined above would seem to suggest that the primary cause of the obesity epidemic might be decreases in physical activity. Unfortunately, data on energy expenditure obtained from activity surveys of individuals do not show this. No national surveys of physical activity have been done across the entire time period of the obesity epidemic using standardized methods. Data from the Minnesota Heart Survey, which examined temporal trends in physical activity between 1980 and the present in the upper Midwest using the Minnesota Leisure Time Physical Activity Questionnaire, however, indicate no change in the reported amount of time (minutes per week) spent on leisure time physical activity over this time period (12, 13). That study, like the USDA studies, also found little or no change in reported energy intakes but did report dramatic increases in weight. More recent data from the Behavioral Risk Factor Surveillance System provide a basis for estimating changes in physical activity nationally between 1990 and the present. These data indicate that the proportion of the population engaging in recommended levels of physical activity increased slightly, from 24.3 to 26.3 per cent, between 1990 and 2003, while the proportion of those reporting no physical activity decreased from 28.7 per cent in 1990 to 24.4 per cent in 2002 (14, 15).

Not surprisingly, the problem of physical inactivity is not limited to the US. In 1990, the World Health Organization cited physical inactivity as one of the top ten risk factors for global health, particularly in terms of cardiovascular disease and mortality risk (16). Physical inactivity contributed to 3.9 per cent of deaths world wide in 1990, a number that was greater than the individual contributions of alcohol or illicit drug use, occupational hazards, unsafe sex, or air pollution (16). Although this report indicated that global data on behaviors that may be linked to morbidity or mortality are sparse, the data that are available suggest a need for action in this area.

Data from Australia provide information on recent trends in physical activity participation at the national level. One study of a broad public health campaign to promote physical activity messages in Australian adults found that, although the messages from the campaign were recognized and physical activity knowledge was improved, actual participation in recommended levels of physical activity decreased from 63 per cent meeting goals in 1997 to 57 per cent meeting goals by 1999 (17). Another mail-based campaign to promote participation in physical activity, conducted in 1998 as part of a randomized trial in the Australian state of New South Wales, found no differences in physical activity participation between intervention and control groups (18). If trends in decreased physical activity and failure to respond to public health messages continue, the observation of a negative impact on obesity levels in Australia, or in other countries world wide, would not be surprising.

Given that the data now available on diet and exercise trends in the population with the most complete data over the last 20 to 30 years (i.e. the US) are unclear about the contribution of eating vs. that of physical inactivity to the obesity epidemic (much less the contribution of more specific behaviors), it is understandable that health-care professionals are not in consensus about where efforts to address the obesity epidemic should be focused. Plausible methodological explanations have been offered for the failure of diet and exercise data to track changes in body weight (9). For example increased under reporting of intake and over reporting of activity over time because of the social stigma associated with being overweight, technical changes in assessment methodologies and trends in food and activity characteristics that are difficult to assess (such as portion sizes or preparation methods in food and energy expenditure in everyday activities) may account for the apparent inconsistencies between measurements in behaviors most responsible for energy balance and changes in body weight (9). The net result, however, is genuine uncertainty in the scientific community about how the energy imbalance leading to increased body weight world wide is occurring.

Food supply

Despite our inability to confidently apportion the responsibility for increased body weights to intake or expenditure, data on temporal trends in the food supply and in opportunities to engage in physical activity provide additional information about how environmental factors that may influence eating and activity have been changing. USDA food disappearance data, which have been collected over a long period of time with seemingly consistent methods, provide an aggregate picture of dietary exposures in the US that may be informative. On an aggregate basis, the per capita availability of food energy in the US follows a time course, both quantitatively and qualitatively, that is fairly consistent with changes in body weight and other diet-related health indices (19, 20). Between 1970 and 1980, per capita energy availability remained stable in the US, which is congruent with the stability of body weight over that time period.

Starting in 1980, however, the per capita availability of food energy gradually increased; it is now 15 per cent higher than it was in 1970. The macronutrient compositions of the foods available in the US marketplace over the time period have also changed. Over the course of the "obesity epidemic", carbohydrate availability in the US food supply increased by 27 per cent. Fat availability increased by only 3 per cent. These changes in the macronutrient composition of the food supply are paralleled with changes in individual intakes in diet surveys and provide an explanation for why we have observed declining serum cholesterol levels and declining cardiovascular disease rates, despite increases in body weights. The US food supply was qualitatively healthier with respect to heart disease in the year 2000 than it was in 1980.

Trends toward increases in one particular carbohydrate in the food supply have also been seen in international food supply data, as discussed by Popkin in Chapter 5. Popkin and colleagues have provided the most comprehensive analysis of international trends and have argued very cogently that increased availability of dietary fats and sugars in international food supplies have been pervasive and likely contributions to the obesity epidemic. They also note interesting variations in different populations that may be revealing, such as greater increases in obesity in men than women in some Asian populations accompanying mechanization of male-dominated employments and greater increases in weight in women than men in Middle Eastern populations where women are more likely to live domestic lives with perhaps more exposure to changes in food supply. One important change is the addition of sugars to the food supply, and particularly inexpensive sweeteners derived from corn.

Because people eat foods rather than nutrients, an examination of temporal trends in the per capita availability of specific foods provides an additional perspective on how environmental exposures to food are changing. The complete list of foods for which longitudinal data on availability can be found is large. For our purposes here, we simply note that over the last 30 years there have been many dramatic changes in the availability of many foods, both upward and downward. Some trends would seem to favor weight increases, and others would seem to favor weight decreases. Examples of food availability changes between 1970 and 2000 in the US seemingly favorable to lower body weight include the following: red meat decreased by 12 per cent; chicken increased by 87 per cent; butter decreased by 8 per cent; whole milk decreased by 63 per cent; fresh fruit increased by 30 per cent; vegetables increased by 27 per cent; refined sugar decreased by 35 per cent; diet soft drinks increased by 287 per cent; and alcohol was unchanged (20). Simultaneously, other changes in food availability seemingly favor increased weight: salad and cooking oil increased by 102 per cent; cheese increased by 99 per cent; corn sweetener increased by 277 per cent; and regular soft drinks increased by 65 per cent (20, 21). As noted above, international trends have highlighted increased availability of edible fats and sugars (especially corn sweeteners). There may be clues in these data to the factors that might contribute to population obesity. However, in the absence of a method for analytically tying time trends in food availability to time trends in body weight, food supply statistics are probably more valuable as a reminder of the complexity and volatility of the food marketplace than they are as a tool for identifying specific foods that are contributing to changes in the prevalence of obesity.

The food environment in the US has changed in many ways over the last quarter century other than in the availability of specific foods. An especially striking trend is the increase in the emphasis on convenience in food availability. Convenience in food availability includes such features as number and proximity of food outlets and how much time is required to purchase and prepare food for consumption. The convenience food industry has been the strongest growth sector in the food distribution economy. Between 1967 and 1997, the number of food stores in the US actually declined by 15 per cent. However, the numbers of locations where ready-to-eat foods can be purchased (e.g. restaurants, cafeterias, and snack bars) more than doubled (22). Americans have dramatically increased the proportion of their food dollars spent away from home (23) and the majority is spent at so called "fast food" restaurant outlets with limited menus, quick service, and the option to take food out to be eaten elsewhere (24). The amount and variety of foods distributed through automated vending machines has also increased (25). Foods available in traditional food stores are also increasingly processed to facilitate ease of preparation. For example sales of prepared meals at grocery stores more than doubled between 1982 and 1992 and were projected to double again by 1997 (26). Overall, it certainly seems plausible that increased availability and convenience in food distribution may have contributed to net increases in per capita food intake relative to energy expenditure in the US The absence of agreed on definitions for terms like "availability" and "convenience", however, is a serious impediment to scientific study of the question. The internationalization of food processing and distribution also mean that the product lines and distribution systems that were originally developed for the US market are now being applied all over the world and might be causally related to the spiraling rates of obesity outside the US.

Temporal trends in exercise exposures

Data on longitudinal trends in population exposures to physical activity are in shorter supply than those on trends on the food supply, which makes an appraisal of these factors for the obesity epidemic more difficult. The availability of recreational opportunities in some areas has increased dramatically. For example the number of commercial health clubs and related recreational facilities is up significantly, as is the number of sporting goods stores (22). The number of homes with exercise equipment has also increased substantially (27). The mix of physical activity has also changed with time. Bowling alleys, bicycling, and rowing machines have declined in popularity in the US, whereas home treadmills and gym sales have increased substantially (22, 27). One area that has clearly seen a reduction in opportunities for physical activity in the US is in public schools.

The amount of curriculum time devoted to physical education is significantly less than it was 20 years ago. Overall, however, it is unclear whether opportunities for recreational activities in the US have declined, increased, or remained unchanged during the period of the obesity epidemic. As with food, there is no agreed definition of overall availability, and there are enough examples to support either side of the argument.

In areas of life that involve non-recreational physical activity, recent trends, for the most part, seem to be consistent with the idea that declining levels of physical activity may contribute to the obesity epidemic. There has been a consistent trend over the last 20 years toward the use of motorized personal transportation world wide and a commensurate decline in the use of public transportation, walking, or bicycling (4).

The hypothesis that inactive forms of entertainment, such as television viewing and home computer use, are contributing to the obesity epidemic is very popular right now, and temporal trends in the availability of these inactive entertainment choices are clearly upward. In the US and much of the developed world, most homes had television sets before 1980 (29). However, videocassette recorders, cable television, and home computers are all technologies that have become widely available to the general population only in the last two decades. The most explosive growth of these technologies has been in the developing world, and within the more affluent countries, multiple electronic entertainment outlets have become normative. In the US, for example, the proportion of households with multiple television sets increased from 35 per cent in 1970 to 75 per cent in 2000. During the same time period, the percentage of households with cable television access increased from 7 to 76 per cent (28).

Many additional labor-saving devices have become available in the last three decades and enthusiastic supporters of increasing physical activity to control body weight are quick to name lawn mowers, garage door openers, television remote controls, keyless entry devices, automatic sprinkler systems, electric pencil sharpeners, and microwave ovens as obesity vectors. Although such devices have clearly proliferated, to the best of our knowledge no studies of the net effects on energy expenditure of having these devices in one's home have been done. Nevertheless, it is certainly plausible that the cumulative effects of labor saving devices like these may contribute, in part, to the steadily declining number of hours that US adults report that they spend on housework (a reduction of 20 per cent since 1965) (29). For better or worse, between 1970 and 1997, there was also a significant increase in the total amount of time that married couples reported that they spent at work in the US, driven in large part by the fact that a larger proportion of households have two full-time working adults (30).

In summary, during the last 20 to 30 years, data on temporal trends in the availability of physical activity choices in the US indicate that trends in access to recreational physical activity choices are mixed, very much like the evidence for food environment exposures. However, changes in activity choices outside the recreational activity area have clearly favored more sedentary lifestyles because of a proliferation of labor saving technologies.

Temporal trends in information

People's diet and activity behaviors, of course, are not only guided by available choices but also by the extent to which they are encouraged to make those choices by social communications from individuals, media, and institutions regarding the most appropriate forms of behavior. In the case of eating, the primary source of public information about what people should eat is, arguably, the food industry. The food industry in the US spends about $50 per person per year to publicize food products. In contrast, the USDA spends about $1.50 per person per year for all types of nutritional education (31). The effects of general food advertising on population consumption trends are seen most clearly in connection with targeted advertising campaigns and products (32). Advertising conducted under the Dairy and Fluid Milk Acts, for example, was estimated to have increased the level of at-home fluid milk consumption by 6 per cent and the level of at-home cheese consumption by 2.3 per cent (33). An experimental study by the Centre for Science in the Public Interest also showed that public advertising of lower fat milk products was associated with a significant increase in the purchase of these products. Trend data also suggest that changes in regulations regarding advertising content may affect both product availability and food consumption patterns. Until 1985, US advertisers of food were limited in the health claims that could be made about foods. When these restrictions were relaxed in the mid 1980s, food was increasingly marketed on the basis of its health-enhancing qualities and many new food products that have been "nutritionally improved" are being marketed (34–36). Emphasis on new products lower in fat and energy is a major trend (35), but the new product introductions also include foods with reduced levels of cholesterol, salt, and sugar, and increased amounts of fiber and calcium. With the recent popularity of the Atkins diet, new food products and advertisements targeting low carbohydrate foods is a striking recent trend. At least two positive population benefits have been accelerated by increased health marketing of foods. These are increased consumption both of high-fiber foods and of lower-fat foods, both of which have been central themes of USDA's dietary recommendations for Americans since the late 1970s (37). Although food industry efforts to promote lower energy foods have not translated into positive trends in population body weight, it is arguable that ambiguity in the federal government's public health messages is partly to blame. Over the years, the Dietary Guidelines for Americans have consistently encouraged the selection of foods with higher nutritional value and discouraged the selection of foods high in fat, cholesterol, sugar, and sodium. They have never recommended eating less (37). The results of low carbohydrate foods and food advertising on health remains to be evaluated.

One of the most talked about food promotion practices over the last two decades has been the promotion of larger portion sizes for small increases in price. Products ranging from soft drinks to bagels are now available in sizes much larger than they were in previous decades (38), and when products are available in multiple sizes, the unit price for larger servings is usually less (32, 39). Some portion sizes that at one time were considered standard (e.g. 177- and 237-ml bottles of Coca Cola) are no longer sold at all and sizes now standard, like the 592 ml soft drink, were unheard of when these products were first introduced. So-called "value pricing" makes sense from a business perspective since the portion size of food is usually a minor determinant of the cost to the marketer. However, adverse effects on consumption seem likely since it has been shown experimentally that portion size has a significant impact on food consumption in single meal settings. Although the overall density of exposure to food advertising and its impact on consumption are difficult to quantify, some evidence suggests that the competition for market share among food providers has become more intense over time, in that the proportion of the purchase price of food attributable to advertising expenditures has systematically increased (40).

Messages about adequate and appropriate physical activity have been clear and consistent since 1965 in the US (i.e. that people should engage in 30 minutes of physical activity three to five times per week), although there has been an increased emphasis on greater frequency and duration of physical activity very recently from a number of sources, including the Centers for Disease Control, Institute of Medicine, and WHO (41). That recommendations about physical activity have not changed much across most of the time period covered by the obesity epidemic parallels our previous discussion that leisure time physical activity has apparently not decreased over the past two decades.

Another form of information about obesity and related behaviors available to the public is the portrayal of personal behavior and body weight in the media. The use of extremely lean models, particularly for women, in the promotion of commercial products, as well as in entertainment media, has been argued to contribute to undesirable eating and exercise behaviors (42, 43). Researchers have tracked time trends in fashionable body shapes for women for several decades. Similar studies of "ideal" body shapes for men are also now available, although for a shorter period of time. For women, fashionable body shapes have gone up and down. They were very thin in the 1920s, became relatively full in the 1950s, became quite thin in the 1960s (i.e. BMIs of 18 to 19 kg/m^2), and have not changed much since then (44). Because women's actual body weights are increasing, the discrepancy between "real" and "ideal" body weights has been widening, which has engendered increasing concern about the media's possible contribution to excessive dieting behaviors. Interestingly, however, male models tend not to be as lean as female models (BMIs of 25 kg/m^2), and over the last decade they have been getting heavier. A recent study of how the media have portrayed eating and exercise behaviors over the last decade or so in the US television programming suggests a mixed picture with respect to influences on weight. Depiction of physically active lifestyles has increased, as has depiction of eating foods high in energy density (45). In summary, although there clearly are some obese celebrities in the US, based on scientific analyses of media depiction of body weight and lifestyle, there seems to be little reason to think that major shifts in social attitudes favoring larger body sizes have taken place over the last 20 years, at least for women. Moreover, available international trends seem to be closely paralleling those in the US.

Associations between environment and weight or weight-related behaviors

A second level of questioning related to environmental factors and obesity is whether there are data that indicate whether people who are exposed to different levels of specific environmental factors have different body weights. A substantial body of data is beginning to emerge showing that people who eat differently and who have different physical activity patterns tend to have different body weights (46). Cross-sectional and longitudinal analyses of the relationships between diet, physical activity, and body weight show that total energy intake and fat intake tend to be associated with higher body weight and that changes in energy and fat intake over time are associated with changes in weight in the same direction (46). Similarly, higher habitual levels of physical activity are associated with lower body weight, and increases and decreases in physical activity over time are associated with weight loss and weight regain, respectively. How often people weigh themselves is inversely related to body weight, however (47). Fewer studies of specific food exposures have been conducted, but those that have suggest that the consumption of some specific high fat foods (e.g. hamburgers and French fries) and of large quantities of sugar (e.g. from soft drinks) tends to be associated with higher body weights in both children and adults (48–51). The frequency of reported eating at fast-food restaurants has also been positively associated with higher body weight (52–54). Reported rates of "dieting" to lose weight and consumption of specific commercially available "diet" foods tend to be higher among more obese persons but, if anything, these behaviors are predictive of weight gain rather than weight loss over time (55–58). One study has shown that if the duration of "dieting" is assessed, individuals reporting that they spend more time intentionally dieting and intentionally exercising for the purpose of controlling weight achieved better weight control over time (58).

Although there has been a good deal of talk about the potential adverse effects of the seemingly ubiquitous availability of convenience food outlets, few systematic studies have been done examining this question. Several studies have shown that the density of convenience food outlets tends to be higher in neighborhoods where people of lower SES live, and it is well known that these individuals, on average, tend to be heavier. Specific links to individuals as opposed to neighborhoods have not been demonstrated, however. A study by the current authors, as yet to be published, suggests that such evidence may be difficult to establish. Using geo-spatial mapping methodologies, the density of "fast food" and other restaurants with respect to the home and work addresses of a population sample was assessed. Reported use of "fast food" restaurants, but not other restaurants, was positively associated with higher body weight. Proximity of "fast food" restaurants to home or work addresses was not related either to reported usage or body weight. Indeed, the only significant association noted in these data between food outlet density and weight was not in the expected direction – men working in higher-density restaurant areas (cities) were leaner than their counterparts in lower-density restaurant areas.

In summary, cross-sectional and longitudinal data on the relationship between food selections or exposures and body weight provide additional support for the idea that the increased availability and convenience of energy dense foods may contribute to obesity. However, research on the consumption of specific foods and body weight is very limited and data on the relationship between environmental exposures and body weight is even scarcer. Thus, conclusions about the unique contribution of specific food items to obesity are highly speculative as are the relationships between consumption and environmental exposures.

Data on exposures to individual environmental factors and physical activity are also quite modest. A substantial literature on urban design, primarily developed by transportation planners, shows that different structural features in communities are associated with higher or lower levels of use of automobiles (59). Communities laid out in rectangular grid patterns tend to be associated with more travel by foot and less travel by automobile. Several longitudinal studies of traffic-calming measures (e.g. speed bumps and other devices introduced to discourage high-speed automobile traffic) have shown increased use of the street by pedestrians after the introduction of such changes (59).

Several recent studies have shown that living in physical-activity-friendly environments is associated with greater reported physical activity. One community survey reported a positive cross-sectional association between the proximity of commercial physical-activity facilities and the levels of physical activity reported by the survey respondents. The proximity of publicly available recreational facilities (such as parks and school athletic fields) was not associated with physical activity, however (60). Another community survey of Australian adults reported positive cross-sectional associations between activity-unfriendly environments (e.g. a highway with limited or no sidewalk access) and excess body weight (61). A major problem methodologically with such studies is that exercise friendliness is highly related to population density, which is related to a host of sociodemographic and economic factors that are very difficult to control for analytically. Additional studies of the effects of proximity on physical activity opportunities have shown positive relationships between the presence of physical-activity equipment in people's homes and their reported levels of physical activity (62). One as yet to be published study has also indicated an inverse, though non-significant, relationship between BMI and hours of physical education in public school children (63).

Television viewing has attracted special attention as a potential obesity promoter. Several studies have now shown that the number of hours of television viewing per week is associated with higher body weights in both children and adults (61, 64–69). Longitudinal relationships between television viewing and body weight change have been less strong, however, and one study of obese children's physical activity preferences before and after successful weight loss has suggested that preference for passive over active forms of entertainment may be a consequence rather than a cause of obesity (70). Interesting, as well, are studies that show a stronger relationship between television viewing and eating than between television viewing and recreational physical activity (71, 72). If true, it suggests that the mechanism connecting television viewing to higher body weights may be through increased eating rather than decreased physical activity. The observation that television advertising represents about three-fourths of food industry advertising expenses is consistent with this idea (31).

Overall, the most extensively studied environmental exposures associated with obesity are those involving television viewing and convenience foods. The associations for both exposures are consistent with the idea of that there is a causal connection, but the associations for both exposures are also subject to question because of inconsistent and sometimes weak associations, especially those trying to establish temporal sequencing. Both exposures also have a strong association with social class that may be difficult to control for statistically. In addition, both television viewing and the consumption of convenience foods are high-frequency behaviors that are almost certainly embedded in larger diet and physical activity patterns. Thus, they may be symbols identifying obesity-promoting lifestyles rather than unique, independent causal agents.

Summary and conclusions

The cause of the obesity epidemic that has affected the world for the last 30 years remains unknown. Although changes in body weight and fatness are surely the result of changes in energy intake and energy expenditure that are mediated by changes in food and activity choices, clear data identifying the specific contribution of energy intake vs. energy expenditure or the specific contributions of specific behavioral choices are not available. It is argued here that consideration of both biological and behavioral aspects of energy intake and utilization strongly favor change in energy intake as the most likely cause. However, the inability of population data on energy intake and energy expenditure to elucidate this issue is a cause for concern.

A point of general agreement is that the cause of the obesity epidemic is most likely to be found in changes in environment rather than changes in biological factors. However, the scientific evidence available at present is so weak that it seems unlikely that a quick consensus will be reached on either what environmental factors are driving the epidemic or, for that matter, how the search for them might best be organized. This review has shown that the state of knowledge in the area is fragmented, of uneven coverage with respect to topics, and very likely of uneven quality as well. Many of the available data simply consist of descriptive information about contemporaneous trends in environmental factors, behaviors, and body weight, which are among the weakest forms of data for making causal inferences.

Cross-sectional and longitudinal studies on the relationship between specific environmental exposures and body weight have provided better insights into the possible importance of a few high profile environmental factors and body weight (e.g. television viewing and convenience foods). The available data are quite limited in scope, however, and causal interpretations are plagued by potential confounders such as social class, by the fact that temporality has at best been weakly demonstrated, and, in many cases, by the absence of data establishing plausible underlying mechanisms.

What further research is needed to improve our understanding of the environment and the obesity epidemic? More research is needed in almost every area. We need better ways to conceptualize and measure the environmental factors that might be related to health behavior, as well as better and more accurate means of surveillance of the eating and exercise habits of the population and environmental changes. We also need more experimental and observational studies that specifically examine environment, behavior, and weight interactions. It is an exciting area and one in need of more research to make progress in halting and reversing the obesity epidemic. It should also be noted that the focus of this review of environmental factors is not meant to discourage investigations into the possibility that socio-cultural factors (such as societal attitudes toward obesity, personal gratification, consumerism, and other factors) are not also worthy of further exploration.

Are there other policy implications that derive from current knowledge about environment and obesity? It would be difficult to look at the existing body of knowledge on environment and obesity and make specific recommendations about actions, in either the public sector or the private sector, that would have a high likelihood of making a substantive impact on the prevalence of obesity in the population. Those strategies with strongest empirical support are politically infeasible now and are inconsistent with the values held by most members of society. The most important policy message that comes from an examination of the current state of affairs with respect to obesity and environment is probably that it is time to open up a candid dialogue among organizations and individuals who are influential in setting environmental factor-related policies worldwide with the objective of reaching consensus that: (i) obesity is an important problem that needs to be addressed; (ii) solution of the obesity epidemic will require society-wide and environmental efforts; and (iii) we need to work together to develop concrete steps that may be taken to develop a solution. There are also several specific areas in which public policy changes are probably feasible and that have good face validity with respect to the obesity epidemic. These are articulated well in current WHO guidelines (3,7) for addressing the obesity epidemic.

Acknowledgments

This research was supported by the University of Minnesota Obesity Prevention Centre, the National Institute of Mental Health (NIMH) grant MH068127, and the National Institute of Diabetes and Digestive and Kidney Diseases (NIDDK) grants DK50456 and DK064596.

References

1. Flegal KM, Carroll MD, Ogden CL, Johnson CL (2002). Prevalence and trends in obesity among US adults, 1999–2000. *JAMA* **288**, 1723–7.

2. Jeffery RW, Utter J (2003). The changing environment and population obesity in the United States. *Obes Res* **11**,12S–22S.

3. World Health Organization (1997). Energy balance and the physiological regulation of body weight. In: *Obesity: preventing and managing the global epidemic,* p. 109. Report of a WHO Consultation on Obesity, Geneva.

4. U.S. Bureau of the Census (2001). *Means of transportation to work for the US (1970, 1980, 1990) and travel time to work for the United States (1990 and 1980).* Journey-to-Work and Migration Statistics Branch, Population Division, U.S. Bureau of the Census, Washington, DC.

5. Nielsen Media Research (2000). *2000 Report on television: the first 50 Years.* AC Nielsen, New York.

6. Chopra M, Galbraith S, Darnton-Hill I (2002). A global response to a global problem: the epidemic of overnutrition. *Bull WHO* **80**, 952–8.

7. WHO/FAO Expert Consultation (2003). *Diet, nutrition and the prevention of chronic diseases.* WHO Technical Report Series, No. 916. Report of a joint World Health Organization/Food and Agriculture Organization of the United Nations Expert Consultation, Geneva.

8. Drewnowski A, Popkin BM (1997). The nutrition transition: new trends in the global diet. *Nutr Rev* **55**, 31–43.

9. Harnack LJ, Jeffery RW, Boutelle KN (2000). Temporal trends in energy intake in the United States: an ecologic perspective. *Am J Clin Nutr* **71**, 1473–84.

10. Popkin BM, Siega-Riz AM, Haines PS, Jahns L (2001). Where's the fat? Trends in U.S. diets 1965–1996. *Prev Med* **32**, 245–55.

11. Wright JD, Kennedy-Stephenson J, Wang CY, McDowell MA, Johnson CL (2004). Trends in intake of energy and macronutrients—United States, 1971–2000. *MMWR* **53**, 80–2.

12. Folsom AA, Jacobs DR, Caspersen CJ, Gomez-Marin O, Knudsen J (1986). Test-retest reliability of the Minnesota leisure time physical activity questionnaire. *J Chronic Dis* **39**, 505–11.

13. Steffen LM, Arnett D, Shaw G, McGovern P, Luepker RV, Jacobs DR (2001). *Trends in leisure time physical activity: the Minnesota Heart Survey, 1980–97.* (Abstract) American Heart Association's Scientific Session 2001, Anaheim, CA.

14. Centers for Disease Control and Prevention (2000). Physical activity trends – United States, 1990–1999. *Food Rev* **23**, 8–15.

15. **Division of Adult and Community Health, National Center for Chronic Disease Prevention and Health Promotion Centers for Disease Control and Prevention.** *Behavioral Risk Factor Surveillance System Online Prevalence Data, 1990–2003.* http://apps.nccd.cdc.gov/brfss/index.asp

16. Murray CJL, Lopez AD (1996). Evidence-based health policy – lessons from the Global Burden of Disease Study. *Science* **274**, 740–3.

17. Bauman A, Armstrong T, Davies J, *et al.* (2003). Trends in physical activity participation and the impact of integrated campaigns among Australian adults. *Aust NZ J Public Health* **27**, 76–9.

18. Marshall AL, Bauman AE, Owen N, Booth ML, Crawford D, Marcus BH (2004). Reaching out to promote physical activity in Australia: a state-wide randomized controlled trial of a stage-targeted intervention. *Am J Health Promotion* **18**, 283–7.

19. Putnam J (2000). Major trends in the US food supply. *Food Rev* **23**, 13.

20. Putnam JJ, Allshouse JE (1999). *Food consumption, prices and expenditures, 1970–97.* Statistical Bulletin No. 965. Food and Consumer Economics Division, Economic Research Service, U.S. Department of Agriculture, Washington, DC.

21. **Putnam J, Allshouse J, Kantor LS** (2002). U.S. per capita food supply trends: more calories, refined carbohydrates, and fats. *Food Rev* **25**, 2–15.

22. U.S. Bureau of the Census (1967, 1977, 1987 and 1997). *Economic census.* U.S. Department of Commerce, Washington, DC.

23. Chain Store Age Industry Data (2001). *Share of income spent for food.* Lebhar-Friedman, New York.

24. National Restaurant Association (1998). *Restaurant industry numbers: 25-Year history, 1970–1995.* National Restaurant Association, Washington, DC.

25. **Sanford T** (1997). 1997 census of the industry. *Vending Times* **37**, 1–66.

26. **Jekanowski M** (1999). Grocery industry courts time-pressed consumers with home meal replacements. *Food Rev* **22**, 32–4.

27. **Carr M, Deters T, Moffatt T, Pitts E** (1998). *Tracking the fitness movement: 1987–1997 A decade of change.* Sporting Goods Manufacturers Association, North Palm Beach, FL.

28. Nielsen Media Research (2000). *2000 report on television: the first 50 years.* AC Nielsen, New York.

29. **Bianchi SM, Milkie MA, Sayer LC, Robinson JP** (2000). Is anyone doing the housework? Trends in the gender division of household labor. *Social Forces* **79**, 191–228.

30. **Jacobs JA, Gerson K** (2001). Overworked individuals or overworked families? Explaining trends in work, leisure, and family time. *Work Occup* **28**, 40–63.

31. **Gallo AE** (1999). Food advertising in the United States. In: Frazao E, ed. *America's eating habits: changes and consequences. Agriculture information bulletin no. 750*, pp. 173–80. Economic Research Service, U.S. Department of Agriculture, Washington, DC.

32. **French SA, Story M, Jefery RW** (2001). Environmental influences on eating and physical activity. *Annu Rev Public Health* **22**, 309–35.

33. **Blisard N** (1999). Advertising and what we eat: the case of dairy products. In Frazao E, ed. *America's eating habits: changes and consequences. Agriculture information bulletin no. 750*, pp. 181–8. Economic Research Service, U.S. Department of Agriculture, Washington, DC.

34. Economic Research Service, U.S. Department of Agriculture (1999). Table 1—Number of new food products bearing nutrient content claims, 1988–97. In: Frazao E, ed. *America's eating habits: changes and consequences. Agriculture information bulletin no. 750*, p. 398. Economic Research Service, U.S. Department of Agriculture, Washington, DC.

35. **Klassen ML, Wauer SM, Cassel S** (1990/1). Increases in health and weight loss claims in food advertising in the eighties. *J Advertising Res* **30**, 32–7.

36. **Mathios AD, Ippolito PM** (1999). Food companies spread nutrition information through advertising and labels. *Food Rev* **21**, 38–43.

37. **Davis C, Saltos E** (1999). Dietary recommendations and how they have changed over time. In: Frazao E, ed. *America's eating habits: changes and consequences. Agriculture information bulletin no. 750*, pp. 35–50. Economic Research Service, U.S. Department of Agriculture, Washington, DC.

38. **Young LR, Nestle MS** (1995). Portion sizes in dietary assessment: issues and policy implications. *Nutr Rev* **53**, 149–58.

39. **Wansink B** (1996). Can package size accelerate usage volume? *J Market* **60**, 1–14.

40. **Troy L** (1993). Report on 'selected operating factors in percentage of net sales: advertising.' In: Troy L, ed. *Almanac of business and industrial financial ratios.* Prentice-Hall, Englewood Cliffs, NJ.

41. U.S. Department of Health and Human Services (1996). *Physical activity and health: a report of the surgeon general.* National Centre for Chronic Disease Prevention and Health Promotion, Centers for Disease Control and Prevention, U.S. Department of Health and Human Services, Atlanta, GA.

42. **Berel S, Irving L** (1998). Media and disturbed eating: an analysis of media influence and implications for prevention. *J Primary Prev* **18**, 415–30.

43. **Thompson JK, Heinberg LJ** (1999). The media's influence on body image disturbance and eating disorders: we've reviled them, now can we rehabilitate them? *J Social Issues* **55**, 39–53.

44. **Spitzer BL, Henderson KA, Zivian MT** (1999). Gender differences in population versus media body sizes: a comparison over four decades. *Sex Roles* **40**, 545–65.

45. **Terre L, Drabman RS, Speer P** (1991). Health-relevant behaviors in media. *J Appl Social Psychol* **21**, 1303–19.

46. **Sherwood NE, Jeffery RW, French SA, Hannan PJ, Murray DM** (2000). Predictors of weight gain in the Pound of Prevention study. *Int J Obes Relat Metab Disord* **24**, 395–403.

47. **Linde J, Jeffery RW, French SA.** (2005). Self-weighing in weight gain prevention and weight loss intervention trials. *Ann Behav Med,* in press.

48. **French SA, Jeffery RW, Forster JL, McGovern PG, Kelder SH, Baxter JE** (1994). Predictors of weight change over two years among a population of working adults: the Healthy Worker Project. *Int J Obes Relat Metab Disord* **18**, 145–54.

49. **Wirfalt AKE, Jeffery RW** (1997). Using cluster analysis to examine dietary patterns: nutrient intakes, gender, and weight status differ across food pattern clusters. *J Am Diet Assoc* **97**, 272–9.

50. **Maskarinec G, Novotny R, Tasaki K** (2000). Dietary patterns are associated with body mass index in multiethnic women. *J Nutr* **130**, 3068–72.

51. **Ludwig DS, Peterson KE, Gortmaker SL** (2001). Relation between consumption of sugar-sweetened drinks and childhood obesity: a prospective, observational analysis. *Lancet* **357**, 505–8.

52. **Jeffery RW, French SA** (1998). Epidemic obesity in the United States: are fast foods and television viewing contributing? *J Am Public Health* **88**, 277–80.

53. **French SA, Jeffery RW** (2000). Fast food restaurant use among women in the Pound of Prevention study: dietary, behavioral and demographic correlates. *Int J Obes Relat Metab Disord* **24**, 1353–9.

54. **McCrory MA, Fuss P, Hays NP,** *et al.* (1999). Overeating in America: association between restaurant food consumption and body fatness in healthy adult men and women ages 19 to 80. *Obes Res* **7**, 564–71.

55. **Crawford D, Jeffery RW, French SA** (2000). Can anyone successfully control their weight? Findings of a three year community-based study of men and women. *Int J Obes Relat Metab Disord* **24**, 1107–10.

56. **French SA, Jeffery RW, Forster JL** (1994). Dieting status and its relationship to weight, dietary intake, and physical activity changes over two years in a working population. *Obes Res* **2**, 135–44.

57. **French SA, Jeffery RW** (1994). Consequences of dieting to lose weight: effects on physical and mental health. *Health Psychol* **13**, 195–212.

58. **French SA, Jeffery RW, Murray D** (1999). Is dieting good for you?: prevalence, duration and associated weight and behavior changes for specific weight loss strategies over four years in US adults. *Int J Obes Relat Metab Disord* **23**, 320–7.

59. **Frank LD, Engelke P, Hourigan D** (2002). *How land use and transportation systems impact public health: an annotated bibliography.* Active Community Environments (ACEs) Working Paper 2. Sponsored by the Centers for Disease Control and Prevention and the Georgia Institute of Technology.

60. **Sallis JF, Hovell MF, Hofstetter CR,** *et al.* (1990). Distance between homes and exercise facilities related to frequency of exercise among San Diego residents. *Public Health Rep* **105**, 179–85.

61. **Giles-Corti B, Macintyre S, Clarkson JP, Pilora T, Donovan R** (2003). Environmental and lifestyle factors associated with overweight and obesity in Perth, Australia. *Am J Health Promotion* **18**, 93–102.

62. Jakicic JM, Wing RR, Butler BA, Jeffery RW (1997). The relationship between presence of exercise equipment in the home and physical activity level. *Am J Health Promotion* **11**, 363–5.

63. Schmitz, K (2004). Personal communication.

64. Dietz WH, Gortmaker SL (1985). Do we fatten our children at the television set? Obesity and television viewing in children and adolescents. *Pediatrics* **5**, 807–12.

65. Tucker LA, Friedman GM (1989). Television viewing and obesity in adult males. *Am J Public Health* **79**, 516–8.

66. Tucker LA, Bagwell M (1991). Television viewing and obesity in adult females. *Am J Public Health* **81**, 908–11.

67. Robinson TN, Hammer LD, Killen JD, *et al.* (1993). Does television viewing increase obesity and reduce physical activity? Cross-sectional and longitudinal analyses among adolescent girls. *Pediatrics* **91**, 273–80.

68. Sidney S, Sternfeld B, Haskell WL, Jacobs DR, Liu K, Hulley SB (1996). Television viewing and cardiovascular risk factors in young adults: the CARDIA Study. *Ann Epidemiol* **6**, 154–9.

69. Crawford DA, Jeffery RW, French SA (1999). Television viewing, physical inactivity and obesity. *Int J Obes Relat Metab Disord* **23**, 437–40.

70. Epstein LH, Smith JA, Vara LS, Rodefer JS (1991). Behavioral economic analysis of activity choice in obese children. *Health Psychol* **10**, 311–6.

71. Crespo CJ, Smit E, Troiano RP, *et al.* (2001). Television watching, energy intake, and obesity in US children. *Arch Pediatr Adolesc Med* **155**, 360–5.

72. Hernandez B, Gortmaker SL, Colditz GA, Peterson KE, Laird NM, Parra-Cabrera S (1999). Association of obesity with physical activity, television programs and other forms of video viewing among children in Mexico City. *Int J Obes Relat Metab Disord* **23**, 845–54.

Chapter 5

The implications of the nutrition transition for obesity in the developing world

Barry M. Popkin

Introduction

Dietary and physical activity patterns around the world have shifted at accelerated rates over the past decade. Rapid increases in the globalization of the food supply and food distribution networks, technology related to work and leisure, and the coverage of modern mass media are key global causal factors. Each of these global forces, along with urbanization and other shifts at the local level, underlie the quickening of the rate of change of diet and activity patterns of large subpopulation groups among most countries in the world. The resultant shifts in dietary patterns and away from energy-intense, market-oriented economic and home production-oriented work, travel, and leisure toward increased sedentarianism and lower overall physical activity levels have occurred concurrently. The nutrition transition stage associated with diet-related non-communicable disease has been reached very quickly by huge segments of the developing world, while other segments in these same countries face an earlier pattern of diet and activity linked with under nutrition. The speed of change in obesity, along with the shifting burden of disease toward the poor, is also discussed briefly. This chapter will highlight data on these dietary trends around the world, with a combination of individual dietary intake analysis and more aggregate consumption analysis. The implications of these trends for public health policy and programs will be discussed.

What is the nutrition transition?

Two historic processes of change occur simultaneously with, or precede, the "nutrition transition". One is the demographic transition: the shift from a pattern of high fertility and mortality to one of low fertility and mortality (typical of modern industrialized countries). The second is the epidemiological transition, first described by Omran (1): the shift from a pattern of high prevalence of infectious disease, associated with malnutrition, periodic famine, and poor environmental sanitation, to one of high prevalence of chronic and degenerative disease, associated with urban–industrial lifestyles (2).

The nutrition transition is closely related to the other two transitions. Large shifts have occurred in diet and in physical activity patterns, particularly in the last few decades of the twentieth century. Modern societies seem to be converging on a diet high in saturated fats, sugar, and refined foods and low in fiber (often termed the "Western diet") and on lifestyles characterized by lower levels of activity. These changes are reflected in nutritional outcomes, such as changes in average stature, body composition, and morbidity.

Human diet, activity patterns, and nutritional status have undergone a sequence of major shifts, defined as broad patterns of food use and corresponding to nutrition-related disease. Over the last three centuries, the pace of dietary and activity change appears to have accelerated, to varying degrees in different regions of the world. Further, dietary and activity changes are paralleled by major changes in health status, as well as by major demographic and socioeconomic changes. Obesity emerges early in the shift, as does the level and age composition of morbidity and mortality. We can think of five broad nutrition stages. They are not restricted to particular periods of human history. For convenience, the stages are outlined as historical developments; however, "earlier" stages are not restricted to the periods in which they first arose, but continue to characterize certain geographic and socioeconomic subpopulations.

Stage 1: collecting food

This diet, which characterizes hunter–gatherer populations, is high in carbohydrates and fiber and low in fat, especially saturated fat (3, 4). In meat from wild animals, the proportion of polyunsaturated fat is significantly higher than in meat from modern domesticated animals (5). Activity patterns are very high and little obesity is found among hunter–gatherer societies. It is important to note that much of the research on hunter–gatherers is based on modern hunter–gatherers as there is much less evidence from prehistoric people.

Stage 2: famine

The diet becomes much less varied and subject to larger variations and periods of acute scarcity of food. These dietary changes are hypothesized to be associated with nutritional stress and a reduction in stature (estimated by some at about 10 cm) (6, 7). During the later phases of this stage, social stratification intensifies, and dietary variation according to gender and social status increases (8). The stage of famine (as with each of the stages) has varied over time and space. Some civilizations are more successful than others in alleviating famine and chronic hunger, at least for their more privileged citizens (9). The types of physical activities changed but there was little change in activity levels during this period.

Stage 3: receding famine

The consumption of fruits, vegetables, and animal protein increases, and starchy staples become less important in the diet. Many earlier civilizations made great progress in reducing chronic hunger and famines, but only in the last third of the last millennium have these changes become widespread, leading to marked shifts in diet. However, famines continued well into the eighteenth century in portions of Europe and remain common in some regions of the world. Activity patterns start to shift and inactivity and leisure becomes a part of the lives of more people.

Stage 4: nutrition-related non-communicable disease (NRNCD)

A diet high in total fat, cholesterol, sugar, and other refined carbohydrates and low in polyunsaturated fatty acids and fiber, often accompanying increasingly sedentary life, is characteristic of most high-income societies (and increasingly of portions of the population in low-income societies), resulting in increased prevalence of obesity and contributing to the degenerative diseases that characterize Omran's final epidemiological stage.

Stage 5: behavioral change

A new dietary pattern appears to be emerging as a result of changes in diet evidently associated with the desire to prevent or delay degenerative diseases and prolong health. Whether these changes, instituted in some countries by consumers and in others also prodded by government policy, will constitute a large-scale transition in dietary structure and body composition remains to be seen (10–12). If such a new dietary pattern takes hold, it may be very important in enhancing "successful aging", that is postponing infirmity and increasing the disability-free life expectancy (13, 14).

Our focus is increasingly on Stages 3 to 5, in particular on the rapid shift in much of the world's low and moderate income countries from the stage of receding famine to NRNCD. Figure 5.1 presents this focus. The concern on this period is so great that the term the Nutrition Transition is synonymous, for many, with this shift from Stage 3 to 4. The changes are all driven by a range of factors, including urbanization, economic growth, technical change, and culture.

Dietary shifts: more fat, more added caloric sweeteners, more animal-source foods

The diets of the developing and developed world are converging on quite common patterns. Nevertheless there are some marked differences in eating patterns between these two worlds so we will discuss, first, higher income countries and then lower and middle income ones.

The higher income "developed world"

There are a large number of higher income countries, in particular the US, Japan, South Korea, and the UK , that have quality dietary monitoring survey systems.

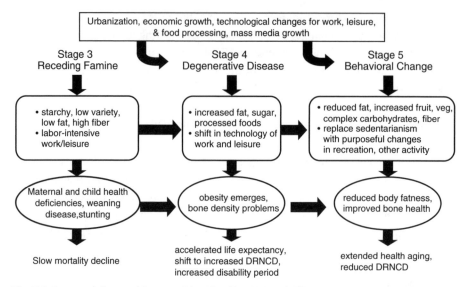

Fig. 5.1 Stages of the nutrition transition (Popkin, 2002a (58)).

The US nationally representative surveys are readily available to the public and are used extensively by this author. The US data will be used here to delineate a number of patterns of dietary change that are relevant. It appears that these countries are further along in the transition toward greater processed food and a diet dominated by away-from-home food consumption.

Overview of US dietary shifts

Overall, daily caloric intake appears to be increasing, primarily from energy-dense, nutrient-poor foods and snacks (15–21). These foods are being eaten in a greater number of daily snacking episodes (17, 18). Additionally, an increasing number of meals are being consumed away from home (15–18, 20). Concurrently, food portion sizes offered in restaurants have increased dramatically (15, 16, 22–24) and weekend eating has taken on greater importance: adults consume 115 extra calories daily from fat and alcohol during the Friday to Sunday period (19).

Many of these dynamic shifts have led to growing concern about diet quality for two reasons. First, fast foods generally are more energy dense but lack many critical nutrients (25, 26). Second, several studies, although correlational rather than causal, suggest a positive association between the frequency of fast food consumption and body fatness, weight gain, and overweight/obesity in adults and adolescents (27–32). Associated with greater accessibility of low-cost foods in fast and convenient food outlets, is a shift in the types of foods being consumed, including significant increases in salty snacks and fast foods (15–18) and a rapid increase in intake of added caloric sweeteners (33, 34). Although availability and intake of fruits and vegetables has been increasing since 1970 (15, 16, 35), the average number of servings per day remains far below the recommended levels (15, 16, 24).

Soft drinks and fruit drinks lead the way! One of these US patterns of dietary change, the rapid increase in caloric sweetener intake, is a global pattern, as we show below. Table 5.1 presents nationally representative weighted US data that shows the key foods responsible for this shift (24). Of the total increase of 83 kcal, 54 kcal per day come from soft drinks and 13 kcal from similar sugared fruit drinks. These figures represent close to 81 per cent of the increase in caloric sweetener intake between 1977 and 1996 for the average US resident aged two and older. Much smaller components of the changes come from desserts (5 kcal) and confectionary (9 kcal). Five major food groups are responsible in the US for most of the shifts in caloric sweetener intake. They are soft drinks, fruit drinks, desserts, sugar and jellies, confectionary, and RTE cereals.

Higher portion sizes. Other dietary changes, such as larger portion sizes, still seem to be phenomena of higher income countries in general, although super sizing of soft drinks is occurring in many countries around the world. For example, in September 2003, the World Cancer Research Fund in the UK started a campaign against big portions in the UK. Portion sizes increased for all key foods (other than pizza) at all locations examined for the total US population aged two and older (21). The size of the increases are large. For instance, over this 19-year period, the quantity of salty snacks increased by 93 kcal (0.6 ounces), soft drinks by 49 kcal (6.8 ounces), hamburgers by 97 kcal (1.3 ounces), French fries by 68 kcal (half an ounce), and Mexican dishes by 133 kcal (1.7 ounces) (see Table 5.2 for details). Certain key portion sizes increased more than others: between 1977 and 1996, the average portion of salty snacks increased from 132 to 225 kcal (1 to 1.6 ounces); the average soft drink consumed increased from 144 to 193 kcal (13.1 to 19.9 fluid ounces), and the average cheeseburger from 397 to 533 kcal (5.8 to 7.3 ounces). Overall portion sizes for all of the selected foods, other than pizza, increased. There were no differing trends within age groups that were statistically significant; however there are age group differences, particularly for the 60 year olds. In 1996, the largest portion sizes for most foods were found at fast food establishments, including salty snacks, soft drinks, fruit drinks, French fries, and Mexican food. For desserts, hamburgers, and cheeseburgers, the largest portion sizes were found at home. Consistently, restaurant portion sizes were smaller across all key foods.

Shifts in eating location. In the US, the trends in location and food sources are almost identical for all age groups (21). Key dietary behavior shifts included: greater away from home consumption; large increases in total energy from salty snacks, soft drinks, and pizza; as well as large decreases in low and medium fat milk and in medium and high fat beef and pork. Total energy intake has increased over the past 20 years, with shifts away from meals to snacks and from at home to away from home.

Table 5.1 Trends in the amount of caloric sweetener intake by specific food groups for Americans aged 2 and above (Popkin and Nielsen, 2003 (24))

Food	% Calories/day from caloric sweetener			Caloric sweetener as % of total energy			Caloric sweetener as % of carbohydrate		
	77–78	89–91	94–96	77–78	89–91	94–96	77–78	89–91	94–96
Soft drinks	52[ab]	74[ac]	105[bc]	2.9[ab]	4.1[ac]	5.3[bc]	6.5[ab]	8.5[ac]	10.4[bc]
Fruit drinks	18[b]	19[c]	31[bc]	1.0[b]	1.1[c]	1.6[bc]	2.3[b]	2.2[c]	3.1[bc]
Desserts	54[ab]	47[ac]	60[bc]	3.0[ab]	2.6[ac]	3.0[bc]	6.8[ab]	5.4[ac]	5.9[bc]
Sugars, jellies	43[ab]	31[a]	31[b]	2.4[ab]	1.7[a]	1.6[b]	5.4[ab]	3.6[a]	3.1[b]
Candy	7[ab]	9[ac]	16[bc]	0.4[ab]	0.5[ac]	0.8[bc]	0.9[ab]	1.0[ac]	1.6[bc]
Ready to eat cereals	7[ab]	11[ac]	14[bc]	0.4[ab]	0.6[ac]	0.7[bc]	0.9[ab]	1.3[ac]	1.4[bc]
Breads	15[ab]	13[ac]	14[bc]	0.8[ab]	0.7[ac]	0.7[bc]	1.9[ab]	1.5[ac]	1.4[bc]
Coffee/tea	7	5[c]	10[c]	0.4	0.3[c]	0.5[c]	0.9	0.6[c]	1.0[c]
All milk, cream products	9[b]	10[c]	12[bc]	0.5[b]	0.6[c]	0.6[bc]	1.1[b]	1.1[c]	1.2[bc]
Low fat fruit/non-citrus fruit juice	8[ab]	6[ac]	4[bc]	0.4[ab]	0.3[ac]	0.2[bc]	1.0[ab]	0.7[ac]	0.4[bc]

P = 0.01

[a] significant difference between 1977–78 and 1989–91.

[b] significant difference between 1977–78 and 1994–96.

[c] significant difference between 1989–91 and 1994–96.

Table 5.2 Trends in energy intake by calories/day of key food items and food location, all Americans ages 2 and up, weighted to be nationally representative for each time period (Nielsen and Popkin, 2003 (21))

Food	Home			Restaurant			Fast Food			Total		
	77–78	89–91	94–96	77–78	89–91	94–96	77–78	89–91	94–96	77–78	89–91	94–96
Salty snacks	127[ab]	189[ac]	206[bc]	113[b]	150	178[b]	160[b]	185	249[b]	132[ab]	199[ac]	225[bc]
Desserts	302[b]	315	324[b]	259[b]	280	306[b]	277[a]	331[a]	302	316[ab]	334[ac]	357[bc]
Soft drinks	130[b]	133[c]	158[bc]	125[b]	126[c]	155[bc]	131[ab]	143[ac]	191[bc]	144[ab]	157[ac]	193[bc]
Fruit drinks	137[ab]	149[ac]	181[bc]	133[b]	125[c]	201[bc]	147[b]	135[c]	210[bc]	139[ab]	152[ac]	189[bc]
French fries	196[ab]	240[a]	236[b]	168[ab]	229[a]	222[b]	171[ab]	260[ac]	284[bc]	188[ab]	247[a]	256[b]
Hamburgers	390	397	608	362	335	362	419[b]	414[c]	497[bc]	389[b]	392[c]	486[bc]
Cheeseburgers	405[b]	465	542[b]	381	425	485	406[ab]	564[a]	537[b]	397[ab]	544[a]	533[b]
Pizza	493[a]	591[ac]	506[c]	628	571	516	538	603[c]	503[c]	487[a]	556[ac]	476[c]
Mexican	452[b]	509	559[b]	396	448	495	410[b]	431[c]	594[bc]	408[b]	446[c]	541[bc]

P = 0.01

[a] a significant difference between 1977–78 and 1989–91.

[b] a significant difference between 1977–78 and 1994–96.

[c] a significant difference between 1989–91 and 1994–96.

Shifts in the number of eating occasions. In other research we have shown a trends towards increased snacking coupled with an overall increase in the number of eating occasions, particularly for youth and young adults (36, 37). In the US, the prevalence of snacking has increased in all age groups. For youth the average size of snacks and energy per snack remained relatively constant, while for young adults the size of the snacks also increased significantly. For all age groups, the number of snacking occasions increased significantly, therefore increasing the average daily energy from snacks. Compared to non-snack eating occasions, the nutrient contribution of snacks has decreased in calcium density and increased in energy density and the proportion of energy from fat. Currently, snacking represents about a fourth of the energy and a fifth of many other nutrients, similar to any other meal occasion. For some US age groups, the increase in nutrient contribution from snacks is primarily due to an increase in the frequency of snacking but for others it is both frequency and the size of each snack that has changed. Moreover, energy density is much higher for snacks than all other foods. The energy density for snacks has increased dramatically between 1977 and 1996 (about 0.14~0.20 kcal/g more).

Overview of US physical activity shifts. Relative to what is known about dietary patterns, our understanding of physical activity (PA) trends is primitive. The only nationally representative US data have been collected from the 1990s onward and are limited to broad patterns of PA. Little is understood about the separate components that constitute an overall activity pattern. Individual scholars study walking or sports participation, but there are no large-scale studies that have collected in-depth PA data on all dimensions in detail (comparable to a 24-hour diet or PA recall). There are excellent measures of overall energy expenditures (albeit very expensive ones) and good measures of overall motion, but it is challenging to apply them to large-scale intervention evaluation or even to population monitoring and surveillance of trends over time.

US research has tended to focus on leisure activities while research in other countries has shown that shifts in PA patterns at work, and travel to work, represent equally critical determinants of obesity among adults (38–40). Both for PA and diet there are poorer patterns found in lower socioeconomic status (SES) and minority subpopulations (41–44) for various ages. One recent study provided useful insights into the changes in PA linked with home production, that is with housework and transportation and movement in buildings. A comparison of old-fashioned labor-intensive activities with modern ones for clothes and dish washing, driving vs. walking, and walking up stairs vs. use of an elevator found reductions in each of these activities with modern technology of 0.75 kcal/min, 0.52 kcal/min, 2.53 kcal/min, and 2.9 kcal/min, respectively (45). Among youth, there is a systematic decline in PA with age. An extensive literature has focused on the contribution of inactivity (IA), in particular TV viewing, to diminished PA in the US. PA tracks from childhood to adulthood, so that PA and IA patterns developed in the earlier years are likely to persist. This is best illustrated by the

Cardiovascular Risk in Young Finns study (42, 46–48) in a review of the epidemiology of PA in youth, that found a consistent decline in PA over the school years, with males decreasing less than females.

The lower and middle income "developing world"

The diets of the developing world are shifting rapidly, particularly with respect to fat, caloric sweeteners, and animal-source foods (33, 49).

Edible oil

In the popular mind, the Westernization of the global diet continues to be associated with increased consumption of animal fats. Yet the shift in the stage of the nutrition transition toward one linked with NRNCDs in developing countries typically begins with major increases in the domestic production and imports of oilseeds and vegetable oils, rather than meat and milk. For example between 1991 and 1996/7, global production of vegetable fats and oils rose from 60 to 71 million metric tons (50). In contrast, the production of visible animal fats (butter and tallow) has remained steady at approximately 12 million metric tons. Principal vegetable oils include soybean, sunflower, rapeseed, palm, and groundnut oil. With the exception of groundnut oil, global availability of each has approximately tripled between 1961 and 1990.

Fat intake increases with income, but there have also been dramatic changes in the aggregate income–fat relationship. These are displayed for the period 1962–90 in Figure 5.2. Most significantly, even poor nations had access to a relatively high-fat diet by 1990, when a diet deriving 20 per cent of energy (kcal) from fat was associated with countries having a GNP of only $750 per capita. In 1962, the same energy diet (20 per cent from fat) was associated with countries having a GNP of $1475 (both GNP values in 1993 dollars).

This dramatic change arose principally from a major increase in the consumption of vegetable fats. In 1990, these accounted for a greater proportion of dietary energy than animal fats for countries in the lowest 75 per cent of the per capita income distribution (all of which have incomes below $5800 per capita). The change in edible vegetable fat prices, supply, and consumption is unique because it affected rich and poor countries equally, but the net impact is relatively much greater on low-income countries (51).

Caloric sweetener

Sugar is the world's predominant sweetener but this is rapidly changing as high fructose corn syrup and other caloric sweeteners become more dominant (24). For this article, however, we use the term caloric sweetener instead of added sugar, as there is such a range of non-sugar products used today. High fructose corn syrup is a prime example as it is the sweetener used in all US soft drinks.

The overall trends show a large increase in caloric sweetener consumed (Table 5.3). In 2000, 306 kcal were consumed per person per day, about a third more than in 1962;

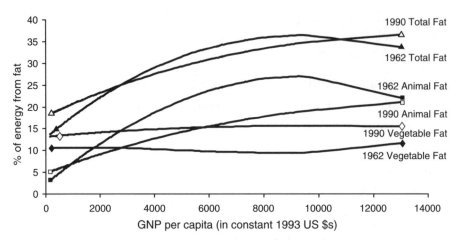

Fig. 5.2 Relationship between the percentage of energy from fat and GNP per capita, 1962 and 1990. (Source: nonparametric regressions run with food balance data from FAOUN and GNP data from the World Bank for 134 countries; Guo *et al.* 2000 (63).)

caloric sweeteners also accounted for a larger share of both total energy and total carbohydrates consumed. Unsurprisingly, Table 5.3 shows that all measures of caloric sweetener increase significantly as GNP per capita of the country and urbanization increase. However, the interaction between income growth and urbanization is important. Figure 5.3 shows the relationship between the proportion of energy from different food sources and GNP, for two different levels of urbanization (see Drewnoswski and Popkin (51) for a description of the analysis). In the less urbanized case (Fig. 5.3a), the share of sweeteners increases sharply with income, from about 5 per cent to about 15 per cent. In the more urbanized case (Figure 5.3b), the share is much higher at lower income (over 15 per cent), and hardly increases with income. The analysis confirms previous observations, that people living in urban areas consume diets distinct from those of their rural counterparts (52).

Animal-source foods

The revolution in animal-source foods (ASF) refers to the increase in demand for and production of meat, fish, and milk in low-income developing countries. Delgado has studied this issue extensively in a number of seminal reports and papers (53, 54). Most of the world's growth in production and consumption of these foods comes from the developing countries. For instance, developing countries will produce 63 per cent of meat and 50 per cent of milk in 2020. It is a global food activity, transforming the grain markets for animal feed. It also leads to resource degradation, rapid increases in feed grain imports, rapid concentration of production and consumption, and social change.

Table 5.3 World trends in caloric sweetener intake for GNP and urbanization quintiles (Popkin and Nielsen, 2003 (24); FAO, FAOSTAT data set for food balance data)

	Quintile 1	Quintile 2	Quintile 3	Quintile 4	Quintile 5	Total
A. Quintiles of GNP (Using 1962 GNP levels for each country)						
Caloric sweetener (kcal/capita/day)						
1962	90	131	257	287	402	232
2000	155	203	362	397	418	306
% Caloric sweetener of total energy						
1962	4.5	6.2	11.9	12.0	13.5	9.5
2000	6.4	8.3	13.4	13.7	12.7	10.9
% Caloric sweetener of total carbohydrates						
1962	6.2	8.5	16.8	17.7	24.4	14.6
2000	9.0	12.1	20.6	22.4	24.6	17.7
GNP						
1962	216	478	983	2817	12234	3282
2000	435	839	2836	5915	28142	7198
% urban						
1962	10.0	21.6	37.3	46.7	66.2	36.1
2000	27.7	41.3	58.7	70.0	78.0	54.9
B. Quintiles of % urban (using 1962 values for each country)						
Caloric sweetener (kcal/capita/day)						
1962	79	131	236	335	389	232
2000	151	201	339	403	441	306
% caloric sweetener of total energy						
1962	3.8	6.3	11.0	13.2	13.8	9.5
2000	6.5	8.1	12.3	13.7	13.9	10.9
% caloric sweetener of total carbohydrates						
1962	5.4	8.5	15.4	20.3	24.1	14.6
2000	6.0	12.1	19.2	22.7	25.7	17.7
GNP						
1962	287	734	1294	4696	9606	3282
2000	653	1798	8798	11739	20568	7198
% Urban						
1962	7.1	20.4	33.9	47.6	73.0	36.4
2000	27.0	42.3	57.6	64.9	84.0	54.9

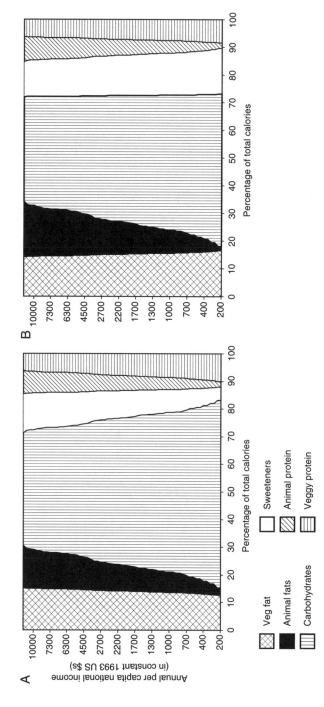

Fig. 5.3 Relationship between the proportion of energy from each food source and gross national product per capita and urbanization, 1990. (a) The proportion of the population residing in urban areas is placed at 25%; (b) the proportion of the population residing in urban areas is placed at 75%. (Source: Drewnowski and Popkin (1997). *Nutrition Reviews* **55**, 31 (51). Food balance data from the FAOUN; GNP data from the World Bank; regression work by UNC-CH.)

China provides a most useful example. This chapter uses the China Health and Nutrition Survey (CHNS) which reported 3 days of weighed and measured dietary intake (55). First, we find that intake of cereals decreased considerably during the past two decades in both urban and rural areas and among all income groups (Table 5.4). During the 8-year period from 1989 to 1997, the total intake of cereals decreased by 127 g/capita/day (67 g for urban residents and 161 g for rural residents). The decrease in the low-income group was the largest, at 196 g/capita, compared with their counterparts in mid- and high-income groups (86 g and 85 g respectively). However, there remains an inverse relationship between income and cereal intake. For example, in 1997, the intake in low-, mid-, and high-income groups was 615 g, 556 g, and 510 g/capita, respectively. The shift away from coarse grain consumption, such as millet, sorghum, and corn, is a key component of this change. CHNS data showed a 38 g decrease in refined cereals between 1989 and 1997, but an even larger decrease in coarse cereal consumption of 89 g.

Second, consumption of animal products increased, more so for the rich than the poor, and for the urban than the rural. As shown in Table 5.4, urban residents' intake of animal foods per capita per day in 1997 was higher than for rural residents (178.2 g for urban vs. 116.7 g for rural) and also showed a larger increase (46.7 g vs. 36.8 g) from 1989 to 1997. The amount and growth of intake of animal foods were positively associated with income levels. The intake level and the increase in the high-income group from 1989 to 1997 were almost three times those in the low-income group.

Third, and partly as a result of this change, data from the CHNS also show a shift in the diet away from carbohydrates to fat (Table 5.5). Energy from carbohydrates fell for all residents, and by over 20 per cent for urban residents. Energy from fat increased sharply, from 19.3 per cent in 1989 to 27.3 per cent in 1997. Other data show that over 60 per cent of urban residents consumed more than 30 per cent of energy from fat in 1997.

Finally, when we specifically examine the combined effect of these various shifts in the structure of rural and urban Chinese diets, we find an upward shift in the energy density of the foods consumed (33). The kcal of energy intake from foods and alcohol per 100 g of food in both urban and rural Chinese adult diets increased by 13 per cent between 1989 and 1997. These are really very rapid shifts.

Critical related reductions in physical activity

There are several linked changes in physical activity. One is a shift away from high energy expenditure activities such as farming, mining, and forestry towards the service sector. Elsewhere we have shown this large effect (56). Reduced energy expenditures in the same occupation are a second change. Other major changes relate to mode of transportation and activity patterns during leisure hours.

China again provides interesting illustrations. Table 5.6 shows that the proportion of urban adults (male and female) working in occupations where they participate in

Table 5.4 Shift in consumption (g/capita/day) in the Chinese diet for adults, ages 20 to 45 (China Health and Nutrition Study, 1989–1997; Du et al., 2002 (57))

Food	Urban		Rural		Low income		Mid income		High income		Total	
	89	97	89	97	89	97	89	97	89	97	89	97
Total grains	556	489	742	581	811	615	642	556	595	510	684	557
Course	46	25	175	54	226	68	98	43	78	30	135	46
Refined	510	465	567	527	585	546	544	513	517	479	549	511
Fresh vegetables	309	311	409	357	436	356	360	357	335	325	377	345
Fresh fruit	14.5	35.9	14.9	16.7	5.5	8.0	13.2	18.1	26.1	37.5	14.8	21.7
Meat, meat products	73.9	96.6	43.9	57.6	36.3	40.2	57.5	63.9	66.5	96.2	53.3	67.8
Poultry, game	10.6	15.5	4.1	11.7	4.1	7.0	6.6	10.2	7.7	20.3	6.1	12.7
Eggs, egg products	15.8	31.6	8.5	19.6	6.0	13.9	10.6	21.7	15.8	31.5	10.8	22.7
Fish, seafood	27.5	30.5	23.2	26.9	11.8	16.4	28.7	26.0	33.4	40.1	24.6	27.9
Milk, milk products	3.7	4.0	0.2	0.9	0.8	0.1	0.2	1.4	3.5	3.6	1.3	1.7
Plant oil	17.2	40.4	14.0	35.9	12.9	32.1	15.8	37.1	16.4	41.5	15.0	37.1

Table 5.5 Shifts in energy sources in the Chinese diet for adults, ages 20 to 45 (China Health and Nutrition Survey, 1989–1997; Du *et al.*, 2002 (57))

	Energy from fat (%)				Energy from carbohydrates (%)			
	89	91	93	97	89	91	93	97
Urban	21.4	29.7	32.0	32.8	65.8	58.0	55.0	53.3
Rural	18.2	22.5	22.7	25.4	70.0	65.6	65.2	62.1
Low income	16.0	19.3	19.7	23.0	72.9	69.2	68.6	64.5
Mid income	20.3	25.2	25.5	27.1	67.5	62.6	62.2	60.3
High income	21.5	30.0	31.5	31.6	65.4	57.5	55.4	54.8
Total	19.3	24.8	25.5	27.3	68.7	63.2	62.1	59.8

vigorous activity patterns has decreased. In rural areas, however, there has been a shift for some towards increased physical activity linked to holding multiple jobs and more intensive effort. For rural women, there is a shift towards a larger proportion engaged in more energy-intensive work, but there are also sections where light effort is increasing. In contrast, for rural men there is a small decrease in the proportion engaged in light work effort.

In China, 14 per cent of households acquired a motorized vehicle between 1989 and 1997. In one study we showed that the odds of being obese were 80 per cent higher ($p<0.05$) for men and women in households which owned a motorized vehicle compared to those which did not own a vehicle (39). Television ownership has also skyrocketed in China, leading to greater inactivity during leisure time (57).

Table 5.6 Chinese labor force distribution among adults, aged 20 to 45, by level of activity (%) (China Health and Nutrition Survey, 1989–1997; Du *et al.*, 2002 (57))

	Light		Vigorous	
	1989	1997	1989	1997
Urban				
Male	32.7	38.2	27.1	22.4
Female	36.3	54.1	24.8	20.8
Rural				
Male	19.0	18.7	52.5	59.9
Female	19.3	25.5	47.4	60.0

The speed of change: obesity shifts provide insights

There is limited research and long-term data to truly allow us to study, in any depth, the rates of change in dietary and physical activity and obesity patterns around the world. In the dietary area, we do not have across the world the depth and breadth of data to allow us to rigorously test if the rates of change have truly sped up (49). Evidence that does exist supports this hypothesis. There are a small number of higher and lower income countries that allow us to examine this topic systematically for obesity and overweight status.

In Figure 5.4 nationally representative, comparable data for a number of countries for current levels of overweight and obesity prevalence and their rates of change are presented. The rate of change in obesity in lower- and middle-income countries is shown to be much greater than in higher-income countries (see Popkin (58) for an overview). Figure 5.4a presents the level of obesity and overweight in several illustrative countries (US, Brazil and Mexico, Egypt and Morocco, South Africa, Thailand, and China). It probably surprises many people that the levels of obesity of several countries, all with much lower income levels than the US, are so high. Figure 5.4b shows how quickly overweight and obesity status has emerged as a major public health problem in some of these countries. Compared with the US and European countries, where the annual increase in the prevalence of overweight and obesity is about 0.25 for each, the rates of change are very high in Asia, North Africa, and Latin America (two to five times greater than in the US).

The burden is shifting world wide towards the poor!

In a series of new papers utilizing data from 36 developing countries, Monteiro and Popkin have shown that the burden of obesity is shifting towards the poor in many of these countries (59, 60). Many countries had high levels of overweight in both urban and rural women. Overweight exceeded underweight in the great majority of countries: the median ratio of over- to underweight was 5.8 in urban and 2.1 in rural areas. Countries with high per capita income and urbanization levels had not only high absolute levels of overweight, but small urban–rural differences in overweight and very high ratios of over- to underweight. However, even many of the poorest countries also had fairly high levels of rural overweight, and ratios of over- to underweight ≥ 1.0.

Traditionally, belonging to the lower SES group confers strong protection against obesity in low-income economies, but it is a systematic risk factor for the disease in upper-middle income developing economies. Using multilevel modeling techniques, Monteiro *et al.* (59) showed that obesity starts to fuel health inequities in the developing world when the GNP reaches a value of about US$2500 per capita. Thus, it is now clear that for most upper-middle income economies and part of the lower-middle income

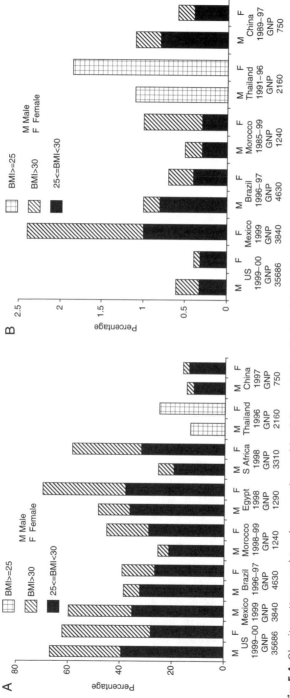

Fig. 5.4 Obesity patterns and trends across the world, adults aged 20 and older. (a) Prevalence rates; (b) obesity trends (annual percentage point increase in prevalence). (Popkin, 2002a (58)).

economies, obesity among adult women is already a relevant booster of health inequities and, in the absence of concerted national public actions to prevent obesity, economic growth will greatly expand the list of developing countries where this situation occurs.

Summary

This overview shows a rapid shift in the dietary, activity, and obesity patterns around the world that is unique in human history. The structures of diet and activity have shifted quite rapidly as was shown by the rapid increases in obesity prevalence in many countries.

How do we understand the causes of the changes that have occurred?

First, economic theory would clearly predict the changes in diet and activity that we see. Obtaining a more varied and tasteful diet and a less burdensome work pattern is an important choice desired by most individuals. The choices being made are rational. Preferences for dietary sugars and fats are regarded by many as an innate human trait. Sweetness, in particular, serves as the major cue for food energy in infancy and childhood, and preferences for sweet taste are observed in all societies around the globe (61). An argument has been made that preferences for dietary fats are also either innate or learned in infancy or childhood (62). References to the desirable qualities of milk and honey (i.e. fat and sugar), cream, butter, and animal fats are found throughout recorded history.

Second, an important factor is the interaction between income and consumption preferences. As we have shown in several studies, not only is income increasing, but the structure of consumption is shifting, and additional higher-fat foods are being purchased with additional income (33, 63).

A third element is lower food prices. Delgado (54) documents the large long-term reduction in the real costs of basic commodities in the developing world over the past several decades. He has shown that inflation-adjusted prices of livestock and feed commodities fell sharply from the early 1970s to the early 1990s, stabilized in the mid-1990s in most cases, and fell again thereafter (64). Others have shown how important cost constraints might be (65, 66).

Fourth, we might point to the centralization of the mass media and the generation of major pushes to promote selected dietary patterns directly and indirectly via these media. There is, as yet, little in the way of rigorous analysis to link shifts in mass media coverage to consumption or work patterns in the developing world, but there is an emerging literature on increased television ownership and viewing (57, 67). There is a profound cultural side not only to the globalization of mass media, but also to the related penetration of Western-style fast food outlets into the developing world. There is some evidence that these changes affect the entire culture of food production and consumption (68, 69).

Fifth, an added push has come from technological factors that affect work and leisure, productivity, and effort. Most of the changes affecting home production (from piped water to electricity to microwave ovens and lower-cost gas and butane ovens) reduce domestic effort. Similarly, the onset of mass transportation, the availability of cheap motor scooters and cycles and buses reduce energy expenditure in transportation. Similar, profound changes affect all types of work. The computer revolution, the availability of small gas-powered systems for ploughing and many others affect the work of farmers and other workers. Importantly, the reduction in the cost of producing and distributing food, and of work-related technology, is affected by urbanization. More dense residential development cuts the costs for marketing, distribution, and even production in many cases.

Finally, there are other changes in household purchasing, preparation, and eating behavior that matter greatly. These include location of the purchase, consumption of food, and the processing of the foods purchased, *inter alia*. Elsewhere we have discussed the rapid shifts in sources of energy away from at-home preparation and consumption to away-from-home purchase and consumption (17, 70, 71). There are few systematic studies of location of preparation and consumption in the developing world; however, it is clear that many important changes are occurring in both the level of processed food consumed at home and the proportion of meals consumed away from home. As the food system changes and as incomes rise, these changes are expected to intensify. Reardon and Berdegué's work on supermarkets in Latin America represents one example of a major shift in the marketing of food in the developing world (72).

How do we move into Stage 5 of the nutrition transition?

Issues to be addressed from the food sector include learning how to increase the intake levels of fruit and vegetables and higher fiber products, and to reduce the intake of caloric sweeteners and fat. We should note that there is great controversy about the need to reduce total fat intake or just the intake of selected types of fats (transfatty acids, erucic acid, saturated fats) (73, 74). Clearly, all agree that the removal of carcinogenic or artherogenic edible oils is important, but the role of total fat is not as clear. Similarly, there is some debate about the role of caloric sweeteners. For instance, an expert committee of the World Health Organization has recommended a maximum of 10 per cent of energy from caloric sweeteners, a level above that of caloric sweeteners consumed in diets in high-, low-, and moderate-income countries (75). In contrast, the US Institute of Medicine conducted the same review and concluded that 25 per cent of energy from caloric sweeteners was appropriate (76).

Similar shifts in the physical environment to enhance physical activity exist. There is a growing body of knowledge that points to the role of a spread of environmental factors ranging from connectivity of streets, to availability of walking options and street safety, to the organization and layout of buildings and communities. Higher density of, and proximity to, opportunities for physical activity, such as recreation facilities (for example private and public facilities, parks, recreation centers, green spaces, shopping centers) and transportation options (for example sidewalks, cycle paths, public transportation, high road connectivity, and lower automobile transportation density) will increase physical activity levels and decrease overweight prevalence. Conversely, constraints to physical activity, such as crime and air pollution, will decrease physical activity and increase overweight prevalence.

For each of the desired changes in the food supply and the physical environment, there are clearly myriad options, some easy to implement and many quite complex. A few countries are already beginning to take some steps forward to address these issues (77–79). There have also been some limited successes in the higher-income world (79).

References

1. **Omran AR** (1971). The epidemiologic transition: a theory of the epidemiology of population change. *Milbank Memorial Fund Quarterly* **49**, 509–38.
2. **Olshansky SJ, Ault AB** (1986). The fourth stage of the epidemiologic transition: the age of delayed degenerative diseases. *Milbank Memorial Fund Quarterly* **64**, 355–91.
3. **Truswell AS** (1977). Diet and nutrition of hunter-gathers. Health and diseases in tribal societies. *Ciba Foundation Symposium* **149**, pp. 213–26. Elsevier, Amsterdam.
4. **Harris DR** (1981). The prehistory of human subsistence: a speculative outline. In: Walcher DN, Kretchmer N, eds. *Food, nutrition and evolution: food as an environmental factor in the genesis of human variability.* Masson, New York.
5. **Eaton SB, Shostak M, Konner M** (1988). *The paleolithic prescription: A program of diet and exercise and a design for living.* Harper and Row, New York.
6. **Eaton SB, Konner M** (1985). Paleolithic nutrition: A consideration on its nature and current implications. *New Eng J Med* **312**, 283–9.
7. **Vargas LA** (1990). Old and new transitions and nutrition in Mexico. In: Swedlund AC, Armelagos GJ, eds. *Disease in populations in transition.* Greenwood, Westport, CT.
8. **Gordon KD** (1987). Evolutionary perspectives on human diet. In: Johnson FE, ed. *Nutritional anthropology*, pp. 3–41. Liss, New York.
9. **Newman LF, Kates RW, Matthews R, Millman S** (1990). *Hunger in history.* Basil Blackwell, Cambridge, MA.
10. **Popkin BM, Haines PS, Reidy KC** (1989). Food consumption of the U.S. women: patterns and determinants between 1977 and 1985. *Am J Clin Nutr* **49**, 1307–19.
11. **Milio N** (1990). *Nutrition policy for food-rich countries: a strategic analysis.* The Johns Hopkins University Press, Baltimore, MD.
12. **Popkin BM, Haines PS, Patterson R** (1992). Dietary changes among older Americans, 1977–78. *Am J Clin Nutr* **55**, 823–30.
13. **Manton KG, Soldo BJ** (1985). Dynamics of health changes in the oldest old: new perspective and evidence. *Health Soc* **63**, 206–85.
14. **Crimmins EM, Saito Y, Ingegneri D** (1989). Changes in life expectancy and disability-free life expectancy in the United States. *Population Dev Rev* **15**, 235–67.

15. French SA, Story M, Jeffery RW (2001a). Environmental influences on eating and physical activity. *Ann Rev Public Health* **22**, 309–35.

16. French S, Story M, Jeffery RW (2001b). Fast food restaurant use among adolescents: associations with nutrient intake, food choice, and behavioral and psychosocial variables. *Int J Obes* **25**, 1823–33.

17. Nielsen SJ, Siega-Riz AM, Popkin BM (2002a). Trends in energy intake in the U.S. between 1977 and 1996: similar shifts seen across age groups. *Obes Res* **10**, 370–8.

18. Nielsen SJ, Siega-Riz AM, Popkin BM (2002b). Trends in food locations and sources among adolescents and young adults. *Prev Med* **35**, 107–13.

19. Haines PS, Hama MY, Guilkey DK, Popkin BM (2003). Weekend eating in the United States is linked with greater energy, fat and alcohol intake. *Obes Res* **11**, 945–9.

20. Jeffery R, Utter J (2003). The changing environment and population obesity in the United States. *Obes Res* **11**, 12S–22S.

21. Nielsen SJ, Popkin BM (2003). Patterns and trends in portion sizes, 1977–1998. *JAMA* **289**, 450–3.

22. Nestle M, Jacobson MF (2000). Halting the obesity epidemic: a public health policy approach. *Public Health Rep* **115**, 12–24.

23. Young LR, Nestle M (2002). The contribution of expanding portion sizes to the US obesity epidemic. *Am J Public Health* **92**, 246–9.

24. Popkin BM, Nielsen SJ (2003). The sweetening of the world's diet. *Obes Res* **11**, 1325–32.

25. Guthrie JF, Lin BH, Frazao E (2002). Role of food prepared away from home in the American diet, 1977–78 versus 1994–96: changes and consequences. *J Nutr Educ Behav* **34**, 140–50.

26. Paeratakul S, Ferdinand DP, Champagne CM, Ryan DH, Bray GA (2003). Fast-food consumption among US adults and children: dietary and nutrient intake profile. *J Am Diet Assoc* **103**, 1332–8.

27. McCrory MA, Fuss PJ, Hays NP, Vinken AG, Greenberg AS, Roberts SB (1999). Overeating in America: association between restaurant food consumption and body fatness in healthy men and women ages 19 to 80. *Obes Res* **7**, 564–71.

28. French SA, Harnack L, Jeffery RW (2000). Fast food restaurant use among women in the Pound of Prevention study: dietary, behavioral and demographic correlates. *Int J Obes Relat Metab Disord* **24**, 1353–9.

29. Gordon-Larsen P, Adair LS, Popkin BM (2003). The relationship of ethnicity, socioeconomic factors, and overweight in US adolescents. *Obes Res* **11**, 121–9.

30. Ma Y, Bertone ER, Stanek EJ 3rd, *et al.* (2003). Association between eating patterns and obesity in a free-living adult population. *Am J Epidemiol* **158**, 85–92.

31. Nicklas TA, Yang SJ, Baranowski T, Zakeri I, Berenson G (2003). Eating patterns and obesity in children: The Bogalusa Heart Study. *Am J Prev Med* **25**, 9–16.

32. Thompson M, Ballew C, Resnicow K, *et al.* (2004). Food purchased away from home as a predictor of change in BMI z-scores among girls. *Int J Obes* **28**, 282–9.

33. Popkin BM, Du S (2003). Dynamics of the nutrition transition toward the animal foods sector in China and its implications: a worried perspective. *J Nutr* **133**, 3898S–906S.

34. Bray GA, Nielsen SJ, Popkin BM (2004). High fructose corn sweeteners and the epidemic of obesity. *Am J Clin Nutr* **79**, 537–43.

35. Li R, Serdula M, Bland S, Mokdad A, Bowman B, Nelson D (2000). Trends in fruit and vegetable consumption among adults in 16 US states: behavioral risk factor surveillance system, 1990–1996. *Am J Public Health* **90**, 777–81.

36. Jahns L, Siega-Riz AM, Popkin BM (2001). The increasing prevalence of snacking among U.S. children and adolescents from 1977 to 1996. *J Pediatr* **138**, 493–8.

37. Zizza C, Siega-Riz AM, Popkin BM (2001). Significant increase in young adults' snacking between 1977–78 and 1994–96 represents a cause for concern! *Prev Med* **32**, 303–10.

38. Bell C, Ge K, Popkin BM (2001). Weight gain and its predictors in Chinese Adults. *Int J Obes* **25**, 1079–86.

39. Bell AC, Ge K, Popkin BM (2002). The road to obesity or the path to prevention? Motorized transportation and obesity in China. *Obes Res* **10**, 277–83.

40. Paeratakul S, Popkin BM, Ge K, Adair LS, Stevens J (1998). Changes in diet and physical activity affect the body mass index of Chinese adults. *Int J Obes* **22**, 424–31.

41. Wolf AM, Gortmaker SL, Cheung L, Gray HM, Herzog DB, Colditz GA (1993). Activity, inactivity, and obesity: racial, ethnic, and age differences among schoolgirls. *Am J Public Health* **83**, 1625–7.

42. Bild DE, Jacobs DR Jr, Sydney S, Haskell WL, Anderssen N, Oberman A (1993). Physical activity in young black and white women. The CARDIA Study. *Ann Epidemiol* **3**, 636–44.

43. Gordon-Larsen P, McMurray RG, Popkin BM (1999). Adolescent physical activity and inactivity vary by ethnicity: The National Longitudinal Study of Adolescent Health. *J Pediatr* **135**, 301–6.

44. Gordon-Larsen P, McMurray RG, Popkin BM (2000). Determinants of adolescent physical activity and inactivity patterns. *Pediatr* **105**, 1–8.

45. Lanningham-Foster L, Nysse LJ, Levine JA (2003). Labor saved, calories lost: the energetic impact of domestic labor-saving devices. *Obes Res* **11**, 1178–81.

46. Raitakari OT, Porkka KV, Taimela S, Telama R, Rasanen L, Viikari JS (1994). Effects of persistent physical activity and inactivity on coronary risk factors in children and young adults. The cardiovascular risk in Young Finns Study. *Am J Epidemiol* **140**, 195–205.

47. Anderssen N, Jacobs DR Jr, Sidney S, *et al.* (1996). Change and secular trends in physical activity patterns in young adults: a seven-year longitudinal follow-up in the Coronary Artery Risk Development in Young Adults Study (CARDIA). *Am J Epidemiol* **143**, 351–62.

48. Sallis JF, Prochaska JJ, Taylor WC (2000). A review of correlates of physical activity of children and adolescents. *Med Sci Sports Exerc* **32**, 963–75.

49. Popkin BM (2002b). The shift in stages of the nutrition transition in the developing world differs from past experiences! *Public Health Nutr* **5**, 205–14. (Republished by the *Malaysian J Nutr* (2002) **8**, 109–24.)

50. US Department of Agriculture (1997). *World Agricultural Supply and Demand Estimates (WASDE-315).* Table: Vegetable oil consumption balance sheets (in million metric tons), FAS Online. USDA, Washington, DC. http://www.fas.usda.gov/oilseeds/circular/1997/97–03/mar97opd2.html

51. Drewnowski A, Popkin BM (1997). The nutrition transition: new trends in the global diet. *Nutr Rev* **55**, 31–43.

52. Mendez M, Popkin BM (2005). Globalization, urbanization and nutritional change in the developing world. *Electronic J Agr Dev Econ* **1**, 220–41.

53. Delgado CL, Rosegrant MW, Steinfeld H, Ehui SK, Courbois C (1999). *Livestock to 2020: the next food revolution.* International Food Policy Research Institute; Food and Agriculture Organization of the United Nations (FAO); International Livestock Research Institute (ILRI), Washington D.C., Rome, Nairobi, Kenya.

54. Delgado CL (2003). Rising consumption of meat and milk in developing countries has created a new food revolution. *J Nutr* **133**, 3907S–10S.

55. Zhai F, Guo X, Popkin BM, *et al.* (1996). Evaluation of the 24-hour individual recall method in China. *Food Nutr Bull* **17**, 154–61.

56. **Popkin BM** (1999). Urbanization, lifestyle changes and the nutrition transition. *World Dev* **27**, 1905–16.

57. **Du S, Lu B, Zhai F, Popkin BM** (2002). The nutrition transition in China: a new stage of the Chinese diet. In: Caballero B and Popkin BM, eds. *The nutrition transition: diet and disease in the developing world*, pp. 205–22. Academic Press, London.

58. **Popkin BM** (2002a). An overview on the Nutrition transition and its health implications: the Bellagio Meeting. *Public Health Nutr* **5**, 93–103.

59. **Monteiro CA, Conde WL, Lu B, and Popkin BM** (2004). *Is obesity fuelling inequities in health in the developing world?* University of North Carolina Manuscript, Chapel Hill, NC.

60. **Mendez MA, Monteiro CA, Popkin BM** (2004). *Overweight now exceeds underweight among women in most developing countries!* University of North Carolina Manuscript, Chapel Hill, NC.

61. **Drewnowski A** (1987). Sweetness and obesity. In: Dobbing J, ed. *Sweetness*. Springer-Verlag, London.

62. **Drewnowski A** (1989). Sensory preferences for fat and sugar in adolescence and in adult life. In: Murphy C, Cain WS, Hegsted DM, eds. *Nutrition and the chemical senses in aging*. Academy of Sciences, New York.

63. **Guo X, Mroz TA, Popkin BM, Zhai F** (2000). Structural changes in the impact of income on food consumption in China, 1989–93. *Econ Dev Cult Change* **48**, 737–60.

64. **Delgado C, Rosegrant M, Meijer S** (2001). *Livestock to 2020: the revolution continues*. Paper presented at the annual meetings of the International Agricultural Trade Research Consortium (IATRC), Auckland, New Zealand, 18–19 January. Available at www.iatrcweb.org/publications/ proceedings Accessed 28 October 2004.

65. **Guo X, Popkin BM, Mroz TA, Zhai F** (1999). Food price policy can favorably alter macronutrient intake in China. *J Nutr* **129**, 994–1001.

66. **Darmon N, Ferguson EL, Briend A** (2002). A cost constraint alone has adverse effects on food selection and nutrient density: an analysis of human diets by linear programming. *J Nutr* **132**, 3764–71.

67. **Tudor-Locke C, Ainsworth BA, Adair LS, Popkin BM** (2003). Physical activity in Filipino youth: The Cebu Longitudinal Health and Nutrition Survey. *Int J Obes* **27**, 181–90.

68. **Jin J, ed.** (2000). *Feeding China's little emperors: food, children, and social change*. Stanford University Press, Palo Alto, CA.

69. **Watson JL, ed.** (1997). *Golden arches east: McDonald's in East Asia*. Stanford University Press, Palo Alto, CA.

70. **Bisgrove E, Popkin BM** (1996). Does women's work improve their nutrition? Evidence from the Urban Philippines. *Soc Sci Med* **43**, 1475–88.

71. **McGuire J, Popkin BM** (1989). Beating the zero sumgame: women and nutrition in the third world. *Food Nutr Bull* **11**, 38–63; Part II **12**, 3–11.

72. **Reardon T, Berdegué JA** (2002). The rapid rise of supermarkets in Latin America: challenges and opportunities for development. *Dev Policy Rev* **20**, 371–88.

73. **Bray GA, Popkin BM** (1998). Dietary fat intake does affect obesity. *Am J Clin Nutr* **68**, 1157–73.

74. **Willett WC** (1998). Is dietary fat a major determinant of body fat? *Am J Clin Nutr* **67** (suppl.), 556S–62S.

75. **WHO/FAO** (2002). *Expert consultation on diet, nutrition and the prevention of chronic diseases, 28 January–1 February Geneva*.

76. Panel on Macronutrients, Subcommittees on Upper Reference Levels of Nutrients and Interpretation and Uses of Reference Intakes, and the Standing Committee on the Scientific Evaluation of Dietary Reference Intakes (2002). *Dietary reference intakes for energy, carbohydrate, fiber, fat, fatty acids, cholesterol, protein, and amino acids (macronutrients)*. National Academy Press, Washington, DC.

77. **Coitinho D, Monteiro CA, Popkin BM** (2002). What Brazil is doing to promote healthy diets and active life-styles. *Public Health Nutr* **5**, 263–7.

78. **Zhai F, Fu D, Du S, Ge K, Chen C, Popkin BM** (2002). What is China doing in policy-making to push back the negative aspects of the nutrition transition? *Public Health Nutr* **5**, 269–73.

79. **Puska P, Pietinen P, Uusitalo U** (2002). Influencing public nutrition for noncommunicable disease prevention: from community intervention to national programme: experiences from Finland. *Public Health Nutr* **5**, 245–51.

Part 2

Chapter 6

Population approaches to promote healthful eating behaviors

Simone A. French

Introduction

A substantial body of research supports the role of diet in contributing to secular increases in population-wide obesity prevalence (1–3). Both dietary composition (4–7) and energy availability (7–13) are implicated in the etiology of weight gain and obesity at the population level. In addition to its role in obesity, dietary intake plays an important role in the etiology and prevention of chronic diseases such as cardiovascular disease, cancer, diabetes, stroke, and osteoporosis (14, 15). Effective community-based interventions to improve dietary quality and food choices could promote population-wide health and substantially reduce the population burden of chronic disease.

This chapter presents an overview of the state of the science research on population-based interventions to promote healthful food choices. An overview of the theoretical models and conceptual and intervention issues is provided first. Intervention strategies are presented by specific settings: worksites, schools, and other community settings. Cross-cutting strategies include individual and environmental level interventions such as: promotion, advertising, and media; food pricing; and availability. The chapter does not aim to present an exhaustive review of the literature. Rather, important state of the science research theories and intervention strategies are presented, and illustrative studies are described that provide strong examples of a particular theoretical or methodological approach. The overall aim is to illustrate the most promising intervention strategies and conceptual models to date, and to define the next steps for developing the most effective research-based interventions to promote population-wide, healthful food choices and dietary intake.

Theoretical conceptualizations of population behavior change

Efforts in the field of epidemiology to promote public health, traditionally, have focused on reducing environmental exposures to health-compromising environmental threats (16, 17). However, disease-oriented theoretical models have included individual-level concepts, illustrated in the classic epidemiologic triad of host (individual), vector (behavior), and agent (environment) (18). By contrast, health promotion efforts originating in the behavioral sciences have focused on changing individual behavior to reduce health risk (19–21). Individual-level behavioral theoretical models have included environmental concepts, illustrated in the widely used Social Cognitive Theory (22), in which behavior is hypothesized to be a function of reciprocal interaction between person, environment, and behavior. However, even interventions focused on changing population behaviors primarily have adopted individual-level strategies, such as education and behavioral change programs, and have not fully utilized environmental change strategies, or have ignored such approaches altogether (19–21).

A social ecology framework provides a conceptual perspective that is perhaps one of the most well suited for developing public health interventions to change population behaviors (23–25). Similar to the epidemiology and behavioral theories, social ecological perspectives conceptualize behavior as an ongoing transaction between environment and individual, with an emphasis on a multilevel perspective and a more complex, multidimensional conceptualization of the environment (23).

Four broad assumptions underlie the social ecological conceptualization of health promotion (23). First, efforts to promote health should include an understanding of both environmental and individual-level variables. Second, environments need to be conceptualized as complex and multidimensional (e.g. physical and social; objective and perceived; proximal and distal). Third, environments can be conceived as nested within different levels, each of which is interdependent with the other levels (e.g. family, worksite, schools, local community, state, country). Fourth, individuals in these environments can be approached at different levels of aggregation (e.g. individuals, families, neighborhoods, social groups, populations). Interventions will be maximally effective to the extent that co-ordination among the different levels of aggregation is fostered (aggregation of people, settings, and environments). Interventions to change behavior will be most effective when the dynamic interplay between different levels is both understood and incorporated into the intervention strategies.

The social ecological perspective emphasizes multicomponent interventions that simultaneously target different levels. A social ecological conceptualization of population eating behaviors is illustrated in Table 6.1. Several dimensions of both individual and environmental variables are shown, with example variables related to eating behavior and food choices. Individual level variables related to food choices and eating behaviors include demographic, psychological, and behavioral factors. Environmental variables related to food choices include physical, social, and macroenvironmental factors.

Obviously, no single study can implement intervention strategies at all levels. To date, most research has focused on a single level (e.g. individual education or behavior change programs), or two levels (individual level, plus local environmental changes). For example a typical school-based intervention to change food choices includes strategies at two levels: individual and environmental. Individual-level strategies typically include classroom curricula (26). Environmental strategies include working with

Table 6.1 Influences on food choices and leverage points for population-based nutrition interventions (Based on Stokols, 1992 (23))

| Demographic/biological | Individual | | Environmental | | |
	Psychological	Behavioral	Physical community	Social community	Macroenvironmental
Gender	Self-efficacy	Behavioral skills	Food availability	Mass media programs	Food-related policies
Age	Outcome expectations	Dietary behaviors	supermarkets farmers'	for nutrition and food	and programs
Education	Values (health)	Physical activity	markets fast food	Community programs	federal state local
Income	Perceived norms	behaviors	convenience stores	for nutrition and food	(e.g. price subsidies,
Race/ethnicity	Perceived barriers	TV viewing	Food prices	Cultural food practices	feeding programs,
Household configuration	Stress	Transportation		Neighborhood	labeling regulations))
Employment number		choices		socioeconomic status	
of hours type of work				Worksite policies and	
				environment	

school food service staff to change the foods available in the school meals and other food and beverage outlets in school, place promotional signage, and change food prices to promote the purchase of healthy foods. Typically, multiple strategies within each level are implemented. Studies that have implemented both environmental and individual-level strategies in tandem typically have shown positive effects on student food choices and dietary quality (26). However, such studies have not been designed to evaluate separately the potentially independent effects of interventions that target each level. Analyses of process evaluation data on implementation and exposure to various intervention components can show associations between these variables and dietary behavior change, and can often provide information about the relative effectiveness of intervention strategies that target different levels (27).

Study design and evaluation issues

Several study design and analysis issues are important to consider in evaluating population-based interventions for dietary and eating behavior change in community settings (28, 29). The first and most challenging is the unit of analysis issue. Most worksite and school-based interventions published in the 1980s and early 1990s randomized worksites but conducted analyses at the individual level (19, 20). Such designs do not account for the nesting of individuals within worksites. Individuals clustered within worksites or schools may be more similar to each other on the behavioral outcome of interest. This similarity among individuals within clusters must be accounted for in the outcome analysis. The strongest study design is to randomize worksites or schools to experimental conditions, and include a sufficient number of worksites or schools to ensure adequate power for the primary outcome analysis at the group level. Studies that use a large number of diverse worksites or schools are quite expensive to fund and are difficult to conduct with good fidelity with respect to intervention implementation and outcome evaluation.

A second methodological issue is that a number of worksite intervention studies focused the evaluation on intervention program participants only and did not evaluate the intervention effects on the broader worksite population. School interventions have typically been more inclusive in their evaluation of the entire student population because many interventions focused on classroom curriculum changes, which target and reach the majority of students attending the school. In worksite interventions, evaluation of the worksite population is particularly important when worksite interventions include environmental changes that potentially can impact workers who do not actively participate in individual-level behavioral or educational program worksite intervention components. In fact, one of the attractive aspects of worksite interventions is the potential to reach and impact the broader workforce population beyond the subset of health-motivated workers who actively choose to participate in specific nutrition programs.

Another important methodological issue regarding population-based nutrition interventions is the multicomponent nature of many intervention programs.

Worksite, school, and community-based nutrition interventions most often comprise a package of several intervention components, some of which target the individual and some of which target the environment. The independent or interdependent nature of the individual intervention component effects on behavior change is impossible to separate in the program evaluation.

Other factors that may be important influences on the implementation and evaluation of community-based nutrition interventions include whether the intervention targets a single or multiple behaviors. Interventions that target a single behavior may be more effective because the intervention message can be focused. For example, are interventions that target increased intake of fruit and vegetables more effective than those that simultaneously target increased intake of fruit and vegetables, high fiber, and whole grain foods, and decreased intake of higher fat foods? Are interventions that focus only on dietary behavior changes more effective than those that also target changes in other health-related behaviors such as physical activity or smoking?

Recent worksite and school-based nutrition interventions conducted since the mid 1990s have addressed many of these methodological issues in their study designs and analysis. Fewer group-randomized trials have been conducted in community settings such as grocery stores, restaurants, faith-based groups, households, and neighborhoods. Current methodological issues of concern have focused on the financial and logistical barriers involved in implementing nutrition interventions in which worksite, school, or other group unit is the unit of randomization, intervention, and analysis. New designs need to be developed that enable fewer worksites, schools, or other social or physical units to be included yet provide adequate statistical power when the analyses control for individual clustering within group (28–30). Additional research methodologies, such as observational studies, qualitative, and dissemination research, could be utilized to move the scientific research base forward (31).

Settings

Population-based interventions to promote healthful eating behaviors have been conducted in diverse settings, including worksites, schools, and other community settings such restaurants and grocery stores. Worksite and school settings have received by far the most research attention, and comprise the most sophisticated research designs, interventions, and evaluations available in the literature. Far less research is available in other community settings, and, in general, available studies are much less sophisticated in their research design and methodology. Research conducted in each of these settings is described below, with an emphasis on worksite and school settings.

Worksites

Worksites are an attractive setting through which to conduct population-based nutrition interventions for several reasons. In the US, for example, about 70 per cent of adults aged 18–65 years are employed; therefore, worksites offer a channel through which to reach a broad and diverse adult population (32). Worksite interventions can be offered on a continuing basis, and thus have the potential to reach employees repeatedly over a sustained time period. The worksite environment offers the potential to support both social and physical environmental interventions that might increase the effectiveness or provide effects independent of the intervention components that target individual-level change. Worksite interventions, particularly those that address the social and physical environment, also may impact the entire worksite population, and thus are not limited in their potential effects to a self-selected subset of motivated individuals who choose to seek out and participate in worksite health promotion programs.

Limitations of worksite-based interventions include the potential difficulty of creating and sustaining programs that have high visibility and participation, and that are intense enough to produce measurable changes in the targeted behavioral outcomes. Worksites most receptive to participation in health promotion interventions may not be representative of the workforce. Employees who are difficult to reach, such as those who work part-time schedules or shift work, may benefit less from worksite based nutrition interventions because they receive less exposure to the intervention components.

Previous reviews of worksite nutrition interventions

An earlier review of worksite nutrition interventions located 10 worksite nutrition interventions published between 1980 and 1995 (19). Six of the 10 studies used non-randomized designs. Only one study randomized worksites to intervention or control group. Most of the studies reported outcomes only for a subset of self-selected program participants, not for the entire employee population. Even among this subset of participants, attrition rates were high, thus jeopardizing the internal validity of the results. Although the non-randomized studies showed some positive behavioral outcomes, the extent to which these are attributable to the intervention, self-selection, social desirability reporting bias, or secular trends is unclear (19).

Since 1995, the results of several worksite nutrition intervention trials that addressed many of the methodological limitations of previous research have been published (Table 6.2) (33–39). Common intervention components across worksite programs included: targeting the entire employee worksite population for behavior change; worksite-wide mass media and educational campaigns; interactive educational activities; taste tests; contests; point-of-purchase signage; and use of employee advisory groups to assist with intervention development and implementation. Common design and evaluation components included randomization of worksites to experimental condition, and evaluation of the entire worksite population to assess intervention effects on behavioral outcomes.

Overall the results of these "second generation" worksite nutrition intervention studies have been modestly positive and suggest that nutrition interventions implemented at the worksite can have positive effects on behavior change in the broader worksite population (Table 6.2). Most studies found small but significant decreases in

Table 6.2 Worksite nutrition interventions, 1992–2001

Author	Outcome	Study design	Intervention	Results
Beresford et al. 2001 (36)	Fruit and vegetable servings/day	Group randomized trial n = 14 intervention n = 14 control 12-month intervention 24-month follow-up evaluation Worksite population evaluated	Individual behavior skill-building activities cooking demonstrations incentives Environmental mass media cafeteria signage and promotion employee advisory board	+0.30 fruit and vegetable servings/day intervention–control difference (p < 0.05)
Buller et al. 1999 (35)	Fruit and vegetable servings/day	Group randomized trial n = 41 intervention cliques n = 41 control cliques 9-month intervention 6-month follow-up evaluation Clique participants only evaluated	Individual behavior 5-A-Day educational materials incentive items Environmental peer educator program	+0.77 fruit and vegetable servings/day
Sorensen et al. 1999 (34)	Fruit and vegetable servings/day	Group randomized trial n = 7 worksite n = 7 worksite + family n = 8 control 5-A-Day (mass media + taste test) 19.5-month intervention Immediate postintervention evaluation Worksite population evaluated	Individual Behavior nutrition education taste tests Environmental mass media point-of-choice labeling fruit and vegetable availability employee advisory board + Family written learn-at-home program mailings family festival	Worksite: +0.2 fruit and vegetable servings/day Worksite + family: +0.5 fruit and vegetable servings/day Control: +0.01 fruit and vegetable servings/day (p < 0.05; worksite + family differs from worksite and control)
Glasgow et al. 1997 (39)	Fat g/day Low fat eating behaviors	Quasiexperimental matched pairs n = 11 intervention n = 11 control 19-month intervention Immediate postintervention evaluation Worksite population evaluated	Individual behavior 12-week behavior change program incentives Environmental employee advisory board menu choice of intervention activities	Fat intake (g/day) (cohort) intervention –3.89 g/day control –1.28 g/day (p < 0.05) Low fat eating behaviors intervention +0.08 control +0.02 (p < 0.02)

continued

Table 6.2 (continued) Worksite nutrition interventions, 1992–2001

Author	Outcome	Study design	Intervention	Results
Sorensen et al. 1996 (34)	Fat percentage Fiber g/day Fruit and vegetable servings/day	Group randomized trial n = 54 intervention n = 54 control 2-year intervention Immediate postintervention evaluation Worksite population evaluated	Individual behavior nutrition education activities/contests Environmental mass media point-of-purchase signage food availability catering policies employee advisory board	−0.37 percent fat (p < 0.03) +0.13 g/1000 kcal fiber (p < 0.06) +0.18 fruit and vegetable servings/day (p < 0.0001)
Tilley et al. 1999 (37)	Fruit and vegetable servings/day	Group randomized trial n = 15 intervention n = 13 control 2-year intervention Immediate postintervention evaluation Worksite population evaluated	Individual behavior nutrition classes self-help materials personalized feedback	Fat percentage (NS) Fruit and vegetable servings/day (NS) Fiber (g/1000 kcal) intervention +0.6 control +0.1 (p < 0.001)
Sorensen et al. 1992 (47)	Fat percentage Fiber (ln) g/day	Group randomized trial n = 8 intervention n = 8 control 12-month intervention Immediate postintervention evaluation Worksite population evaluated	Individual behavior nutrition education food demonstrations Environmental point-of-choice labeling employee advisory board	Fat percentage intervention −1.20 control −0.50 (p < 0.01) Fiber (ln) intervention +0.03 control +0.01 (NS)

dietary fat intake (34, 39), increases in servings of fruit and vegetables (33–36), or increases in fiber intake (34, 37). Observed changes in the dietary variables were small, but meaningful from a population perspective (16, 17).

Current state of the science

The largest and most comprehensive worksite nutrition intervention study conducted to date is the Working Well Trial (34). That study examined changes in fruit, vegetable, fiber, and fat intake among employees in 108 worksites over a 2-year intervention period. Worksites were randomized to a multicomponent intervention or to a no-treatment control group. Outcomes were measured using a food frequency questionnaire administered to a cross-sectional sample of employees at each worksite at baseline and follow-up (postintervention).

The intervention was developed based on several theoretical models, including the stage of change trans-theoretical model (an individual-level theoretical framework) (40), and organizational and community activation theories (34). Individual-level intervention strategies aimed to increase individual awareness, to provide behavioral skills training, and skills development around maintenance of behavior change. Activities included kick-off events, posters and brochures, interactive activities, self-help materials, contests, and direct education classes. Environmental change intervention components included changes in the foods available from worksite cafeterias and vending machines, changes in worksite catering policies, and increases in the availability of worksite nutrition education opportunities. Community participatory intervention components included the formation of an employee advisory group at each worksite. The employee advisory group comprised four to 12 members and included workers and management staff. The employee advisory group provided: assistance with tailoring some intervention components to the unique needs and culture of the individual worksite; generating enthusiasm for and awareness of the program among employees; and assisting with the development and implementation of some intervention activities.

Results showed a significant but modest decrease in per cent fat energy, and significant but modest increases in fruit and vegetable servings and fiber intake among workers in the intervention worksites compared to workers in the control sites (34). Process evaluation data showed 82 per cent of the nutrition intervention implementation objectives were attained; 96 per cent of the worksites implemented a kick-off activity; 88 per cent delivered a self-assessment activity; 78 per cent delivered a self-help program; and 69 per cent delivered a multisession direct education program. Results of the employee survey data showed significantly greater awareness and participation in nutrition-related worksite programs and activities among intervention worksites compared to control worksites (41). Compared to control worksites, key informants at intervention worksites were significantly more likely to report an increase in the use of point-of-purchase vending machine labeling, "any" vending machine changes and "any" food service changes (42). No significant differences were observed in worksite catering policy changes, increased nutrition labeling in cafeteria, or availability of lower fat or higher fiber foods in the worksite cafeteria or the vending machines.

The Working Well Trial represents a second generation, state of the science worksite nutrition intervention. It was a theory-based intervention, included both individual-level and environmental intervention components, evaluated outcome changes in the worksite population, and randomized worksites and analyzed the data at the appropriate level of analysis. Results were modest but positive and provide some guidance for improving the next generation of worksite-based nutrition interventions. The extent to which the environmental intervention components were implemented is unclear, since the process measure of implementation relied on retrospective self-reports of the food service and vending machine service staff. Memory or social desirability concerns may jeopardize the validity of the reports regarding the extent to which the environmental changes were implemented.

Results of other second generation worksite nutrition intervention studies have shown similar positive effects on nutrition outcomes such as dietary fat, fruit and vegetable servings, and fiber (Table 6.2). Several worksite interventions funded as part of the Five-A-Day research program have shown success in increasing fruit and vegetable intake among worksite employees (34, 36, 47).

The worksite interventions conducted to date have largely focused on educational and behavior change intervention strategies that are individually-oriented, but applied on a larger scale in the worksite setting. Potential worksite intervention strategies that have not yet been fully implemented or carefully evaluated include environmental strategies that change the social and or physical environment. A notable innovative intervention designed and implemented specifically using social networks within worksites did observe significant increases in fruit and vegetable servings over an 18-month period (35). Social networks were identified at worksites of 10 public employers. Workers identified by their social network peers as central in their social network were trained to implement fruit and vegetable promotion and communication activities among the members of their social network. Compared to those who received an information-only Five-A-Day promotional campaign, social network members who received a peer-delivered intervention significantly increased their fruit and vegetable servings per day (35). This innovative approach is notable because of its potential to be effective and feasible for implementation among overlooked worker populations (see below) or among workers who have no physical worksite location (such as bus, truck and taxi cab drivers, traveling sales workers, housecleaning or janitorial workers), and who instead rely upon social networks for informational, instrumental, and social support related to healthful dietary behaviors.

Strengthening the environmental intervention components can strengthen future worksite nutrition interventions. One way to accomplish this is to have research intervention staff be more actively involved in working with food service and vending service staff to implement changes in food availability, nutrition labeling at the point-of-purchase, and promotional efforts. Specific goals could be set in collaboration with the food service and vending staff regarding the number and type of food and beverages offered. Intervention staff could also take responsibility for implementing and maintaining nutrition signage. In addition, food pricing strategies are another environmental intervention that has shown promise for promoting healthier food choices in the worksite cafeteria and vending machines (43–45, 53, 58). Price incentives represent an environmental intervention strategy with established effectiveness and warrant additional evaluation in worksite nutrition intervention research. Interventions could be strengthened by more fully incorporating worksite social networks into the intervention as a means both to disseminate and deliver the intervention, and as a means of social influence to promote the desired behavior changes (46). The local neighborhood environment also could be included as an environmental intervention target (46). Worksite nutrition interventions could incorporate neighborhood fast food and other restaurants, grocery stores, and convenience stores in intervention components related to nutrition education, availability, pricing, and promotion strategies.

Evaluation of interventions that creatively use different sources of social and environmental resources is needed. For example, to strengthen social influences, partnerships with labor unions could be utilized to develop and implement environmental and policy interventions to promote healthful food environments and eating behaviors at worksites (31). Worksite policies related to schedules and break time, work shifts, health promotion program availability, and health care insurance coverage are often negotiated between labor unions and management. These work structure policies can directly affect workers' health behaviors, including eating behaviors and nutrition. Labor and management collaborations could lead to the development and enforcement of worksite policies that support healthful eating behaviors (46).

The next generation of worksite nutrition interventions should focus on the development of innovative programs to target "invisible" and mobile worker populations (46). Invisible worker populations include night shift, temporary, and contract workers. Mobile populations include transportation workers such as truck, bus, and taxi cab drivers, whose "worksite" is their vehicle, and workers such as sales people, home healthcare aids, and housecleaners, who travel from site to site. These worker populations comprise a large and growing segment of the workforce, and are at higher than average risk for unhealthful dietary behaviors. To our knowledge, no nutrition intervention research has targeted these difficult-to-reach workers. Strategies that rely on social networks may be one potentially effective approach, since no regular physical workplace location may be available in which to implement educational interventions or intervention components that target the physical environment of the worksite.

Schools

Schools are an optimal setting in which to reach children and adolescent populations from diverse socioeconomic and racial/ethnic backgrounds. In the US, for example, over 95 per cent of youth aged 5–17 years attend school (48). Children typically eat one or two meals per day at school, or about 30 per cent of their total daily energy. Thus, nutrition interventions that target the school food environment have the potential to substantially impact students' dietary intake and eating behaviors. In addition to providing classroom-based nutrition education, schools provide an environment in which students observe social norms and role models for eating behaviors.

The majority of nutrition intervention studies that have targeted youth have been implemented in school settings. Methodological issues similar to those for worksites have provided challenges to the design, implementation, and evaluation of school-based nutrition interventions. Randomization of schools as the unit of intervention and analysis, evaluation of the school-wide student population, implementation of intervention activities using trained research staff vs. school staff, and evaluation of multicomponent programs involving both individual-level behavioral and environmental components are some examples of the methodological challenges faced by school-based nutrition interventions. Below, the results of school-based nutrition intervention research are briefly summarized. Several methodologically outstanding or innovative studies are highlighted. Research directions that offer promising potential for moving the field forward are outlined.

Previous reviews of school-based nutrition interventions

School-based nutrition intervention studies to date have focused on several different outcomes. A large number of research studies have targeted changes in food choices and eating behaviors as the primary outcome. Several recent obesity prevention studies have targeted change in body weight or body fatness as the primary outcome, and have included changes in food choices and eating behaviors as a secondary outcome. Overall, the results of school-based studies that targeted food choices and eating behaviors have been positive. However, obesity prevention studies have not been very successful in changing body weight or fatness, but have shown some success in changing dietary intake.

Six elements of successful youth-targeted nutrition education programs were identified based on a review of the evaluated empirical literature (49): (1) behaviorally based programs developed based on behavior change theory; (2) family involvement for programs that target elementary-school-aged children; (3) self-assessment activities for programs that target middle and senior high-school-aged children; (4) programs that include intensive instruction time; (5) programs that include intervening in the school environment; and (6) programs that include intervening in the community environment. Another recent review of 16 school-based cardiovascular risk factor prevention intervention studies found that studies were most effective in changing cognitive variables such as self-efficacy and outcome expectations, and were least effective in changing physiological variables such as body fatness (50). However, these studies are difficult to compare because of the diversity of their intervention components and the primary outcomes targeted. Some interventions were only based on classroom curricula, while others included the school food environment and or physical education classes. Some interventions targeted behaviors such as nutrition, physical activity, or smoking, while others targeted physiological variables such as serum cholesterol, blood pressure, or body fatness.

The most comprehensive school-based intervention to date that included dietary intervention components was the Child and Adolescent Trial for Cardiovascular Health (CATCH) (51). A more recent behavioral intervention for obesity prevention that also targeted dietary intake and eating behaviors was Pathways (52). These studies implemented interventions that included both environmental and individual behavior change components, with classroom curricula, food service and physical education changes, and a family home component, and are described in greater detail below. Both interventions were successful in changing dietary intake, but they did not have significant effects on physiological variables such as body weight or serum cholesterol. It has been suggested that school-based interventions should target behavioral variables only, such as food choices, or their hypothesized cognitive precursors, such as knowledge, attitudes, and skills (50). CATCH (51), Pathways (52), and other recent school-based nutrition interventions (53), have been successful in changing the school food environment. These environmental changes have resulted in changes in student food purchases and eating behaviors (50, 53). Targeting environmental changes in school-based nutrition interventions may represent an effective strategy to strengthen the intervention impact on eating behaviors (26, 53–57). Specific environmental intervention strategies that show promise for changing student food choices include food pricing, availability, and promotion (26, 43–45, 53, 56–58).

Current state of the science

Multicomponent interventions. Multicomponent school-based studies have demonstrated positive effects on student food choices and dietary intake. The largest, most comprehensive school-based intervention conducted to date was CATCH (51). The aim of the CATCH intervention was to lower serum cholesterol among third through fifth grade students through a classroom behavioral curricula based on Social Cognitive Theory (22) and changes in the school food service meals and the structure of the physical education (PE) classes. Ninety-six schools in four US states were randomized to the intervention or to a no-intervention control group for a 3-year period. The school food environmental intervention component included training the food service staff in specific food preparation behaviors designed to lower the fat and sodium content of the school meals. Food service staff were also encouraged to promote healthful foods to students and to place point-of-purchase promotional signage in the school cafeteria. Results showed no significant effects on students' serum cholesterol, the primary outcome. However, significant intervention-related reductions in the per cent energy from fat were observed in the school meals (food environment).

Student-level dietary recalls showed significant intervention-related decreases in energy and per cent fat intake. These findings show that a multicomponent intervention that includes an individual-level behavioral classroom curriculum in tandem with environmental changes in the cafeteria and the school meal nutritional content can produce positive significant effects on students' dietary intake.

Pathways (51) aimed to prevent obesity among third, fourth, and fifth grade American Indian school children. Forty-one schools serving American Indian communities in Arizona, New Mexico, and South Dakota were randomized to a 3-year intervention or to a no-treatment control group. The multicomponent intervention package was similar to the CATCH intervention, and included a behavioral curriculum component and environmental changes that targeted food service and PE classes. The primary outcome was change in body fatness, and secondary outcomes were changes in dietary intake and physical activity. Results were not significant for change in body fatness. Significant reductions in the per cent energy from fat were observed for the school meals. Changes in student-level intake were significant for total energy and per cent energy from fat when measured by 24-hour recall. Observations of student food intake at lunch showed significant intervention-related reductions in fat intake but not total energy.

The results of these two large, multicenter trials are consistent in demonstrating that significant changes can be made in the school food environment, particularly in the school meals. These school food environment changes are associated with reductions in students' energy and fat intake. These changes were achieved in the context of intervention trials that were not specifically designed with dietary changes as the primary outcome. The interventions did not target changes in specific foods, but rather focused on a broad range of changes in dietary intake, including choosing lower fat foods, preparing foods to lower the fat content, and increasing intake of foods such as fruits and vegetables. The interventions did include an individual-level classroom educational component.

A second major program of school-based nutrition intervention studies was initiated and funded by the US National Cancer Institute to examine strategies to increase fruit and vegetable intake among youth (26, 59). Five school-based studies were evaluated: three randomized trials targeted fourth and fifth grade students (60–62); one quasiexperimental study targeted fourth and fifth grade students (63); and one randomized study targeted high school students (64). Social Cognitive Theory was the predominant theoretical framework guiding the intervention (22). Intervention programs were 2 to 3 years in duration. All studies included a classroom curriculum component of some type. Three studies included a food service intervention component (60, 61, 64); and four studies included a parent home component (60–62, 64). Overall, four of the five studies reported significant intervention effects for increasing fruit and vegetable intake (60–63). Significant intervention effects were more often observed for fruit intake compared to vegetable intake (26).

Several innovative intervention components were implemented and some unique results were observed in each of these Five-A-Day studies. For example Reynolds *et al.* (60) observed significant intervention-related changes among parents' fruit and vegetable intake. Although the mechanism is not clear, if school-based nutrition interventions could produce changes in parent food choices and eating behaviors, they might considerably strengthen their effects on the targeted children. Parents serve as role models for healthful food choices; influence home food availability through food purchases; and are responsible for home food policies and practices that affect their children's food choices.

In another Five-A-Day study, Foerster *et al.* (63) evaluated a school-based fruit and vegetable intervention with and without a community intervention component. The intervention provides a model for the types of study designs called for to intervene at multiple levels and through multiple channels in the community and is currently a rare example of such an approach that also includes a separate evaluation of the community component. Although the school-only and the school-plus-community intervention conditions did not differ in their effects on fruit and vegetable intake, both produced significantly greater increases in fruit and vegetable intake compared to the control schools.

Finally, the only Five-A-Day study to examine an intervention among high school students did not find significant changes in fruit and vegetable intake (64). The pattern of change observed was a significant increase in the intervention schools during the first intervention year, followed by a "catch-up" among the control schools. Although no supporting data are reported, the authors attribute the increase in fruit and vegetable intake in the control schools to a district-wide change in the school food service aimed to meet the national guidelines for school meals. If this were the case, the study results show the powerful effects that policy changes can produce on diet. Such changes could far surpass the effects of school-based behavioral curricula and or cafeteria-based interventions.

The results of CATCH (51), Pathways (52), and the Five-A-Day school-based interventions (26) show that multicomponent interventions can produce positive effects on food choices and dietary intake. A limitation of these studies is that the components cannot be evaluated separately. Therefore, it is not known whether behavioral curricula targeting individual knowledge and behavior, or changes in the school food environment are each independently effective, or whether both are necessary to change behavior. Studies that are designed to directly evaluate the separate and combined effects of individual-level and environmental interventions are clearly needed and would provide useful information about the size of the effects on behavior associated with intervention strategies that target different levels of influence.

Environmental interventions: food pricing, availability, and promotion

Empirical data are available from a series of several well-designed school-based interventions that targeted only environmental factors to change students' food choices, without a classroom educational component. These interventions have changed the pricing, availability and promotion of targeted foods and evaluated their effects on food choices and dietary intake.

Food pricing

Changes in food prices have been examined in several school-based studies for their effect on food purchases. CHIPS (Changing Individuals' Purchase of Snacks) (43) is methodologically the strongest study to date to examine the effects of pricing strategies on food choices. The aim of CHIPS was to increase the purchase of lower fat snacks from vending machines in 12 high schools and 12 worksites by lowering prices on the targeted snacks. In addition to price changes, the independent effect of point-of-purchase promotion was evaluated. Four pricing levels (low fat and high fat snacks at equal price, −10, −25, and −50 per cent low fat snack price reduction) and three promotional signage levels (no sign; low fat label only; low fat label plus a promotional sign) were crossed in a Latin square design, with each of the 12 experimental conditions implemented in a random order in each school or worksite for a 1-month period. Results showed that sales of the lower fat snacks significantly increased in direct proportion to the magnitude of the price reduction. Price reductions of 10, 25, and 50 per cent were associated with 9, 39 and 93 per cent increases in the proportion of lower fat snacks sold. Under equal prices, low fat snacks comprised about 11 per cent of all vending snacks sold. Under the 50 per cent price reduction condition, lower fat snacks comprised about 21 per cent of all snacks sold. Promotional signage in combination with lower fat labels had small but independent significant effects on sales of lower fat snacks.

In a study that served as one of several pilot studies for CHIPS, prices on fresh fruit and vegetables were reduced by 50 per cent for a 3-week period in two high school cafeterias (58). Minimal promotional activity was implemented (small signs near the fruit/vegetable area). Results showed a four-fold increase in sales of fresh fruit and a two-fold increase in sales of baby carrots during the price reduction period. Sales returned to baseline levels when prices were returned to usual.

One issue to consider in the food pricing interventions is the effect of price reductions on sales volume. For example, in the CHIPS study (43), aggregate sales data were tracked, but data on individual purchases were not collected. While a price reduction of 10 per cent did not increase the total volume of lower fat snacks sold, price reductions of 25 and 50 per cent did increase the total volume of lower fat snacks sold. This suggests that with smaller price reductions, customers may change their snack choice to a more healthful snack. With larger price reductions, however, it is possible that customers may purchase additional snack items at the reduced price. This may result in increasing their total energy intake, an unintended and undesirable effect. Depending on the food type (e.g. fresh fruit or vegetables vs. vending machine snack foods), the amount of the price reduction needs to be considered in terms of its potential effect on food choice and amount or number of foods purchased. Another strategy that warrants evaluation is concurrent increases in the prices of less healthful foods and decreases in prices of healthful foods (65). Further research is needed on the effects of price increases and decreases implemented in tandem on food purchases and revenues.

Food availability

A second environmental intervention that has been evaluated with positive results is increasing the availability of healthful food choices in the school cafeteria (53, 56, 57, 66). Four studies (three in elementary schools and one in high schools) found increases in student choice of targeted foods when availability of the targeted foods was increased. In TACOS (Trying Alternative Cafeteria Options in Schools) (53), 20 high schools were randomized to an intervention or control group for a 2-year period. In intervention schools, the availability of lower fat foods in school cafeteria *a la carte* areas was increased, and school-wide promotional activities were implemented by student groups to promote the lower fat *a la carte* foods. Sales of lower fat *a la carte* foods were measured continuously using the computerized point of sales data collected from the school food service. After 2 years, the availability of lower fat foods in *a la carte* areas increased 51 per cent in intervention school cafeterias, and decreased 5 per cent in control school cafeterias. Sales of lower fat foods significantly increased by 10 per cent during year one in intervention schools, compared with a 2.8 per cent decrease in control schools.

Whitaker *et al.* (56) increased the availability of lower fat meals in school lunches in 16 elementary schools in the US during a single school year. During a baseline period of 6 months, a lower fat meal was available on 23 per cent of school lunch days. During the subsequent eight months, the lower fat meal was available on 71 per cent of the school lunch days. No educational signage or promotional activities were implemented. Results showed that during the baseline period, 39 per cent of the students selected the lower fat meal. During the increased availability period, 29 per cent of the students selected the lower fat meal. However, the fat content of the average student meal decreased from 36 to 30 per cent calories from fat. In a follow-up study (57), the incremental effects of a promotional newsletter targeting students' parents was evaluated. Sixteen elementary schools were randomized to an "availability only" or to an "availability plus parent newsletter" condition. Low fat meals were available as one of two choices daily in all schools. After a 5-month baseline period, intervention schools received a promotional program. School lunch menus that children carried home highlighted the lower fat meals, and parents received a mailed copy of the school menu, plus nutrition information and a letter requesting them to encourage their child to select the lower fat meal at school. Results showed a significant increase in the proportion of students who selected the lower fat meal in schools assigned to the availability plus promotion condition (35.5 per cent) compared to the availability-only condition (32.2 per cent).

Perry *et al.* (66) randomized 26 elementary schools to a no-treatment control group or to an intervention in which the availability of fruits and vegetables in the school lunch meal was increased and food service staff verbally encouraged students to choose and consume fruits and vegetables from the lunch line. Taste tests and contests were held in the lunchroom periodically during the 2-year intervention. Based on observations of lunchtime food intake, the intervention significantly increased students' intake of fruit and vegetable servings (without potatoes).

The results of these school-based randomized trials provide strong evidence that increasing the availability of healthful foods such as lower fat meals, fruit and vegetables, or lower fat *a la carte* foods, is effective in increasing students' choice of the targeted foods. All four studies were methodologically strong in study design, implementation and evaluation, and are consistent in the pattern of results obtained across studies. The results were consistent across a variety of food types, in both the school meal and the *a la carte* food settings, and among both elementary school and high school age groups. Several cross-sectional school-based studies further suggest that greater availability of higher fat foods is associated with lower intake of more healthful foods (67, 68). The effect of simultaneous increases in the availability of healthful foods and decreases in the availability of less healthful foods on food purchases warrants evaluation.

Food promotion

Most of the school-based nutrition interventions reviewed above, both the environmental interventions alone and the multicomponent interventions that included a school cafeteria component, included a food promotion component. Promotional activities most often consist of promotional or informational signage, at the point-of-purchase or elsewhere in the cafeteria, posters, table tents, taste tests, contests, coupons, or fliers. Promotional activities have been implemented in tandem with the food pricing and the availability strategies described above, and the effects of each strategy are impossible to evaluate separately. However, the studies that were designed to evaluate the independent effects of promotional activities and pricing (43) or promotional activities and availability (56) did find small but independent and significant effects for promotion on student food choices. Promotional activities are easy and inexpensive to implement, consistently show positive effects on food choices, and should be implemented broadly to support healthful food choices.

The results of the environmental interventions described above provide consistent empirical support for the effectiveness of food pricing, availability, and promotion strategies to promote healthful food choices in school settings. Additional research is needed to further develop these promising intervention strategies. Simultaneous increases and decreases in food prices or food availability, and identification of the most effective promotional strategies warrant further careful evaluation.

Communities

Community-based public health interventions to promote healthful food choices range from targeting entire communities through mass media, health screening, and other community-wide intervention strategies, to changing food-related policies at the local, state, or federal level, to implementing interventions in restaurants, grocery stores, churches, health care providers, and community groups. Research on food-related policies is addressed elsewhere in this book. Although less evaluated research has been conducted, community-based interventions offer the potential for a broad and substantial population impact. Many of the strategies included in community-based interventions are similar to those used in worksite and school-based interventions, such as food availability, pricing, point-of-purchase promotion, and mass media campaigns.

Previous community interventions

The most well-known community interventions that included food choices in the intervention program were the pioneering studies of North Karelia, Finland (70); the Stanford Three Community Study (71); the Stanford Five Community Study (72); the Minnesota Heart Health Program (69); and the Pawtucket Heart Health Program (47, 73). These non-randomized studies assigned matched communities to an intervention or control group. The intervention included components such as community mass media, health screenings, and educational programs such as grocery store shelf labeling, restaurant menu nutrition labeling, and educational classes held in worksites or adult education centers. The North Karelia and the Stanford Five Community studies found significant positive results on eating behaviors. The other three community studies did not find significant results for dietary intake or eating behaviors.

Mass media campaigns

Mass media campaigns implemented either by themselves or in conjunction with other community interventions have shown some positive effects on food choices. In the US, the Five-A-Day for Better Health campaign is an example of a state level, public–private partnership that was successfully expanded to the national level and has shown some success in impacting its target outcome of fruit and vegetable intake in the general population (59, 74). The 1 Per cent or Less campaign is a second example of a local community mass media campaign that produced positive changes in the targeted outcome of low fat milk purchases (75).

Five-A-Day for Better Health. The Five-A-Day for Better Health program was established in 1991 by the National Cancer Institute and the Produce for Better Health Foundation to increase fruit and vegetable consumption in the US (59, 74, 76). The Five-A-Day program has media, retail, community, and research components (59, 76, 77). The national media campaign is implemented at the local level in co-operation with health, educational, agricultural, and voluntary organizations working with private sector groups (77). The National Cancer Institute has licensed 51 state and territorial health departments to co-ordinate Five-A-Day efforts in local areas (77).

Results of population-based national surveys conducted in 1991 before the Five-A-Day program began, and in 1997 after its implementation, showed a significant increase in both the population mean fruit and vegetable intake and in the percentage of the population who reported eating five or more fruit and vegetable servings per day (74). The mean daily fruit and vegetable servings in 1997 was 3.98 servings per day, vs. 3.75 servings per day in 1991. Twenty six per cent of US adults reported eating five or more servings of fruit and vegetables per day in 1997, compared to 23 per cent in 1991 (74). Unfortunately, these increases were not significant when adjusted for population demographic changes (e.g. age, sex, ethnicity, education, income) during the 1991–1997 period. Program message awareness was significantly higher in 1997 (17.8 per cent) compared with 1991 (2.0 per cent), among the total population and among all demographic subgroups examined. Program awareness was significantly positively correlated with reported fruit and vegetable servings per day (74).

1 Per Cent or Less. The 1 Per Cent or Less campaign evaluated the effects of a community mass media campaign to promote the purchase of low fat milk instead of high fat milk on sales of milk in three West Virginia (US) communities (75). Two small cities in West Virginia were assigned to the intervention and one other city served as the control. The intervention was implemented over a 7-week period and consisted of paid advertisements (television, radio, and newspaper), and other community education activities. Milk sales data were collected for a 1-month period, three times during the study (before, after, and 6 months postintervention). Results showed significant increases in sales of low fat milk in the intervention cities postintervention and 6 months postintervention. Baseline low fat milk sales were 1404 gallons (5314 litres) per store per month. Postintervention, low fat milk sales were 3730 gallons (14118 litres) per store per month. The low fat milk market share was 18 per cent at baseline and 40 per cent at postintervention. Low fat milk sales and market share remained stable in the control city between baseline and postintervention. Sales of high fat milk significantly decreased in both the intervention and control cities from baseline to postintervention. Overall milk sales increased in the intervention cities and did not significantly change in the control cities between baseline and postintervention.

The results of these two mass media campaigns are consistent and suggest that a mass media campaign that targets an entire community and focuses its message on a specific food group has a significant and positive impact on food choices. Although other factors, such as the price of the targeted foods, may exert powerful influences on food choices, the results suggest that mass media promotion campaigns that are very focused and specific with respect to the target food choice recommended can have an effect on population food choices. The independent effects of promotion and price have been demonstrated in controlled studies in community settings (43). Given the relatively inexpensive cost of mass media advertising, relative to multicomponent educational interventions that target individuals, mass media campaigns warrant further evaluation as a population-based food choice intervention strategy. Future research should examine the effects of media dosage over time, channel of media delivery, message type (specific food categories vs. broader nutrition messages), and the independent effects of promotion vs. food price or availability.

Restaurants and grocery stores

Interventions to influence food choices in restaurants and grocery stores have used similar strategies to those discussed above, including point-of-purchase nutrition labels, pricing strategies, increased availability of targeted foods, and media promotion (78, 79). Research studies in these settings have not used the group-randomized design, and have typically included only a limited number of sites. Although research in these settings is very difficult to design, implement, and evaluate, restaurants and grocery stores represent important settings for interventions to influence population food choices. In 1995 in the US, for example, people purchased and consumed 34 per cent of their total daily energy from restaurants, a greater proportion than ever before (5). Restaurants remain an optimal setting to implement strategies such as increasing the availability of healthful food choices, promoting healthful foods through advertising and pricing strategies, and influencing food choices through food labeling.

Recently, there has been a call from public health and nutrition groups for legislation to require restaurants to provide nutrition labels for their foods. In the US, restaurants currently are exempt from the federal Nutrition Labeling and Education Act that requires food labels on all packaged food sold in grocery stores and most other food outlets (other than restaurants) (70). Innovative intervention approaches include experimenting with labeling formats such as labels that provide information about the number of fruit and vegetable servings a food provides, or the amount of physical activity (minutes or steps) needed to expend the energy provided in a serving or package of a food item. Increasing the availability of healthful menu items and implementing pricing strategies that eliminate incentives for the purchase of larger portion sizes are strategies that also have received attention and are being advocated with the aim to promote healthful food choices and portion sizes (11–13, 81). Research is needed to further evaluate the effectiveness of these strategies in restaurant settings. One barrier is the difficulty of working with commercial restaurant establishments that may be reluctant to implement labeling, pricing, or promotional interventions without assurances that such strategies will not decrease business revenues or customer satisfaction. Cross-marketing promotions are also an idea that could be evaluated, such as offering a free or discounted piece of fresh fruit with the sale of newspapers or magazines. Bundling fruit or vegetables with other items such as value meals is more common today, but data are needed on the effects of these innovative marketing strategies.

Perhaps because they are such complex environments in which to implement and evaluate interventions, little data are available on the effectiveness of nutrition intervention strategies implemented in grocery stores. An innovative study conducted in the Netherlands in grocery stores run by the researchers showed that increased access to lower fat food items was effective in reducing energy intake and per cent fat energy (82). Normal weight individuals from the community were randomized to shop at one of two researcher-operated grocery stores. The grocery stores both offered the same foods, but the foods differed in fat content (lower fat items with 52 per cent less fat, or full fat items). Participants could take as many items as they wished, and were not charged for the foods. The experimental food items included frozen meals, meats, cheese, desserts, pizza, salads, and comprised about 37 per cent of total energy among the control (full fat) group participants and 30 per cent of energy among the reduced fat group participants. The study results are intriguing, and demonstrate that simple availability, or change in the food supply, can reduce energy and fat intake. It is notable that participants did not receive any nutrition education or instruction, and were not attempting to lose weight or otherwise change their diet.

One factor that was not explored in the Dutch grocery store study, although it was held constant across the two conditions, is the effect of food prices on food choices. In the study, the food items were provided free of charge. However, in real community settings, food prices are reportedly one of the main influences on food purchases (83–85). Healthful foods, such as fruits and vegetables, or reduced fat prepackaged products, are perceived as more expensive than less healthful foods. Much more research is needed to examine the relative importance of food promotion, availability, and prices and how they interact to influence food purchases. This is an important but especially complex area, given that the influence of price may vary by food category or type (e.g. fruit and vegetables vs. meat, poultry or fish vs. prepackaged snack foods or sweets). Both prices and availability may differ among neighborhoods and among grocery stores catering to people of different income and demographic groups.

While much more research is needed to evaluate pricing, availability, and promotion strategies in grocery store settings, grocery stores represent a setting in which the majority of the population access the food they consume, and a diverse demographic population cross-section could be examined. Furthermore, the computerized scanners currently used in most grocery stores offer the potential to examine both aggregate and individualized sales data at the specific food level. Potentially, food choices, energy, and nutrients could be tracked in aggregate at the store level and among a cohort of customer patrons to examine environmental and individual-level changes in food purchasing in response to specific interventions.

Other community settings

Other community settings that deserve mention as potential settings for nutrition interventions include churches and community groups such as after-school programs, and girls and boys clubs. A small but growing body of research has examined nutrition interventions delivered in these settings (86–90). Although limited in number, initial studies have show positive results in feasibility of implementation, in reaching new population segments, and in positively impacting food choices and dietary intake. The intervention strategies examined have been similar to those examined in other community settings. Innovative strategies are needed to take advantage of the unique environments provided by these previously untapped settings. For example does the cohesive social network present in some church settings offer a potential for an intervention to capitalize on such highly integrated networks? Can an intervention be designed to tap this unique environmental component? Do churches bring a spiritual or religious dimension that could be utilized in some way to strengthen an intervention component or to develop a unique approach to an intervention for healthful eating behaviors? Similar questions need to be addressed in interventions based in girls and boys clubs. Is there something unique about this community social group or setting that lends itself to a different intervention strategy, perhaps one that is designed to take advantage of the social integration of the organization, or the greater access to a network of parents who are socially integrated within the group to allow greater provision of and access to resources for the participating children?

Summary and future research directions

There remains much to learn about the most effective intervention strategies to promote healthful food choices in the population. Based on the literature to date, it is clear that both environmental intervention strategies and individual-level strategies implemented in tandem will be most effective in promoting healthful eating behaviors in the population. Environmental strategies offer potential for behavior changes of large magnitude and may be implemented with relatively low cost. Social environmental interventions, such as those involving social networks to promote behavior change, may be most promising to reach invisible and mobile population subgroups. Interventions that target environmental variables such as food availability and food prices warrant further research to evaluate their impact on food choices. Smaller, more intensive interventions are needed to examine dose-response impacts on the magnitude of behavior change. Studies are needed that co-ordinate interventions at several levels in the community, such as schools, worksites, grocery stores, and households. Policy change is an understudied but potentially powerful intervention strategy that warrants more extensive evaluation, perhaps using a community organizing approach.

References

1. World Health Organization (2004). *Diet, nutrition and the prevention of chronic diseases.* WHO, Geneva.
2. World Health Organization (1999). *Obesity: Preventing and managing the global epidemic: Report of the WHO consultation.* WHO technical report series 894. WHO, Geneva.
3. World Health Organization. (2000). *Obesity: Preventing and managing the global epidemic: Report of the WHO consultation.* WHO technical report series 894. WHO, Geneva.

4. **Drewnowski A, Popkin BM** (1997). The nutrition transition: new trends in the global diet. *Nutr Rev* **55**, 31–43.

5. **Guthrie JF, Lin B-H, Frazao E** (2002). Role of food prepared away from home in the American diet, 1977–78 versus 1994–96: changes and consequences. *J Nutr Educ Behav* **34**, 140–50.

6. **Kant AK, Graubard BI** (2004). Eating out in America, 1987–2000: trends and nutritional correlates. *Prev Med* **38**, 243–9.

7. **Kant AK** (2000). Consumption of energy dense, nutrient poor foods by adult Americans: nutritional and health implications. The third National Health and Nutrition Examination Survey, 1988–1994. *Am J Clin Nutr* **72**, 29–36.

8. **Harnack LJ, Jeffery RW, Boutelle KN** (2000). Temporal trends in energy intake in the United States: an ecologic perspective. *Am J Clin Nutr* **71**, 1478–84.

9. **Nielsen SJ, Siega-Riz AM, Popkin BM** (2002). Trends in energy intake in US between 1977 and 1996: similar shifts across age groups. *Obes Res* **10**, 370–8.

10. **Koplan JP, Dietz WH** (1999). Caloric imbalance and public health policy. *JAMA* **282**, 1579–81.

11. **Nestle M** (2003). Increasing portion sizes in American diets: more calories, more obesity. *J Am Diet Assoc* **103**, 39–40.

12. **Young LR, Nestle M** (2002). The contribution of expanding portion sizes to the US obesity epidemic. *Am J Public Health* **92**, 246–9.

13. **Rolls BJ** (2003). The supersizing of America: portion size and the obesity epidemic. *Nutr Today* **38**, 42–53.

14. World Cancer Research Fund/American Institute for Cancer Research (1997). *Food, nutrition, and the prevention of cancer: A global perspective*. World Cancer Research Fund/American Institute for Cancer Research.

15. **Potter JD, Steinmetz K** (1996). Vegetables, fruit, and phytoestrogens as preventive agents. In: Stewart BW, McGregor D, Kleihues P, eds. *Principles of chemoprevention*, pp. 61–90. International Agency for Research on Cancer Scientific Publications no. 139. IARC, Lyon.

16. **Rose G** (1985). Sick individuals and sick populations. *Int J Epidemiol* **14**, 32–8.

17. **Rose G** (1992). *The strategy of preventive medicine*. Oxford University Press, New York.

18. **Kelsey JL, Whittemore AS, Evans AS, Thompson WD** (1996). *Methods in observational epidemiology*, 2nd edn, pp. 22–44. Oxford University Press, New York.

19. **Glanz K, Sorensen G, Farmer A** (1996). The health impact of worksite nutrition and cholesterol intervention programs. *Am J Health Promot* **10**, 453–70.

20. **Glanz K, Rimer BF, Lewis FM** (2002). *Health behavior and health education*, 3rd edn. Jossey Bass, San Francisco.

21. **Jeffery RW** (1989). Risk behaviors and health: Contrasting individual and population perspectives. *Am Psychol* **44**, 1194–202.

22. **Bandura A** (1986). *Social foundations of thought and action*. Prentice Hall, Englewood Cliffs, NJ.

23. **Stokols D** (1992). Establishing and maintaining health environments: Toward a social ecology of health promotion. *Am Psychol* **47**, 6–22.

24. **Sallis JF, Owen N** (2002). Ecological models of health behavior. In: Glanz K, Rimer BF, Lewis FM, eds. *Health behavior and health education*, 3rd edn, pp. 462–84 . Jossey Bass, San Francisco.

25. **Cohen DA, Scribner RA, Farley TA** (2000). A structural model of health behavior: A pragmatic approach to explain and influence health behaviors at the population level. *Prev Med* **30**, 146–54.

26. **French SA, Stables G** (2003). Environmental interventions to promote fruit and vegetable consumption among youth in school settings. *Prev Med* **37**, 593–610.

27. **McGraw SA, Stone EJ, Osganian SK, *et al.*** (1994). An overview of process evaluation on CATCH: The Child and Adolescent Trial for Cardiovascular Health. *Health Educ Q* **25** (suppl), S5–26.

28. **Murray DM** (1998). *Design and analysis of group-randomized trials.* Oxford University Press, New York.

29. **Murray DM, Varnell SP, Blitstein JL** (2004). Design and analysis of group-randomized trials: A review of recent methodological developments. *Am J Public Health* **94**, 423–32.

30. **Hennrikus DJ, Jeffery RW** (1996). Worksite intervention for weight control: A review. *Am J Health Promot* **10**, 471–98.

31. **Sorensen G, Emmons K, Hunt MK, Johnston J** (1998). Implications of the results of community intervention trials. *Annu Rev Public Health* **19**, 379–416.

32. **US Bureau of Labor Statistics. Division of Current Employment Statistics. Washington DC.** *Employment Situation.* Available at www.bls.gov. Accessed on 5 August 2004.

33. **Sorensen G, Stoddard A, Peterson K, et al.** (1999). Increasing fruit and vegetable consumption through worksites and families in the Treatwell 5-A-Day Study. *Am J Public Health* **89**, 54–60.

34. **Sorenson G, Thompson B, Glanz K, et al.** (1996). Work site-based cancer prevention: Primary results from the Working Well Trial. *Am J Public Health* **86**, 939–47.

35. **Buller DB, Morrill C, Taren D, et al.** (1999). Randomized trial testing the effect of peer education at increasing fruit and vegetable intake. *J Natl Cancer Inst* **91**, 1491–500.

36. **Beresford SA, Thompson B, Feng Z, et al.** (2001). Seattle 5 a Day worksite program to increase fruit and vegetable consumption. *Prev Med* **32**, 230–8.

37. **Tilley BC, Glanz K, Kristal AR, et al.** (1999). Nutrition intervention for high-risk auto workers: Results of the Next Step Trial. *Prev Med* **28**, 284–92.

38. **Glasgow RE, Terborg JR, Hollis JF, et al.** (1994). Modifying dietary and tobacco use patterns in the worksite: The Take Heart Project. *Health Educ Q* **21**, 69–82.

39. **Glasgow RE, Terborg JR, Strycker LA, Boles SM, Hollis JF** (1997). Take Heart II: Replication of a worksite health promotion trial. *J Behav Med* **20**, 143–61.

40. **Prochaska JO, DiClemente CC** (1992). Stages of change in the modification of problem behaviors. *Prog Behav Modif* **28**, 183–218.

41. **Patterson RE, Kristal AR, Glanz K, et al.** (1997). Components of the Working Well Trial intervention associated with adoption of healthful diets. *Am J Prev Med* **13**, 271–6.

42. **Biener L, Glanz K, McLerran D, et al.** (1999). Impact of Working Well Trial on the worksite smoking and nutrition environment. *Health Educ Behav* **26**, 478–94.

43. **French SA, Jeffery RW, Story M, et al.** (2001). Pricing and promotion effects on low-fat vending snack purchases: The CHIPS study. *Am J Public Health* **91**, 112–7.

44. **French SA, Jeffery RW, Story M, Hannan P, Snyder MP** (1997). A pricing strategy to promote low fat snack choices through vending machines. *Am J Public Health* **87**, 849–51.

45. **Jeffery RW, French SA, Raether C, Baxter JE** (1994). An environmental intervention to increase fruit and salad purchases in a cafeteria. *Prev Med* **23**, 788–92.

46. **Sorensen G, Linnan L, Hunt MK** (2004). Worksite-based research and initiatives to increase fruit and vegetable consumption. *Prev Med* **39**, 94–100.

47. **Sorensen G, Morris DM, Hunt MK, et al.** (1992). Work-site nutrition intervention and employees' dietary habits: The Treatwell program. *Am J Public Health* **82**, 877–80.

48. **US Department of Education. National Center for Education Statistics.** *Digest of Education, Statistics, Tables and Figures.* Accessed on August 8, 2004. Available at www.nces.ed.gov/programs/digest/d02/tables/df041.asp.

49. **Lytle L, Achterberg C** (1995). Changing the diet of America's children: what works and why? *J Nutr Educ* **27**, 250–60.

50. **Resnicow K, Robinson TN** (1997). School-based cardiovascular disease prevention studies: Review and synthesis. *Ann Epidemiol* **S7**, S14–31.

51. Luepker RV, Perry CL, McKinlay SM, *et al.* (1996). Outcomes of a field trial to improve children's dietary patterns and physical activity: the Child and Adolescent Trial for Cardiovascular Health (CATCH). *JAMA* **275**, 768–76.

52. Caballero B, Clay T, Davis SM, *et al.* (2003). Pathways: a school-based, randomized controlled trial for the prevention of obesity in American Indian schoolchildren. *Am J Clin Nutr* **78**, 1030–8.

53. French SA, Story M, Fulkerson JA, Hannan PJ (2004). An environmental intervention to promote lower-fat food choices in secondary schools: outcomes of the TACOS study. *Am J Public Health* **94**, 1507–12.

54. French SA, Story M, Jeffery RW (2001). Environmental influences on eating and physical activity. *Annu Rev Public Health* **22**, 309–35.

55. Wechsler H, Devereaux RS, Davis M, Collins J (2000). Using the school environment to promote physical activity and healthy eating. *Prev Med* **31**, S121–37.

56. Whitaker RC, Wright JA, Finch AJ, Psaty BM (1993). An environmental intervention to reduce dietary fat in school lunches. *Pediatrics* **91**, 1107–11.

57. Whitaker RC, Wright JA, Koepsell TD, Finch AJ, Psaty BM (1994). Randomized intervention to increase children's selection of low fat foods in school lunches. *J Pediatrics* **125**, 535–40.

58. French SA, Story M, Jeffery RW, *et al.* (1997). Pricing strategy to promote fruit and vegetable purchase in high school cafeterias. *J Am Diet Assoc* **97**, 1008–10.

59. Heimendinger J, Van Duyn A, Chapelsky D, Foerster S, Stables G (1996). The national 5 a day for better health program: a large-scale nutrition intervention. *J Public Health Manage Pract* **2**, 27–35.

60. Reynolds KD, Franklin FA, Binkley D, *et al.* (2000). Increasing the fruit and vegetable consumption of fourth-graders: results from the High 5 Project. *Prev Med* **30**, 309–19.

61. Perry CL, Bishop DB, Taylor G, *et al.* (1998). Changing fruit and vegetable consumption among children: the 5-A-Day Power Plus Program in St.Paul, Minnesota. *Am J Public Health* **88**, 603–9.

62. Baranowski T, Davis M, Resnicow K, *et al.* (2000). Gimme 5 fruit, juice, and vegetables for fun and health: outcome evaluation. *Health Educ Behav* **27**, 96–111.

63. Foerster SB, Gregson J, Beall DL, *et al.* (1998). The California children's 5-A-Day Power Play! campaign: evaluation of a large-scale social marketing initiative. *Fam Community Health* **21**, 46–64.

64. Nicklas TA, Johnson CC, Myers L, Farris RP, Cunninham A (1998). Outcomes of a high school program to increase fruit and vegetable consumption: gimme 5 – a fresh nutrition concept for students. *J Sch Health* **68**, 248–53.

65. Hannan PJ, French SA, Story M, Fulkerson JA (2002). A pricing strategy to promote sales of lower fat foods in high school cafeterias: acceptability and sensitivity analysis. *Am J Health Promot* **17**, 1–6.

66. Perry CL, Bishop DB, Taylor GL, *et al.* (2004). A randomized school trial of environmental strategies to encourage fruit and vegetable consumption among children. *Health Educ Behav* **31**, 65–76.

67. Kubik MY, Lytle LA, Hannan PJ, Perry CL, Story M (2003). The association of the school food environment with dietary behaviors of young adolescents. *Am J Public Health* **93**, 1168–73.

68. Cullen KW, Eagan J, Baranowski T, Owens E, deMoor C (2000). Effect of a la carte and snack bar foods at school on children's lunchtime intake of fruits and vegetables. *J Am Diet Assoc* **100**, 1482–6.

69. Luepker RV, Murray DM, Jacobs DR, *et al.* (1994). Community education for cardiovascular disease prevention: risk factor changes in the Minnesota Heart Health Program. *Am J Public Health* **84**, 1383–93.

70. Puska P, Salonen JT, Nissinen A, *et al.* (1983). Change in risk factors for coronary heart disease during 10 years of a community intervention programme (North Karelia project). *BMJ* **287**, 1840–4.

71. Fortmann SP, Williams PT, Hulley SB, Haskell WL, Farquhar JW (1981). Effect of health education on dietary behavior: the Stanford three community study. *Am J Clin Nutr* **34**, 2030–8.

72. Farquhar JW, Fortmann SP, Maccoby N, *et al.* (1985). The Stanford Five-City Project: design and methods. *Am J Epidemiol* **122**, 323–34.

73. Carleton RA, Lasater TM, Assaf AR, Feldman HA, McKinlay S (1995). The Pawtucket Heart Health Program: community changes in cardiovascular risk factors and projected disease risk. *Am J Public Health* **85**, 777–85.

74. Stables GJ, Subar AF, Patterson BH, *et al.* (2002). Changes in vegetable and fruit consumption and awareness among US adults: results of the 1991 and 1997 5 A Day for Better Health Program surveys. *J Am Diet Assoc* **102**, 809–17.

75. Reger B, Wootan MG, Booth-Butterfield S, Smith H (1998). 1% or less: a community-based nutrition campaign. *Public Health Rep* **113**, 410–9.

76. Heimendinger J, Van Duyn MA, Chapelsky D, Foerster S, Stables G (1996). The National 5 A Day for Better Health Program: a large-scale nutrition intervention. *J Public Health Manage Pract* **2**, 27–35.

77. Heimendinger J, Van Duyn MAS (1995). Dietary behavior change: the challenge of recasting the role of fruit and vegetables in the American diet. *Am J Clin Nutr* **61** (Suppl), 1397S–401S.

78. Glanz K, Hoelscher D (2004). Increasing fruit and vegetable intake by changing environments, policy and pricing: restaurant-based research, strategies and recommendations. *Prev Med* **39** (Suppl 2), S88–S93.

79. Glanz K, Yaroch AL (2004). Strategies for increasing fruit and vegetable intake in grocery stores and communities: policy, pricing and environmental change. *Prev Med* **39** (Suppl 2), S75–S80.

80. House of Representatives (1990). *Nutrition labeling on education Act of 1990.* House Report 101–538, Washington, DC.

81. Nestle M (2003). *Food politics: how the food industry influences nutrition and health.* University of California Press, Berkeley, CA.

82. Westrate JA, van het Hof KH, van den Berg H, *et al.* (1998). A comparison of the effect of free access to reduced fat products or their full fat equivalents on food intake, body weight, blood lipids and fat-soluble antioxidants levels and haemostasis variables. *Eur J Clin Nutr* **52**, 389–95.

83. Glanz K, Basil M, Maibach E, Goldberg J, Snyder D (1998). Why Americans eat what they do: taste, nutrition, cost, convenience and weight control concerns as influences on food consumption. *J Am Diet Assoc* **98**, 1118–26.

84. French SA, Story M, Hannan P, *et al* (1999). Cognitive and demographic correlates of low-fat vending snack choices among adolescents and adults. *J Am Diet Assoc* **99**, 471–5.

85. Drewnowski A (2003). Fat and sugar: an economic analysis. *J Nutr* **133**, 838S–40S.

86. Campbell MK, Demark-Wahnefried W, Symons M, *et al.* (1999). Fruit and vegetable consumption and prevention of cancer: the Black Churches United for Better Health Project. *Am J Public Health* **89**, 1390–6.

87. Havas S, Anliker J, Damron D, Langenberg P, Ballesteros M, Feldman R (1998). Final results of the Maryland WIC 5-A-Day Program. *Am J Public Health* **88**, 1161–7.

88. French SA, Story M, Fulkerson JA, *et al.* (in press). Increasing weight-bearing physical activity and calcium-rich foods to promote bone mass gains among 9–11 year old girls: outcomes of the CAL-Girls study. *Int J Behav Nutr Physical Activity.*

89. Baranowski T, Baranowski J, Cullen KW, *et al.* (2002). 5 a Day achievement badge for African-American boy scouts: pilot outcome results. *Prev Med* **34**, 353–63.

90. Ievers-Landis CE, Burant C, Drotar D, *et al.* (2005). A randomized controlled trial of an intervention for the primary prevention of osteoporosis among preadolescent females: one-year outcomes from a behavioral program with Girl Scouts. *J Pediatr Psychol* **30**, 155–65.

Chapter 7

Population approaches to increasing physical activity among children and adults

Jo Salmon and Abby C. King

Introduction

> The greatest pitfall in evolutionary thinking stems from the keenness of hindsight. For example, we know that long ago, over a long period of time, our own ancestors abandoned the trees for the ground and developed effective machinery for bipedal locomotion. This seems beyond dispute, because the pre-hominoid primates were arboreal and we ourselves are bipedal ground walkers. But when we ask why this change, we must remember that our ancestors of the time were not striving to become human. They were doing what all animals do: trying to stay alive (1).

Along with the evolution of the technological industry, the last 100 years have seen incredible transitions at the industrial, social, and cultural levels of society. Unlike our ancestors of long ago, however, our current adaptations to changes in our environment may not be as favorable to our survival as a species. Cars and machinery have reduced the need for physical labor both at home and in the workforce. Living in sprawling suburban housing developments that do not make it easy to walk, concerns about traffic and safety from personal crime, being time-poor, and a lack of individual confidence and motivation are all potential contributors to people being more likely to drive their cars rather than walk or bicycle to most destinations.

There has also been a dramatic increase in opportunities to be sedentary during our recreational time. New technologies allow us to play (e.g. electronic games) and socialize (e.g. via internet chat rooms) without having to leave our homes, or in the case of many adolescents, our bedrooms. In Australia, for example, access to pay television has increased from 5 per cent in 1996 to 19 per cent in 2000 (2). Further, 82 per cent of adolescents in Australia had a home computer in 2001 (a 13 per cent increase since 1999), 61 per cent of households owned two or more television sets, and 87 per cent of households owned one or more video cassette recorders (2).

Social transformations have also resulted in changes to family structure over recent decades. In Australia, for example, there are fewer nuclear families and there have been reductions in the average family size, increased divorce rates, and an increase in the number of single parent families (3). In 2003 in the US, 68 per cent of children less than 19 years of age lived with two married parents; a 9 per cent decrease since 1980 (4). In 1996 in the US, over 22 per cent of adults had been divorced (5). In Australia, more mothers are working than ever before with 44.5 per cent of lone mothers and 58.5 per cent of couple mothers employed (6), while in the US, 61 per cent of children aged under 6 years received non-parental childcare on a regular basis (4). At the other end of the age spectrum, there are higher proportions of older adults who are living longer. In the US over the past 20 years, for example, there has been an increase in the proportion of adults aged 65 years or older in the population (7). While empirical data linking these sociocultural and environmental changes to physical activity levels and increases in overweight and obesity are poor, the challenge for public health is to respond to these changes and to develop strategies to promote physical activity at the population level.

The aim of this chapter is to provide a selected overview of the latest evidence for population approaches to increasing physical activity in different population segments (children, adolescents, young, mid-life, and older adults). This evidence will be considered within a social ecological context. Emerging issues and directions in the field will also be presented.

Social ecological models

To intervene effectively and to make informed judgments about how to measure the success of interventions, health professionals should have an understanding of how health behaviors are adopted and sustained, and the motivating and constraining factors that influence, mediate, and moderate change. There are many behavioral theories and models that have been developed in and effort to help understand this process. In the physical activity field, individual-level psychological theories have been applied more frequently than others (8). However, as described in Chapter 6, social ecological models provide a useful framework for public health interventions that target health behavior change in the population. These models recognize not only individual-level influences on behavior and mechanisms of health behavior change, but also include the sociocultural and environmental level influences. The interactions between social systems, public policy, and the physical environment with individual cognitions and behaviors are a unique characteristic of social ecological models (9, 10).

It has recently been argued that children's health behaviors and health outcomes (e.g. childhood obesity) develop within an 'ecological niche', with the family environment playing a major role in this developmental process (11). Ecological systems theory proposes that factors such as a child's health behaviors (dietary intake, physical activity, sedentary behavior), parenting practices and family characteristics, sibling influences, family television viewing habits, and access to recreational facilities are important influences on the development of childhood obesity (11). Figure 7.1 presents

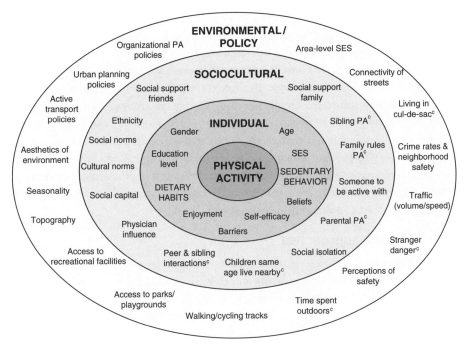

Fig. 7.1 Social ecological model of physical activity. Adapted from Davison and Birch, (11). [c] relevant to children.

an adaptation of that ecological model and illustrates a potential social ecological framework for physical activity.

While social ecological models acknowledge the multifaceted contexts that influence how we live our daily lives and in which physical activity behaviors are shaped and maintained, we currently have a poor understanding of the ecological influences on physical activity across the lifespan. The following section will provide an overview of the recent evidence for promoting physical activity among children and adolescents and will consider this evidence within a social ecological framework.

Review of physical activity intervention literature in children and adolescents

While significant proportions of children and adolescents could benefit from increasing or at least maintaining their current physical activity levels and reducing time spent being sedentary, most interventions have focused only on increasing physical activity. There is, however, an expanding body of evidence on strategies to reduce sedentary behavior among children and adolescents (12–14). While the focus of those studies has been on reducing television viewing, it should be noted that sedentary behaviors are far more extensive than just television viewing (e.g. computer use, electronic games, reading, etc.). Most physical activity and sedentary behavior interventions targeting children and adolescents have been delivered via school settings.

Settings-based approaches have the potential to reach large portions of these groups in the population. A setting is typically a geographical area or institution containing a large "captive" audience (i.e. children and adolescents) whereby physical activity messages and/or programs can be efficiently delivered (10). However, a setting could also be cultural or contextual, for example the family setting. There are a number of settings that are relevant to physical activity and sedentary behavior among children and adolescents including: schools, families, transport, healthcare, and community settings. This section will provide an overview of recent evidence of physical activity approaches among children and adolescents in such settings.

School-based approaches

School-based approaches to promoting physical activity have typically employed three types of strategies including curriculum-based educational strategies, environmental-level strategies, and policy-based strategies. Stone *et al.* (15) reviewed 22 school-based studies and found that most interventions: utilized individual-level behavior change strategies; focused on social influences; and incorporated the program into the academic and physical education (PE) curriculum. Several recent curriculum-based strategies in schools have achieved mixed outcomes in relation to children's physical activity (12, 13, 16, 17).

A recent study by Neumark-Sztainer and colleagues ("New Moves") aimed to increase physical activity and reduce television viewing among adolescent girls by offering a 16-week curriculum-based program as a credit subject to low active girls (17). At postintervention and at 4-months follow-up, there were no significant differences in self-reported physical activity between the intervention and control schools. There were, however, significant improvements in physical activity stages of change for girls in the intervention schools compared with the controls, such that girls in the intervention progressed in their stage of behavioral change for physical activity between baseline and follow-up. Interestingly, a recent curriculum-based intervention that targeted the mediators of physical activity (based on Social Cognitive Theory) among adolescent girls in 24 high schools in the US reported that the intervention had direct effects on self-efficacy for physical activity, and self-efficacy was shown to partially mediate the effects of the intervention on physical activity (18).

There have been several interventions to reduce sedentary behavior and prevent unhealthy weight gain in children and youth. These studies have focused on reducing TV viewing rather than reducing other types of sedentary behavior, such as computer use and electronic games. Robinson (12) recruited one control and one intervention school and targeted children in grades three and four. The intervention strategies were based on principles from Social Cognitive Theory (19). The study used a curriculum-based approach and included behavior change strategies such as self-monitoring and budgeting of TV use. No alternative activities to TV viewing were promoted to the children. Robinson's study demonstrated that reduced TV viewing in the intervention group was significantly associated with relative decreases in BMI, triceps skinfold thickness, and waist and hip circumference over a 6-month period. There was an adjusted difference in mean BMI for the intervention group relative to the control group of $-0.45\,kg/m^2$. There were no significant differences in self-reported physical activity between the two groups.

Another intervention to reduce TV viewing and prevent unhealthy weight gain among children in grades six to eight was evaluated by Gortmaker and colleagues (13). As with Robinson's study, the intervention was primarily delivered via the curriculum, using comprehensively developed intervention materials based on Behavioral Choice (20) and Social Cognitive theories that were blended through the key learning areas (e.g. mathematics, health, English, etc). In addition to providing participants with strategies for reducing TV viewing, Gortmaker's study incorporated educational components teaching children about healthy eating and physical activity. In this 2-year intervention, it was found that reduced TV viewing was most strongly linked to decreases in obesity in girls. Evaluation conducted postintervention showed that the prevalence of obesity among girls in the intervention schools was reduced compared with controls, but was unchanged in boys. In addition, there was greater remission of obesity among intervention girls vs. control girls.

Interestingly, neither of the two studies just described was successful in increasing physical activity. In both the Gortmaker (13) and Robinson (12) studies, a limitation was the reliance on self-reported physical activity rather than using an objective activity measure. It may be that there were increases in incidental or informal types of physical activity that were not detected using self-report. Furthermore, children were only followed-up for a 6-month period, and thus data are only available on the short-term effects of the intervention. It may also be that these studies did not achieve increases in physical activity because children and adolescents did not have the skills or confidence to be active once they reduced their TV viewing.

A recently completed randomized controlled trial conducted in Australia, "Switch-Play" (21), aimed to reduce children's television viewing and also increase children's mastery of fundamental motor skills (FMS). The 12-month follow-up of that study has just been completed and the outcomes will be available shortly. However, initial process evaluation indicates favorable responses from children in the program with approximately 80–90 per cent reporting they had little difficulty in reducing their television viewing, and between 40–60 per cent reporting they played outside instead of watching their usual television shows (21).

Few studies have focused primarily on environmental-level changes to the school setting to promote physical activity. In one experimental study, fluorescent markings were painted on the school playground in an intervention school to promote children's physical activity and used heart rate monitoring to compare activity levels with children in a control school (22, 23). There was an 18-minute increase in moderate- to vigorous-intensity physical activity in the experimental group compared with a 7-minute increase in the control group during recess. However, the impact of this intervention on children's overall physical activity levels and whether these changes were maintained was not reported.

Other school-based interventions (e.g. M-SPAN, APPLES) have used more comprehensive ecological approaches including policy-level changes, curriculum changes, and increased resources (e.g. equipment, staff development) (24–26). The findings from these interventions were not strong, with the US study, M-SPAN, showing a significant increase in physical activity among boys, but not among girls (24). The UK study, APPLES, reported no differences in physical activity between intervention and control schools, and a significant increase in sedentary behavior among overweight children in the intervention schools compared with overweight children in the control schools (25). It was concluded that although environmental level changes were successfully made in the schools, this did not appear to affect children's health behavior. In the US intervention M-SPAN, it was concluded that a better understanding of the barriers and difficulties in fully implementing health policies in schools is required (24).

One of the few long-term studies to report on-going success in promoting physical activity and health behaviors is the study of 24 intervention schools and 16 control schools in Crete, Greece (27, 28). This was a multistrategy intervention combining a curriculum program, two structured physical education sessions per week, workbook exercises completed with parents, and parents' educational meetings on modeling behavior. At the 3- and 6-year follow-ups there were greater increases in children's moderate- to vigorous-intensity physical activity and fitness in the intervention schools compared with the control schools.

In summary, curriculum approaches on their own appear to have mixed effects in promoting physical activity and rarely demonstrate long-term maintenance of behavior change. Strategies to reduce sedentary behaviors delivered via the school curriculum, however, show promise and have been found to prevent unhealthy weight gain, but did not result in increased physical activity. Innovative strategies that manipulate the school physical environment show promise; however, policy-based interventions did not seem to be effective at the behavior change level. The most effective approach reported in the literature to date is one that has used a multistrategy whole-of-school approach that included classroom educational strategies, parental involvement, and changes to the teaching program (increased PE sessions). Few studies have incorporated curriculum, policy, and environmental changes in the school setting (the full social ecological model) to promote physical activity in children and adolescents.

Family-based approaches

Most of the family-based intervention studies that have incorporated physical activity have tended to focus on prevention of unhealthy weight gain among children, or on the treatment of children who are obese. Epstein and colleagues (29) recruited 90 families with obese children between 8 and 12 years of age, through physician referrals, newspaper articles, and advertising. Using behavioral economic techniques, families were assigned to one of four groups that varied treatment conditions (increases to physical activity or decreases to sedentary behavior) and dose (low vs. high). Using praise, reciprocal contracts, and goal setting behavioral modification techniques over a 24-month period, it was found that there were significant increases in physical activity and decreases in sedentary behavior within the respective groups. The study also reported a significant decrease in per cent overweight and body fat over a 2-year period; however, conclusions regarding the efficacy of the intervention are limited by the fact that there was no control group with whom to compare these changes.

More recently, the Girls Health Enrichment Multi-Site project (GEMS) conducted a series of pilot intervention studies targeting health behaviors among African-American girls in the US (30). Several strategies were piloted including: parent vs. child focused program delivery (31); promoting dancing among adolescent girls and reduced family television viewing (32); and an after school program reinforced with regular family contacts (30). The focus of these interventions in the family setting included targeting modifiable family behaviors (e.g. reducing television viewing), parents' educational strategies (e.g. sending informational 'take home packs' to parents via girls once a week), and parent/child interactive strategies (e.g. parents and girls sharing popular dances of their respective generations). All of these strategies appeared to be feasible and effective for promoting physical activity and preventing unhealthy weight gain in this target group. A recent pilot study that compared two 12-week home and centre based physical activity programs for mothers and daughters in the US found both groups had significant improvements in health-related fitness (33). Given the cost-effectiveness of home-based strategies this is an encouraging finding.

Strategies to promote physical activity in the family setting appear to be effective for promoting physical activity, particularly among adolescent girls. As adolescent girls are one of the most "at risk" groups for declines in physical activity during childhood (34), this is an encouraging finding. Furthermore, evidence suggests that a dual focus on school and family settings results in the most effective outcomes.

Primary-care approaches

While the primary-care setting has increasingly been used to promote physical activity among adults (35, 36), fewer studies have targeted children or youth in this setting. However, there have been a small number of primary-care interventions published in the last few years. A quasiexperimental study, Patient-centered Assessment and

Counseling for Exercise plus Nutrition (PACE+), recruited 117 children and youth aged 11–18 years from four pediatric and adolescent outpatient clinics (37). Participants completed a computerized screening and goal setting survey in the clinic waiting room, and discussed their plan with their health care provider (nurse or physician). Participants were randomized to one of four groups: no contact; frequent mail; infrequent mail and telephone contact; or frequent mail and telephone contact. At the end of the 4-month trial, significant increases in moderate-intensity physical activity were identified. However, there were no differences in physical activity between participants who received just the initial computerized screening and counseling compared with those who had extended contact. In contrast, an adaptation of PACE+ on behavioral weight control among 44 overweight adolescents found that those who received the extended contact through mail and telephone displayed better weight control efficacy compared with the one-off screening and counseling group (38).

A recent primary-care setting intervention promoted physical activity on three occasions over a 12-month period to 448 Spanish adolescents (39). Significantly greater increases in the proportion of active adolescents, and higher frequency, intensity and duration of physical activity were reported among the intervention group compared with the controls. In a novel pilot intervention aimed at reducing television viewing among 7–12-year-old African-Americans, families were randomized to receive counseling (e.g. potential problems associated with excessive television viewing and accompanying brochures from the American Academy of Pediatrics), or counseling and behavioral modification (e.g. monitoring and budgeting television viewing, and an electronic television time manager) (40). Both groups reported reduced television viewing time, and the behavioral management group reported significantly higher participation in organized physical activity for the child and increases in time spent playing outside.

The available research suggests that general practitioners and other primary care physicians have an important role to play in the prevention, recognition, and treatment of childhood obesity. Although only a small number of studies have been published to date, the use of primary-care settings to promote physical activity and reduce sedentary behaviors among children and adolescents appears to be a promising approach.

Community-based approaches

There have been a small number of community-based approaches to promoting physical activity in children and adolescents in the last few years. "Active Winners" was a community-based quasi-experimental study promoting physical activity among 436 adolescents based in two rural communities in the US (41). The program targeted students' out-of-school-hours and summer vacation time over an 18-month period and used strategies including: an intensive summer and after-school physical activity program; newsletters for families; formation of committees to improve school environment; and community newspaper articles and physical activity at local events.

The study, however, was not found to be effective in increasing physical activity and was also reported to be extremely resource intensive for very low exposure to the program. Further, there were reported difficulties in recruiting and training staff and peer leaders. The investigators conclude that these results are consistent with other community-based physical activity interventions.

A community-based obesity intervention (GO GIRLS!) tested the feasibility of promoting physical activity and healthy eating among 57 low-income African-American adolescents recruited from public housing developments (42). In the absence of a control group, high vs. low attendees (<50 per cent of program completed) were compared. Whilst there were some significant differences in eating behaviors, there were no differences in physical activity. The investigators report few difficulties in recruiting adolescent girls to the study, however, as with Active Winners (41), attendance and adherence to the program was quite poor (average attendance 43 per cent of the sessions).

Another of the GEMS initiatives (described earlier) employed a combined community- and family-based approach in which 35 girls and their parents were assigned to a treatment or control group (43). This was a two-part intervention with 4 weeks of summer camp to promote physical activity and healthy eating, followed by an 8-week home-based internet intervention for girls and parents. After 12-weeks, there were no differences in objectively assessed physical activity between groups. Unlike the studies by Pate (41) and Resnicow (42), attendance at the summer day camp by the intervention group was high (>90 per cent); however, the internet component of the intervention was not well-attended (<50 per cent of the intervention group logged onto the Website).

The small number of recently published, community-based physical activity interventions reviewed here suggests that there are varied and complex challenges associated with approaches in this setting. Retention and adherence appear to be the most common difficulty in interventions in these settings.

Active transport approaches

Active transport to school has been shown to be a potentially important contributor to children's overall physical activity (44). In developed countries, there are currently many physical activity initiatives being undertaken to promote children's walking and cycling to school (e.g. Walking School Bus). Few, however, have been systematically evaluated. In a cluster randomized controlled trial of 41 primary schools in the UK, Rowland et al. (45) conducted a 1-year intervention that consisted of 16 hours of expert assistance from a school travel co-ordinator to develop and implement school travel plans. Although the intervention was successful in achieving an increased production of travel plans across the schools, there were no effects on children's travel patterns to school, nor on parent's safety concerns. In addition, the investigators reported that few schools were willing to participate. The school travel plan implementation required urban planning activity and it was apparent that for such an intervention to be effective, partnerships with planning departments are necessary.

The Safe Routes to School program in Marin County, California, US currently reaches 4665 students in 15 schools (46). Initiated by two local residents who wished to increase the proportion of children walking and cycling to school, the program includes: mapping safe routes to school; walk or cycle to school days (some schools do this weekly, others monthly); frequent rider miles, where children have "tally cards" and earn points for walking, cycling, catching public transport, or car pooling; a curriculum-based educational program on safety and transport choices; walking school buses and bicycle trains where children engage in active transport in groups; and newsletters and promotions. Between 2000 and 2002, there were significant increases in the proportion of children who were walking to or from school (64 per cent increase), cycling to or from school (114 per cent increase), and car pooling (91 per cent increase), and a corresponding decrease in the number of families driving their child to school unaccompanied by others (39 per cent decrease). The investigators concluded that parental involvement, community volunteers, and community support are essential elements to successful physical activity intervention in future studies.

In summary, few studies have examined the effectiveness of promoting children's active transport to school. These suggest that to have a substantial impact on children's walking and cycling to school it is important to involve parents and the broader community. Urban design issues should also be considered. For example it is important to consider where schools are placed within newly developed neighborhoods in terms of access to schools, safe routes (e.g. pedestrian crossings and sidewalks), travel plans (e.g. public transport routes), and mixed land use (e.g. a mix of shops, homes, and offices). Without involvement of these other sectors, it is unlikely that active transport initiatives will be as effective.

Review of physical activity intervention literature in young, mid-life, and older adults

Personal level approaches

During the past three decades we have witnessed an escalating amount of intervention research aimed at promoting physical activity in young, mid-life, and older adults (47, 48). The majority of this research has occurred on the intra- and interpersonal levels of influence. Drawing primarily from psychosocial and behavioral theoretical perspectives (19, 49–51), investigators from behavioral science, exercise science, and public health fields have targeted demographic, cognitive, and emotional factors, as well as behavioral attributes and skills, in developing programs aimed at inactive or irregularly active individuals (52). Undertaken in either individual or group-based formats, interventions focused on augmenting physical activity-related self-efficacy, self-regulatory skill building, and regular social support for an active lifestyle have been shown to increase physical activity levels for periods spanning 2 years (53–55). The strength of the cumulative literature in this area has led the US Task Force on Community Preventive Services to strongly recommend such individually adapted behavior change programs as well as social support-based interventions delivered in community settings (e.g. behavioral contracts, buddy systems, walking groups) as useful strategies for increasing physical activity behaviors in the population (48).

Although such personal-level interventions appear to be reasonably effective in promoting increased physical activity levels in the research settings in which they have been tested, less is known concerning methods for enhancing the reach and delivery of such interventions across broader segments of the adult population. One promising direction aimed at enhancing program reach involves the use of mediated communication channels for delivering the cognitive, behavioral, and social strategies that constitute the essential elements of such programs (56, 57). Effective physical activity interventions have been developed using individualized print media (56, 58), the telephone (59), and automated communication and information technologies (60–62). The development of physical activity interventions using the internet has also begun (63, 64). Although still in its infancy, systematic efforts to translate scientifically vetted interventions for use by community organizations and other entities have begun to emerge (65, 66).

While the types of personal-level interventions noted above clearly have a place in population-wide efforts to promote regular physical activity, they are constrained by the often reasonably large amounts of time and human resources required for their delivery on an ongoing basis. In addition, they are typically "choice-intensive", requiring individuals to take action and proactively plan for their implementation on a regular basis, which can over time prove to be difficult for many individuals to accomplish (8).

Social, cultural, and organizational level approaches

A substantial amount of research on the correlates of physical activity participation in adults has emphasized the importance of social, cultural, and organizational factors in influencing individuals to be physically active or not (52, 67). Among such potential influences are advice and influence from physicians, social support from family members, friends, coworkers, and peers, and cultural beliefs related to physical activity, health, and well-being (68–74). Yet, surprisingly few well-controlled studies have been conducted that focus specifically on changing the social or organizational aspects of community settings frequented by adults to increase their impact on physical activity behavior. For example while a majority of adults will spend a number of years in work settings, a large proportion of physical activity interventions undertaken at worksites focus primarily, or exclusively, on personal-level approaches (75). Combining personal-level approaches with broader social, organizational, and policy-level strategies could enhance both the initiation and longer-term maintenance of physical activity in both advantaged as well as under-served worksite populations (76–80). Exploring methods of facilitating active commuting to work is another means of harnessing the worksite for promotion of physical activity (81). In addition, several studies have shown the potential promise of culturally-sensitive strategies for promoting physical activity in ethnic minority communities (73, 82–84). Clearly, such efforts require more systematic attention if all segments of the irregularly active or inactive population are to be reached.

The primary care setting and similar health settings also merit continued systematic study, in light of the large proportion of mid-life and older adults who visit their health-care providers on a regular basis (35, 36). Systematic efforts to intervene in primary care settings have met, to date, with mixed results (85–88). These mixed results may stem, in part, from methodological differences among studies (e.g. types of primary care offices that were targeted; extent of patient screening and assessment that occurred as part of eligibility for the study; extent to which organizational or office-based strategies were combined with personal-level strategies). When the target of intervention is the older adult, recent reports have stressed the importance of using the health-care provider as a physical activity advocate who promotes physical activity, as opposed to the more traditional gatekeeper charged with extensively screening the older adult prior to beginning an exercise program (89). The latter role has been judged increasingly to be both unrealistic and often inappropriate for many older adults (89, 90).

While for older adults, retirement communities, assisted living facilities, and other senior residential settings offer potentially useful venues for enacting social and organizational interventions, few systematic research endeavors have occurred in such settings (91, 92). Although a growing number of such settings are being built with an eye towards enhancing choice and safety related to physical activity, through such physical amenities as on-site fitness and activity centers, organized fitness classes, wider streets, gently sloping and clearly marked curbs, streetlights, and carefully constructed intersections, it is currently unclear how such amenities may impact residents' physical activity levels. We do not know, for example, whether selection bias is at work in choosing to live in such settings (i.e. already active individuals seek out neighborhoods and settings which are conducive to their active lifestyles, while inactive individuals do not).

The physical environment and physical activity interventions

Of all of the levels of intervention available to public health researchers, the level of the physical environment may hold the greatest promise for influencing population-wide physical activity levels, yet it is the physical environment that, to date, has received the least amount of systematic attention in the physical activity field. This is rapidly changing, however, as new paradigms are being investigated that emphasize the importance of understanding individual behavior within the context of the larger environments in which people live (54, 93, 94). Such paradigms call for new partnerships with disciplines that historically have had little influence on physical activity research, including urban planning, architecture, transportation, and environmental design (94). As physical activity researchers strive for cross-fertilization with experts from these and related fields, new terms, ideas, and transdisciplinary perspectives are beginning to emerge (8, 95).

Currently the research materializing from such cross-disciplinary discussions and collaborations consists largely of cross-sectional and, to a somewhat lesser degree, prospective observational studies aimed at exploring which aspects of the physical environment may be particularly influential with respect to the physical activity levels of different population groups.

Among the features of the built environment that have received growing attention by physical activity researchers are the density and intensity of urban development, the mix of land uses (e.g. the distance from each house in a neighborhood to the nearest store), connectivity of the street network (i.e. the directness and availability of different routes from one point to another within a street network), the scale of streets in a locale (e.g. how far back buildings are set from streets; street widths), and the aesthetic qualities of a locale or neighborhood (e.g. landscaping, lighting, public benches) (94). Travel behavior has also received increasing attention recently from physical activity researchers, given the potential utility of walking and bicycling as forms of transport, although the primary focus of the transportation literature has been on automobile travel (96). Research suggests, for instance, that people located within older and "walkable" communities (i.e. communities with greater density, a greater mix of land uses, greater street connectivity, and positive aesthetic qualities) make more walking trips than their suburban counterparts (97). Similarly, living in environments that offer convenient access to recreational opportunities has been found to decrease the likelihood of inactive lifestyles (98). In contrast, living in impoverished neighborhoods has been associated with a significant decline in physical activity levels over time, even after adjustment for other behavioral and demographic factors (99).

In addition to its focus on the automobile, much of the transportation and urban planning literature has focused on individuals under the age of 65. It is quite possible, however, that aspects of the physical environment could have a particular impact on the physical activity levels of older adults, who may be especially vulnerable due to physical, economic, and/or social limitations. For example one cross-sectional study found that older adults in Portland, Oregon who lived in more socially cohesive neighborhoods reported higher levels of neighborhood walking than low socially cohesive neighborhood residents (100). Additional neighborhood factors of more recreation facilities, higher senior resident density, and higher proportion of low-income households were also related to higher neighborhood walking (100). Neighborhood safety was not related to neighborhood walking among this elderly sample. Collectively, neighborhood variables accounted for 84 per cent of between-neighborhood variance, underscoring the potential explanatory capability of such environmental variables with respect to older adults' physical activity patterns (100). A second cross-sectional study, involving a randomly selected sample of Australian adults aged 60 years and older, found that in addition to high levels of self-efficacy and regular support and encouragement from friends and family to be active, perceived safety of sidewalks and access to recreational facilities were significantly associated with being active (101).

Similar to the Portland study described above, perceived neighborhood safety was not differentially related to physical activity levels. These studies underscore the potential importance of physical environmental factors on the physical activity levels of older adults.

Although urban planning and related macroenvironmental perspectives hold promise as a means of increasing regular physical activity and decreasing sedentariness among the population at large, it is becoming apparent that such influences must be understood within the context of the individual–environment interface. For example a recent study by Giles-Corti and colleagues evaluating the relative impacts of personal, social, and physical environmental influences on physical activity in a Western Australia community found that the physical environment's direct influence on exercising regularly was perceived to be secondary to individual and social environmental factors (102). The community survey responses suggested that supportive physical environments may be insufficient to increase physical activity in and of themselves, but may require complementary personal and social influences to have a significant impact on people's physical activity levels. Thus, it is critically important that personal, social/ cultural, and environmental factors be studied in concert with one another, to allow for a fuller picture of influences to emerge (103). A potential example of such a person–environmental interface is represented by the promising studies that have used simple "point-of-decision" signage at public choice points involving taking the escalator or the stairs to encourage stair use (104–106). It would be useful to explore how current information technologies could be used to tailor the "point-of-decision" messages to increase stair use among target groups at particular risk for inactivity.

In summary, the recent attention being paid to physical environmental factors in conjunction with personal, social, and cultural factors is a positive step towards the development of innovative new models for understanding and promoting long-term increases in physical activity among youth and adult populations alike.

Emerging issues and directions in the physical activity field

The need to apply the full social ecological model in physical activity interventions

Historically, theories that involve multiple levels of influence (e.g. Social Cognitive Theory, Social Ecological Models) have been applied in a partial or incomplete manner in this field. To significantly advance the field, it is important to apply the full models in development of intervention strategies and approaches. In Chapter 6, French has argued that full implementation of the social ecological model in an intervention would be extremely challenging if not impossible. Furthermore, a recent commentary by Duncan and colleagues argues that appropriate multilevel statistical techniques must be employed in social ecological approaches (107). Certainly, application of the full social ecological model may require new collaborations with experts from different fields (e.g. environmental or urban planning), as well as the continued development of terms and concepts reflecting the more complex relationships and approaches that such collaborations will undoubtedly engender. Only by doing so will we be able to fully understand not just which interventions work, but for whom and within which environmental, social, and cultural contexts.

A better understanding of the mediating and moderating influences on behavior change

In addition to applying the full social ecological model when promoting physical activity, there is a need to better understand the mediating and moderating influences on behavior change. In describing intervention outcomes, very few studies have reported the mechanisms of, or barriers to, change. A better understanding of the social and ecological predictors of physical activity throughout the lifespan will aid in the identification of potential mediators and moderators, which in turn should guide the development of more effective interventions.

Continue efforts aimed at the combined study of physical activity and dietary behaviors

We have inherited a long history of compartmentalizing behavioral risk factors for chronic disease into separate fields for study, training, and program development purposes. Yet, it is currently clear that significant advances in the development of effective approaches for tackling the major public health challenges of our time, among them obesity, Type 2 diabetes, and disablement as we age, will only occur through the study of multiple health behaviors in concert with one another. Chief among such health behaviors are physical activity and dietary patterns. While the physiological synergy between these two important health behaviors has been extensively studied, we remain ignorant of the possible areas of behavioral synergy that may be potentially harnessed in interventions aimed at changing both. The recent emergence of scientific journals and professional organizations focused on combining these two health behaviors is a positive step that should be extended to the formal training of health professionals in both the dietary and physical activity fields. By thoroughly familiarizing health professionals with both health behaviors, we will increase our chances of arriving at the major breakthroughs so desperately needed in areas such as energy balance and other chronic conditions and states.

A focus on reducing sedentary behaviors

Evidence continues to emerge that supports the notion of independent health effects from participation in sedentary behaviors (108–110). New evidence suggests that not only is TV viewing positively associated with an increased likelihood of overweight or obesity among mid-life and older adults, there are also associations with impaired glucose tolerance and type 2 diabetes (108). Very few interventions, however, have been developed to reduce sedentary behaviors among adults. This is an area of tremendous potential that needs to be further explored. Strategies to reduce sedentary behaviors in children have been shown to be effective in preventing unhealthy weight gain. However, a challenge for these interventions among children and youth is that although they are primarily delivered via the school setting (some have been delivered via the primary care setting), the targeted behavior change (typically to reduce TV viewing) occurs mainly within the home. The challenge for interventions to reduce sedentary behaviors will be to not just focus on individual-level behavior change strategies, but to also focus on the social, family, and environmental influences that might mediate or moderate the effects of the intervention outside school hours.

Strive to understand how life-course issues may be harnessed to promote healthful physical activity (and dietary) behaviors

Research in the physical activity field has uncovered specific developmental "milestones" or junctures during the life course when there may be natural tendencies for physical activity levels to either increase or decrease. Such potentially important life-course junctures or transitions include puberty, entering the work force, marriage, child-rearing, retirement, and informal family caregiving for loved ones with infirmities (111–117). It is important to broaden our understanding of how such transitions may differentially affect men and women, and to develop targeted interventions to take advantage of natural changes in physical activity and other health behaviors occurring during those time periods.

The challenge of promoting physical activity in populations where overweight and obesity are already widespread

Although physical activity was the primary outcome of interest in this chapter, some of the interventions reviewed targeted healthy weight maintenance as an outcome. Few studies, however, systematically evaluated the feasibility or effectiveness of approaches to promote physical activity among overweight vs. non-overweight groups. Epidemiological evidence underscores the fact that overweight and obese adults tend to be less active as a group than their leaner peers (57), and also tend to have poorer physical activity success rates in formal programs in which they do enroll (115). These results serve to emphasize the importance of targeting youth who are currently overweight or at risk for overweight as adults, given that research suggests that overweight children are likely to naturally increase their physical activity levels if the right environmental contingencies are in place (14, 29).

There are also challenges, however, in delivering physical activity programs that are appropriate for overweight or obese children, with research showing an inverse relationship between body fatness and fundamental motor skills among boys (118), and overweight children reporting more negative perceptions associated with endurance types of physical activity compared with their non-overweight peers (119). Further, a study of more than 500 fifth through to eighth grade children in the US found that perceived weight criticism during physical activity was associated with reduced enjoyment of physical activity (120). These results serve to highlight the importance of continuing to explore methods of systematically tailoring physical activity programs to meet the particular needs and preferences of overweight children and adults. Programs should incorporate physical activities in which overweight or obese individuals can comfortably participate. Issues such as self-consciousness about being physically active in public places and in social situations also need to be considered.

The relative importance of personal, social, and environmental factors on physical activity is likely to vary between overweight and non-overweight individuals. With a substantial proportion of children, adolescents, and adults already overweight it is important to consider such differences in the development and delivery of physical activity programs.

Conclusions

This selective review indicates that a number of promising intervention approaches aimed at increasing physical activity have been developed for children, adolescents, young, mid-life, and older adults (Table 7.1). Personal level approaches among children (e.g. curriculum-based educational strategies) and among adults (e.g. individually-tailored behavioral modification strategies) have been shown to be effective for increasing physical activity. Approaches that involve multiple settings and multilevel strategies (i.e. application of the social ecological framework) appear to have the greatest effect on physical activity behavior change. Among youth, there are promising approaches in primary care settings for the prevention of unhealthy weight gain through reductions in sedentary behavior. Evidence of the effectiveness of promoting physical activity among adults in worksites is equivocal; however, most worksite interventions have employed personal-level strategies to increase physical activity. Active transport interventions among children show promise, and a greater focus on active transport to and from work is a further potential strategy that could increase opportunities for physical activity among working populations.

In summary, this review suggests that there remains tremendous potential to develop innovative programs to increase physical activity and reduce sedentary behavior. This is particularly the case with respect to environmental and systems level interventions, which may have the greatest potential for reaching the increasingly large segment of the population who are under-active and therefore at risk for overweight/ obesity.

Table 7.1 Summary table of the strength of current evidence from the physical activity intervention literature

Age group	Intervention type	Strength of current evidence
Childhood, adolescence	School settings:	
	curriculum only	+
	environmental only	0
	multiple strategies	+
	(e.g. curriculum and environmental)	
	Family settings	+
	School and family settings	++
	Primary care settings	+
	Community settings	0
	Active transport	+
Young adulthood	Personal level approaches	++
	Worksites	?
	Primary care settings	0
	Physical environment	0
	Person–environment interface	++
	(e.g. point-of-decision signage to use the stairs)	
Mid-aged adults	Personal level approaches	++
	Worksites	?
	Primary care settings	?
	Culturally tailored	+
	Physical environment	0
	Person–environment interface	++
	(e.g. point-of-decision signage to use the stairs)	
Older adults	Personal level approaches	++
	Primary care settings	?
	Culturally tailored	+
	Physical environment	0
	Person–environment interface	0
	(e.g. point-of-decision signage to use the stairs)	

? mixed evidence; + some evidence; ++ consistent evidence; 0 no evidence

References

1. **Hockett CF, Ascher R** (1992). The human revolution. *Curr Anthrop* **33** Supp, 7–45.
2. **ACNielsen MI** (2001). *Australian TV trends 2001.* AC Nielsen Co., Sydney.
3. **Wise S** (2003). *Family structure, child outcomes and environmental mediators. An overview of the development in diverse families study.* Australian Institute of Family Studies, Melbourne.
4. Federal Interagency Forum on Child and Family Statistics. *America's children: key national indicators of well-being.* Available from http://childstats.gov/americaschildren/index.asp. Accessed on 27 July 2004.

5. US Census Bureau (1996). *Marital history for people 15 years old and over by age, sex, race and ethnicity: Fall 1996.* Available from http://www.census.gov/population/socdemo/marital-hist/p70–80/tab01.pdf. Accessed on 28 October 2004.

6. **Gray M, Qu L, de Vaus D, Millward C** (2002). *Determinants of Australian mothers' employment. An analysis of lone and couple mothers.* Australia Institute of Family Studies – Commonwealth of Australia.

7. National Center for Health Statistics (NCHS). *Monitoring the Nation's Health.* Available from http://209.217.72.34/aging/eng/TableViewer/wdsview/dispviewp.asp Accessed on 27 July 2004.

8. **King AC, Stokols D, Talen E, Brassington GS, Killingsworth R** (2002). Theoretical approaches to the promotion of physical activity: forging a transdisciplinary paradigm. *Am J Prev Med* **23**, 15–25.

9. **Stokols D** (1996). Translating social ecological theory into guidelines for community health promotion. *Am J Health Promot* **10**, 282–98.

10. **Sallis JF, Owen N** (2002). Ecological models of health behaviour. In: Glanz K, Lewis FM, Rimer BK, eds. *Health behaviour and health education. Theory, research and practice*, 3rd edn, pp. 462–84. Jossey-Bass, San Francisco.

11. **Davison KK, Birch LL** (2001). Childhood overweight: a contextual model and recommendations for future research. *Obes Rev* **2**, 159–71.

12. **Robinson T** (1999). Reducing children's television viewing to prevent obesity: A randomized controlled trial. *JAMA* **282**, 1561–6.

13. **Gortmaker SL, Peterson K, Wiecha J, et al.** (1999). Reducing obesity via a school-based interdisciplinary intervention among youth: Planet Health. *Arch Pediatr Adolesc Med* **153**, 409–18.

14. **Epstein LH, Valoski AM, Vara LS, et al.** (1995). Effects of decreasing sedentary behavior and increasing activity on weight change in obese children. *Health Psychol* **14**, 109–15.

15. **Stone EJ, McKenzie TL, Welk GJ, Booth ML** (1998). Effects of physical activity interventions in youth. Review and synthesis. *Am J Prev Med* **15**, 298–315.

16. **Harrell JS, McMurray RG, Gansky SA, Bangdiwala SI, Bradley CB** (1999). A public health vs a risk-based intervention to improve cardiovascular health in elementary school children: the cardiovascular health in children study. *Am J Pub Health* **89**, 1529–35.

17. **Neumark-Sztainer D, Story M, Hannan PJ, Rex J** (2003). New Moves: a school-based obesity prevention program for adolescent girls. *Prev Med* **37**, 41–51.

18. **Dishman RK, Motl RW, Saunders R, et al.** (2004). Self-efficacy partially mediates the effect of a school-based physical-activity intervention among adolescent girls. *Prev Med* **38**, 628–36.

19. **Bandura A** (1986). *Social foundations of thought and action: A social cognitive theory.* Prentice Hall, Englewood Cliffs, NJ.

20. **Rachlin H** (1989). *Judgement, decision, and choice: a cognitive/ behavioral synthesis.* WH Freeman, New York.

21. **Salmon J, Ball K, Crawford D, et al.** (2005). Reducing sedentary behaviour and increasing physical activity among 10-year old children: Overview and process evaluation of the "Switch-Play" intervention. *Health Promot Int* **20(1)**, 7–17.

22. **Stratton G** (2000). Promoting children's physical activity in primary school: an intervention study using playground markings. *Ergonomics* **43**, 1538–46.

23. **Stratton G, Leonard J** (2002). The effects of playground markings on the energy expenditure of 5–7-year-old school children. *Pediatr Exerc Sci* **14**, 170–80.

24. **Sallis JF, McKenzie TL, Conway TL, et al.** (2003). Environmental interventions for eating and physical activity: a randomized controlled trial in middle schools. *Am J Prev Med* **24**, 209–17.

25. Sahota P, Rudolf MCJ, Dixey R, Hill AJ, Barth JH, Cade J (2001). Randomised controlled trial of primary school based intervention to reduce risk factors for obesity. *BMJ* **323**, 1–5.

26. Sahota P, Rudolf MCJ, Dixey R, Hill AJ, Barth JH, Cade J (2001). Evaluation of implementation and effort of primary school based intervention to reduce risk factors for obesity. *BMJ* **323**, 1–4.

27. Manios Y, Moschandreas J, Hatzis C, Kafatos A (1999). Evaluation of a health and nutrition education program in primary school children of Crete over a three-year period. *Prev Med* **28**, 149–59.

28. Manios Y, Moschandreas J, Hatzis C, Kafatos A (2002). Health and nutrition education in primary schools of Crete: changes in chronic disease risk factors following a 6-year intervention programme. *Br J Nutr* **88**, 315–24.

29. Epstein LH, Paluch RA, Gordy CC, Dorn J (2000). Decreasing sedentary behaviors in treating pediatric obesity. *Arch Pediatr Adolesc Med* **154**, 220–6.

30. Story M, Sherwood NE, Himes JH, *et al.* (2003). *An after-school obesity prevention program for African-American girls: the Minnesota GEMS pilot study.* Ethn Dis **13**, S54–64.

31. Beech BM, Klesges RC, Kumanyika SK, *et al.* (2003). Child- and parent-targeted interventions: the Memphis GEMS pilot study. *Ethn Dis* **13**, S40–53.

32. Robinson TN, Killen JD, Kraemer HC, *et al.* (2003). Dance and reducing television viewing to prevent weight gain in African-American girls: the Stanford GEMS pilot study. *Ethn Dis* **13**, S65–77.

33. Ransdell LB, Taylor A, Oakland D, Schmidt J, Moyer-Mileur L, Shultz B (2003). Daughters and mothers exercising together: effects of home- and community-based programs. *Med Sci Sports Exerc* **35**, 286–96.

34. Kimm SY, Glynn NW, Kriska AM, *et al.* (2002). Decline in physical activity in black girls and white girls during adolescence. *N Engl J Med* **347**, 709–15.

35. Simons-Morton DG, Calfas KJ, Oldenburg B, Burton NW (1998). Effects of interventions in health care settings on physical activity or cardiorespiratory fitness. *Am J Prev Med* **15**, 413–30.

36. Eaton CB, Menard LM (1998). A systematic review of physical activity promotion in primary care office settings. *Br J Sports Med* **32**, 11–6.

37. Patrick K, Sallis JF, Prochaska JJ, *et al.* (2001). A multicomponent program for nutrition and physical activity change in primary care: PACE+ for adolescents. *Arch Pediatr Adolesc Med* **155**, 940–6.

38. Saelens BE, Sallis JF, Wilfley DE, Patrick K, Cella JA, Buchta R (2002). Behavioral weight control for overweight adolescents initiated in primary care. *Obes Res* **10**, 22–32.

39. Ortega-Sanchez R, Jimenez-Mena C, Cordoba-Garcia R, Munoz-Lopez J, Garcia-Machado ML, Vilaseca-Canals J (2004). The effect of office-based physician's advice on adolescent exercise behavior. *Prev Med* **38**, 219–26.

40. Ford BS, McDonald TE, Owens AS, Robinson TN (2002). Primary care interventions to reduce television viewing in African-American children. *Am J Prev Med* **22**, 106–9.

41. Pate RR, Saunders RP, Ward DS, Felton G, Trost SG, Dowda M (2003). Evaluation of a community-based intervention to promote physical activity in youth: lessons from Active Winners. *Am J Health Promot* **17**, 171–82.

42. Resnicow K, Yaroch AL, Davis A, *et al.* (2000). GO GIRLS!: results from a nutrition and physical activity program for low-income, overweight African American adolescent females. *Health Educ Behav* **27**, 616–31.

43. Baranowski T, Baranowski JC, Cullen KW, *et al.* (2003). The Fun, Food, and Fitness Project (FFFP): the Baylor GEMS pilot study. *Ethn Dis* **13**, S30–9.

44. Cooper AR, Page AS, Foster LJ, Qahwaji D (2003). Commuting to school: are children who walk more physically active? *Am J Prev Med* **25**, 273–6.

45. Rowland D, DiGuiseppi C, Gross M, Afolabi E, Roberts I (2003). Randomised controlled trial of site specific advice on school travel patterns. *Arch Dis Child* **88**, 8–11.

46. Staunton CE, Hubsmith D, Kallins W (2003). Promoting safe walking and biking to school: the Marin County success story. *Am J Public Health* **93**, 1431–4.

47. U.S. Department of Health and Human Services (1996). *Physical activity and health: a report of the Surgeon General.* U.S. Department of Health and Human Services, Centers for Disease Control and Prevention, National Center for Chronic Disease Prevention and Health Promotion, Atlanta, GA.

48. U.S. Department of Health and Human Services (2001). *Increasing physical activity: a report on recommendations of the task force on community preventive services.* Centers for Disease Control and Prevention (CDC).

49. Ajzen I (1991). The theory of planned behavior. *Organizational Behavior And Human Decision Processes* **50**, 179–211.

50. Prochaska JO, DiClemente CC (1984). *The transtheoretical approach: Crossing traditional boundaries of change.* Dorsey Press, Homewood, IL.

51. Biddle SJH, Nigg CR (2000). Theories of exercise behavior. *Int J Sport Psychol* **31**, 290–304.

52. Bauman AE, Sallis JF, Dzewaltowski DA, Owen N (2002). Toward a better understanding of the influences on physical activity: the role of determinants, correlates, causal variables, mediators, moderators, and confounders. *Am J Prev Med* **23**, 5–14.

53. Dunn AL, Marcus BH, Kampert JB, Garcia ME, Kohl HW, Blair SN (1999). Comparison of lifestyle and structured interventions to increase physical activity and cardiorespiratory fitness: a randomized trial. *JAMA* **281**, 327–34.

54. King AC, Jeffery RW, Fridinger F, *et al.* (1995). Environmental and policy approaches to cardio-vascular disease prevention through physical activity: issues and opportunities. *Health Educ Q* **22**, 499–511.

55. Kriska AM, Bayles C, Cauley JA, LaPorte RE, Sandler RB, Pambianco G (1986). A randomized exercise trial in older women: increased activity over two years and the factors associated with compliance. *Med Sci Sports Exerc* **18**, 557–62.

56. Marcus BH, Bock BC, Pinto BM, Forsyth LH, Roberts MB, Traficante RM (1998). Efficacy of an individualized, motivationally-tailored physical activity intervention. *Ann Behav Med* **20**, 174–80.

57. Marcus BH, Nigg CR, Riebe D, Forsyth LH (2000). Interactive communication strategies: implications for population-based physical-activity promotion. *Am J Prev Med* **19**, 121–6.

58. Napolitano MA, Marcus BH (2002). Targeting and tailoring physical activity information using print and information technologies. *Exerc Sport Sci Rev* **30**, 122–8.

59. Castro CM, King AC (2002). Telephone-assisted counseling for physical activity. *Exerc Sport Sci Rev* **30**, 64–8.

60. Jarvis KL, Friedman RH, Heeren T, Cullinane PM (1997). Older women and physical activity: using the telephone to walk. *Womens Health Issues* **7**, 24–9.

61. Pinto BM, Friedman RH, Marcus B, Ling T, Tennstedt S, Gillman M (2000). Physical activity promotion using a computer-based telephone counseling system. *Ann Behav Med* **22**, S212.

62. King AC, Friedman R, Marcus BH, Napolitano MA, Castro C, Forsyth L (2004). Increasing regular physical activity via humans or automated technology: 12-month results of the CHAT trial. *Ann Behav Med* **26**, suppl. S044.

63. Napolitano MA, Fotheringham M, Tate D, *et al.* (2003). Evaluation of an internet-based physical activity intervention: a preliminary investigation. *Ann Behav Med* **25**, 92–9.

64. Marshall AL, Leslie ER, Bauman AE, Marcus BH, Owen N (2003). Print versus website physical activity programs: a randomized trial. *Am J Prev Med* **25**, 88–94.

65. Hooker SP, Shoemaker W, Seavey W, Weidner C (2000). California Active Aging Project: Putting science into practice to promote physical activity for older adults. *Gerontologist* **40**, 260.

66. Hooker SP (2002). California Active Aging Project. *J Aging Physical Activity* **10**, 354–9.

67. Brawley LR, Rejeski WJ, King AC (2003). Promoting physical activity for older adults: the challenges for changing behavior. *Am J Prev Med* **25**, 172–83.

68. Damush TM, Stewart AL, Mills KM, King AC, Ritter PL (1999). Prevalence and correlates of physician recommendations to exercise among older adults. *J Gerontol A Biol Sci Med Sci* **54**, M423–7.

69. Hovell M, Sallis J, Hofstetter R, *et al.* (1991). Identification of correlates of physical activity among Latino adults. *J Community Health* **16**, 23–36.

70. Clark DO (1999). Physical activity and its correlates among urban primary care patients aged 55 years or older. *J Gerontol B Psychol Sci Soc Sci* **54**, S41–8.

71. Oka RK, King AC, Young DR (1995). Sources of social support as predictors of exercise adherence in women and men ages 50 to 65 years. *Womens Health* **1**, 161–75.

72. Yancey AK, Miles O, Jordan AD (1999). Organizational characteristics facilitating initiation and institutionalization of physical activity programs in a multiethnic urban community. *J Health Educ* **30**, S44–S51.

73. Pargee D, Lara-Albers E, Puckett K (1999). Building on tradition: Promoting physical activity with American Indian community coalitions. *J Health Educ* **30**, S37–S43.

74. Eyler AA, Matson-Koffman D, Vest JR, *et al.* (2002). Environmental, policy, and cultural factors related to physical activity in a diverse sample of women: The Women's Cardiovascular Health Network Project-summary and discussion. *Women Health* **36**, 123–34.

75. Dishman RK, Oldenburg B, O'Neal H, Shephard RJ (1998). Worksite physical activity interventions. *Am J Prev Med* **15**, 344–61.

76. Blair SN, Piserchia PV, Wilbur CS, Crowder JH (1986). A public health intervention model for work-site health promotion. Impact on exercise and physical fitness in a health promotion plan after 24 months. *JAMA* **255**, 921–6.

77. King AC, Carl F, Birkel L, Haskell WL (1988). Increasing exercise among blue-collar employees: the tailoring of worksite programs to meet specific needs. *Prev Med* **17**, 357–65.

78. Knadler GF, Rogers T (1987). Mountain climb month program: a low-cost exercise intervention program at a high-rise worksite. *Fitness in Business*, October, 64–7.

79. Hammond SL, Lomg DM, Fowler K, Ryan C, Volansky M (1997). *Centers for Disease Control and Prevention 1996 Director's Physical Activity Challenge Evaluation Report*. Centers for Disease Control and Prevention, Atlanta.

80. Campbell MK, Tessaro I, DeVellis B, *et al.* (2002). Effects of a tailored health promotion program for female blue-collar workers: health works for women. *Prev Med* **34**, 313–23.

81. Oja P, Vuori I, Paronen O (1998). Walking and cycling to work: their utility as health-enhancing physical activity. *Patient Educ Couns* **33**, S87–S94.

82. Grassi K, Gonzales MG, Tello P, He G (1999). La Vida Caminando: a community-based physical activity program designed by and for rural Latino families. *J Health Educ* **30**, S13–S17.

83. Foo MA, Robinson J, Rhodes M (1999). Identifying policy opportunities to increase physical activity in the Southeast Asian community in Long Beach, California. *J Health Educ* **30**, S58–S63.

84. Taylor WC, Baranowski T, Young DR (1998). Physical activity interventions in low-income, ethnic minority, and populations with disability. *Am J Prev Med* **15**, 334–43.

85. Bull FC, Jamrozik K, Blanksby BA (1999). Tailored advice on exercise-does it make a difference? *Am J Prev Med* **16**, 230–9.

86. Goldstein MG, Pinto BM, Marcus BH (1999). Physician-based physical activity counseling for middle-aged and older adults: a randomized trial. *Ann Behav Med* **326**, 793–8.

87. Writing Group for Activity Counseling Trial Research Group (2001). Effects of physical activity counseling in primary care: the Activity Counseling Trial: A randomized controlled trial. *JAMA* **286**, 677–87.

88. Elley CR, Kerse N, Arroll B, Robinson E (2003). Effectiveness of counselling patients on physical activity in general practice: cluster randomised controlled trial. *BMJ* **326**, 793.

89. Morey MC, Sullivan RJ, Jr. (2003). Medical assessment for health advocacy and practical strategies for exercise initiation. *Am J Prev Med* **25**, 204–8.

90. Gill TM, DiPietro L, Krumholz HM (2000). Exercise stress testing for older persons starting an exercise program. *JAMA* **284**, 2591.

91. King AC, Kiernan M, Ahn DK, Wilcox S (1998). The effects of marital transitions on changes in physical activity: results from a 10-year community study. *Ann Behav Med* **20**, 64–9.

92. Mihalko SL, Wickley KL (2003). Active living for assisted living: promoting partnerships within a systems framework. *Am J Prev Med* **25**, 193–203.

93. Sallis JF, Owen N (1997). Ecological models. In: Glanz K, Lewis FM, Rimer BK, eds. *Health behavior and health education: theory, research, and practice*, pp. 403–24. Jossey-Bass, San Francisco.

94. Handy SL, Boarnet MG, Ewing R, Killingsworth RE (2002). How the built environment affects physical activity: views from urban planning. *Am J Prev Med* **23**, 64–73.

95. Frank LD, Engelke PO, Schmid TL (2003). *Health and community design: The impact of the built environment on physical activity.* Island, Washington DC.

96. Frank LD, Stone B, Bachman W (2000). Linking land use with household vehicle emissions in the Central Puget Sound: Methodological framework and findings. *Transp Res* **5**, 173–96.

97. Frank LD, Pivo G (1994). Impacts of mixed use and density on utilization of three modes of travel: single-occupant, transit, and walking. *Transp Res Record* **1466**, 44–52.

98. Centers for Disease Control and Prevention (1998). Self-reported physical inactivity by degree of urbanization – United States, 1996. *MMWR* **47**, 1097–100.

99. Yen IH, Kaplam GA (1998). Poverty area residence and changes in physical activity level: evidence from the Alameda County study. *Am J Public Health* **88**, 1709–12.

100. Fisher KJ, Li F, Michael Y (in press). The influence of social cohesion on neighborhood walking: an exploratory study using a multilevel analysis. *J Am Planning Association.*

101. Booth ML, Owen N, Bauman A, Clavisi O, Leslie E (2000). Social-cognitive and perceived environment influences associated with physical activity in older Australians. *Prev Med* **31**, 15–22.

102. Giles-Corti B, Donovan RJ (2002). The relative influence of individual, social and physical environment determinants of physical activity. *Soc Sci Med* **54**, 1793–812.

103. Satariano WA, McAuley E (2003). Promoting physical activity among older adults: from ecology to the individual. *Am J Prev Med* **25**, 184–92.

104. Brownell KD, Stunkard AJ, Albaum JM (1980). Evaluation and modification of exercise patterns in the natural environment. *Am J Psychiatry* **137**, 1540–5.

105. Blamey A, Mutrie N, Aitchison T (1995). Health promotion by encouraged use of stairs. *BMJ* **311**, 289–90.

106. Andersen RE, Franckowiak SC, Snyder J, Bartlett SJ, Fontaine KR (1998). Can inexpensive signs encourage the use of stairs? Results from a community intervention. *Ann Intern Med* **129**, 363–9.

107. **Duncan SC, Duncan TE, Strycker LA, Chaumeton NR** (2004). A multilevel approach to youth physical activity research. *Exerc Sport Sci Rev* **32**, 95–9.

108. **Dunstan D, Salmon J, Owen N, et al.** (2004). Independent association of television time and physical activity with 'undiagnosed' abnormal glucose metabolism. *Diabetes Care* **27**, 2603–9.

109. **Salmon J, Bauman A, Crawford D, Timperio A, Owen N** (2000). The association between television viewing and overweight among Australian adults participating in varying levels of leisure-time physical activity. *Int J Obes Relat Metab Disord* **24**, 600–6.

110. **Cameron AJ, Welborn TA, Zimmet PZ, et al.** (2003). Overweight and obesity in Australia: the 1999–2000 Australian Diabetes, Obesity and Lifestyle Study (AusDiab). *Med J Aust* **178**, 427–32.

111. **Brown WJ, Trost SG** (2003). Life transitions and changing physical activity patterns in young women. *Am J Prev Med* **25**, 140–3.

112. **Calfas KJ, Sallis JF, Nichols JF, et al.** (2000). Project GRAD: two-year outcomes of a randomized controlled physical activity intervention among young adults. Graduate Ready for Activity Daily. *Am J Prev Med* **18**, 28–37.

113. **King AC** (1991). Community intervention for promotion of physical activity and fitness. *Exerc Sport Sci Rev* **19**, 211–59.

114. **King AC, Brassington G** (1997). Enhancing physical and psychological functioning in older family caregivers: the role of regular physical activity. *Ann Behav Med* **19**, 91–100.

115. **King AC, Rejeski WJ, Buchner DM** (1998). Physical activity interventions targeting older adults. A critical review and recommendations. *Am J Prev Med* **15**, 316–33.

116. **Umberson D** (1987). Family status and health behaviors: social control as a dimension of social integration. *J Health Soc Behav* **28**, 306–19.

117. **Williamson DF, Kahn HS, Remington PL, Anda RF** (1990). The 10-year incidence of overweight and major weight gain in US adults. *Arch Intern Med* **150**, 665–72.

118. **Raudsepp L, Jurimae T** (1996). Relationship between somatic variables, physical activity, fitness and fundamental motor skills in prepubertal boys. *Biol Sport* **13**, 279–89.

119. **Worsley A, Coonan W, Leitch D, Crawford D** (1984). Slim and obese children's perceptions of physical activities. *Int J Obes* **8**, 201–11.

120. **Faith MS, Leone MA, Ayers TS, Heo M, Pietrobelli A** (2002). Weight criticism during physical activity, coping skills, and reported physical activity in children. *Pediatrics* **110**, e23.

Chapter 8

Population approaches to obesity prevention

Robert W. Jeffery and Jennifer A. Linde

Introduction

The body of intervention research directed towards the modification of eating and physical activity behaviors in the population is quite substantial. However, considerably less research has specifically focused on population obesity prevention. The purpose of this chapter is to present a conceptualization of the causes of population obesity, to discuss the implications of this conceptualization for public health interventions, and to review empirical work that has attempted to address obesity treatment and/or prevention in entire populations.

Definition of obesity

Obesity is defined as an unhealthy amount of body fat. Following conventions in clinical practice, it is usually discussed as if it is a discrete entity that is clearly distinct from non-obesity. In point of fact, however, body fatness, like most biological variables, is continuously distributed in the population as a whole. Thus, defining obesity as a distinct entity involves dichotomizing a continuously distributed variable and, regardless of the science behind the choice of cut-off point, it is fundamentally arbitrary, at least in the implicit assumption that individuals on one side of the obesity cut-off point are fundamentally different from those on the other side. The definition of obesity has changed over time, partly because the quantity and quality of empirical data relating to the health risk of obesity have grown and partly because the judgment of scientists and practitioners as to what constitutes an acceptable amount of health risk has changed. The most widely accepted obesity yardstick for both research and clinical purposes worldwide is now body mass index (BMI; body weight (kg)/ height (m)^2). For statistical and epidemiological purposes BMI is an excellent measure. Average population BMI is strongly related to the proportion of a population that will fall above any selected obesity cut-off point (obesity prevalence). Nevertheless, the precision of BMI in identifying individual per cent body fat or individual risk related to fatness is not nearly so precise.

In this chapter we will focus on population rather than individual obesity. We may sometimes talk about obesity prevalence and sometimes about the mean BMI in populations. As noted above, we are comfortable in doing so because the two are highly related. BMI cut-off points for defining obesity are traditionally based on the association of BMI with death rates. In considering the definition of obesity, it is well to keep in mind that the choice of health endpoints used in crafting the definition is important. If one used diabetes rates rather than total death rates to define obesity, the definition cut-off point would probably be lower and apparent population obesity rates higher because diabetes is the health condition most strongly related to body weight. If cancer risk were the defining criteria for obesity, on the other hand, obesity rates would probably be lower since cancer is more weakly related to BMI.

The BMI associated with lowest death rates is not entirely consistent across populations but tends to be in the range of 20 to 23 (1). Death or mortality rates rise slowly with increasing BMI above this point until a BMI of about 30 to 35. Beyond this point mortality rates rise more rapidly. The current WHO classification of obesity based on BMI considers a BMI of 25 as the cut-off point for "overweight" and a BMI of 30 as the cut-off point for clinical obesity (2).

Development of obesity

In populations as a whole, mean BMI and obesity prevalence typically increase slowly from childhood through middle age and then decline late in life (see Chapter 1 for a more detailed review). For the most part, obesity increases with age at a fairly constant rate, although there are sizeable differences between populations. Researchers have had some success in identifying biological and psychosocial transitions that are associated with differential risks of weight gain. These include biological transitions such as the period of intrauterine development prior to birth, the adiposity rebound period in early childhood, puberty, childbirth, and menopause (3). They also include stressful life events such as moving away from home, marriage, divorce, and psychological distress (4). Overall, however, from a population perspective, age itself is the most powerful risk factor. Within populations, there are also both biological and psychosocial risk factors for individual obesity risk. Without attempting an exhaustive review here, the most consistently observed have been genetic susceptibility (i.e. family history) (5), social class/ ethnicity effects (6–8), and gender effects (9). Within populations, these individual difference factors are very powerful and persist independent of historical trends in population obesity. As the average BMI of a population increases with age, the individuals within that population tend to stay in the same relative rank with each other. It has been noted that there is a lot of variability in weight over time (e.g. nearly one person in three gains or loses 5 kg in any given year). Trends, however, in within-person correlations in BMI over periods of time up to 30 or 40 years are remarkably high (10–12). In other words, half or more of the differences between people in fatness are due to individual difference factors.

In addition to individual sources of variance in populations, however, there are also factors between populations that have profound effects on population obesity rates. These include population affluence (globally, more affluent populations are more obese) (2, 13), urbanization (the higher proportion of a population living in urban environments, the higher the prevalence of obesity) (14), diets dominated by energy-dense foods (particularly sugar and fat) (15), low levels of habitual physical activity (16), and, perhaps, cultural values toward fatness and fitness. Culture here refers to some-what hazily understood differences between populations in customary activities that affect energy balance. For example there are different rates of obesity in men compared to women in many populations but not always in the same direction. These differences are most likely due to differences in gender roles in different population subgroups. There are also substantial differences in obesity rates in very similar population subgroups for which easily articulated cultural variable explanations are not so readily available (e.g. different countries in Western Europe).

General considerations relating to population strategies for obesity management

What do data on the behavioral epidemiology of population obesity tell us about which strategies for obesity might be most effective at a population level? Two questions come to mind immediately. The first is whether population strategies for obesity prevention should be targeted at individuals at highest need (i.e. those with identifiable individual risk factors) or whether strategies should be universal and, in effect, target everyone in the entire population? The answer to this question depends on the extent to which it is possible to identify people in greatest need and on the extent to which treatments are available that would work in high-risk persons. Based on the behavioral epidemiology of obesity, it certainly is possible to identify individuals at higher risk. Risk factors include lower social class, minority ethnicity, membership of family in which obesity is common, and perhaps psychological characteristics such as depression. The answer to the question of whether we have obesity treatments available that would be effective for individuals at high risk is more problematic, however. Examination of the literature on obesity treatment clearly indicates that the same factors that put people at risk for developing obesity also put people at greatest risk for failing in treatment. Family and personal history of obesity, lower social class, and psychological distress are all strongly related to treatment failure.

It is also clear from population data that the fact that some people are at greater risk for development of obesity than others does not imply that obesity risk is highly concentrated. Excluding those suffering from energy malnutrition, there are no subgroups of modern societies where increasing rates of obesity have not been seen in recent years (see Chapter 1). Increasing rates have been strongly upward in the rich and the poor, the young and the old, in men and in women. There is also little evidence supporting the idea that interventions applied at different life transition points would be particularly effective compared to interventions applied at other points in time. The only data, of which the present authors are aware, that suggest there are some critical moments in people's lives that would be most amenable to obesity treatment, is data related to obesity treatment in children. Evidence from a variety of studies, spanning several decades, have indicated that treating obesity before puberty may have more enduring effects on relative weight long term than providing similar treatment after puberty or in adulthood (17). The precise cause of the greater durability of treatment in preadolescence is not known. It is also certainly not the case, from a general population perspective, that adolescence is a critical threshold point beyond which individuals are unlikely to develop obesity at all. Indeed, most obese people were not obese as children or adolescents and nevertheless became obese as adults. Even so, a focus on younger age groups is justifiable empirically.

Other critical periods in life have not, to the best of the current authors' knowledge, yet been demonstrated to be associated with more favorable prognosis for long-term weight management. Treatment at any time in life, arguably, has a net benefit. Two recent studies have shown that weight losses of 5 or 10 per cent of body weight over a relatively short period of time (e.g. 1 year) have residual benefits on the trajectory of weight gain over time that lasts 5 years or longer (18, 19). People typically lose 10 per cent of their body weight in the best non-surgical clinical programs for example. This weight is usually regained in its entirety over the course of several years. Nevertheless, people who have lost weight intentionally, on average, are better off in terms of long-term weight trajectory than people who have never lost weight at all.

Casting the argument about treatment strategies in terms of clinical management targeted toward those most at need is an interesting intellectual exercise. However, it greatly neglects two important truisms. First, the number of people affected by obesity is enormous in populations most affected, such as the US, Australia, the UK, and elsewhere in Europe, where one-third to two-thirds of the population may be involved. Second, clinical treatments that are now available for obesity are far too expensive to apply to numbers of that magnitude. Thus, the cost of identifying the minority of people for whom obesity risk is low is probably not worth the effort.

In conclusion, it is argued here that targets for population obesity intervention should be universal, that is entire societies, including people at every age and regardless of individual risk characteristics. We have too little data available on effective ways to identify and manage individual obesity risks to justify a population strategy that would devote resources to sorting people by risk or readiness levels.

Obesity prevention interventions in youth

In a recent literature review of obesity prevention interventions, the present authors identified 17 studies of 6 months or more in duration that targeted obesity prevention or related diet and physical activity behaviors in youth. All of these studies were done in school settings and involved a variety of intervention targets including: increase in physical activity, improvements in diet, nutrition education, and reduction in television viewing. Each will be described briefly here. A study by Robinson in 1999 in San Jose, CA, US, involved 192 children in grades three and four in two elementary schools (20). One of the schools was randomized to receive a classroom curriculum that focused particularly on reducing television-viewing time. The parents of children in the intervention group also received electronic television time managers to use in their homes to facilitate parental control of television viewing. The intervention was applied for 2 months with follow-up at 8 months. Significantly smaller increases were seen in BMI, triceps skinfold thickness, and waist circumference in the intervention compared to the control students.

Gortmaker applied a more extensive program over a long period of time that also included a television-viewing component (21). Study participants were children in grades six to eight in Boston, MA, US. Ten schools were randomized to either treatment or control. The control sites received no intervention. The treatment sites received a 32-lesson, multitargeted, educational intervention that was incorporated into four major academic subjects and also into physical activity classes. The target of the intervention was: decreasing sedentary behavior, including television viewing; decreasing high-fat food consumption; increasing fruit and vegetable intake; and increasing moderate to vigorous physical activity. Over a 2-year period, the per cent of female students who met criteria for the definition of obesity decreased in the intervention schools compared to the control schools. No differences were seen in male students, however.

Mo-Suwan reported the results of a physical-activity-based obesity prevention program in schools in southern Thailand (22). Two hundred ninety-two kindergarten children in eight classes were randomized either to receive 1 hour of physical education class plus 15 minutes of walking and 20 minutes of aerobic dance three times per week or to a control group that received a 1-hour weekly physical education class only. Over about a 6-month period, the investigators reported a marginally significant reduction in the per cent of students with triceps skinfold thicknesses greater than the 95th percentile in the intervention group. A reduction was also seen in the control group, but it was not significant.

Donnelly conducted a 2-year study in rural Nebraska schools (US) with children in grades three to five that included very specific nutrition education curriculum and 30–40 minute physical activity sessions three times per week (23). The program also included reduced fat and sodium in school lunches. The control group received the existing lunch program and a team-oriented sports activity program. After 2 years, no significant differences were seen between the two groups in mean body mass index (BMI).

We identified three studies that targeted physical activity, but did not specifically target obesity. Sallis reported a study in which 955 children in grades four to five, in seven elementary schools, were randomized to receive a physical activity intervention for 2 years or the existing physical education curriculum (24). The intervention, called SPARK, included physical activity classes three times per week, behavior change skills education, homework, and monthly newsletters to parents with incentives for goal achievement. Using mean sum of skinfolds as the marker for obesity, no significant differences were seen in either boys or girls in rate of obesity increase over time.

A study reported by Dwyer *et al.* from South Australia, randomized 510 fifth grade students to one of three physical activity programs for a period of 14 weeks with a follow-up 2 years later (25). The three program conditions were control (30 minutes of traditional physical activity three times a week), skill-focused physical education (PE) in 75-minute daily classes, and fitness-focused PE with 75-minute daily endurance-focus classes. After the 14-week class, there was a significant difference between groups and change in sum of the skinfolds, primarily driven by substantial decrease in fatness in the fitness-focused intervention condition. Repeated measurements 2 years later in schools that adopted the combination of an endurance-focused physical activity and a skills-focused physical activity curriculum showed a significantly lower sum of skinfolds in the intervention condition.

Only one study was identified that attempted to do nutrition-only interventions for youth. This was a study done by Simonetti *et al.* in Italy (26). Children aged 3–9 years in three schools were randomized, one school per treatment condition, to one of two nutrition education conditions or a control condition. After 1 year, larger absolute changes were seen in the more intensive of the two nutrition education conditions in reduction of per cent obesity relative to the other two conditions. However, statistical significance was not reported in these investigations.

Finally, nine studies were identified that involved multicomponent interventions over a sustained period of time. None of these studies specifically targeted weight, but the nutrition–physical activity interventions were very similar to those that one would presumably do in a weight-focused program. The largest of these studies was the CATCH study (27). Five thousand one hundred six students in 96 elementary schools, in grades three–five, were randomized to one of three study conditions. A school intervention included a classroom instructional program, changes in physical activity curriculum, and changes in the school food service to reduce the fat and sodium content of school lunches. A family involvement intervention included the school intervention and in addition had 19 activity packets and family fun nights to encourage family involvement. Control schools received usual physical activity, food service, and health education. After 3 years, significant changes in the hypothesized direction were seen in school lunches, PE class curricula, and self-reported dietary fat intake. There were no differences between treatment conditions in BMI increase however.

Van Dongen reported a study from Western Australia involving 971 children, aged 10–12 years, in 30 schools that were randomized to one of five treatment conditions (28). The treatment conditions included: six classes focusing on fitness and 15 minutes of daily physical activity; school nutrition comprised 10 lessons to improve knowledge, attitudes, and eating habits; home nutrition comprised five nutrition messages delivered through comic books and take-home information for parents; school and home nutrition, which was a combination of the above noted conditions; fitness and school nutrition including the fitness and school nutrition components; and, finally, a control group receiving no treatment. After 1 year, significant differences were seen in skinfold measures of body fatness in boys and girls for the combined fitness and school nutrition program vs. control. No significant differences were seen in body mass index.

Five studies have been published on the Know Your Body program, a school-based curriculum developed originally by Ken Resnicow at the American Health Foundation. The studies, by Resnicow *et al.* (29), Lionus *et al.* (30), Tamir *et al.* (31), Bush *et al.* (32), and Walter *et al.* (33), included two studies in New York City, one in Washington, DC, one in Jerusalem, and one in Crete. Duration ranged from one school year to 5-years follow-up. The program included a multicomponent health education curriculum, school cafeteria modifications, and a variety of skills activities. Control schools all received usual counseling. None of the US-based programs had effects on measures of obesity in children. Significant beneficial effects were seen in the Greek study for BMI, but not sum of the skinfolds; and in the Israeli study, significant beneficial effects in BMI were seen in Arab boys and girls but not Jewish boys and girls.

Alexandrov conducted a health education study among 4213 students, 11 years of age, in two administrative districts of Moscow (34). One district was assigned to a health education program that was largely educational. The other received the usual education. After 3 years, positive effects were reported in a skinfold measure of obesity in boys but not girls. No differences were seen in either gender for BMI.

Finally, Tell and Vellar conducted a study of students, age 10–15, in six schools in Oslo, Norway (35). Four schools were randomized to treatment and two to control. The intervention consisted of a nutrition education and intervention program modified from the Know Your Body program. Nutritionists also made home visits with parents and the physical education program in the school was modified to increase physical activity. After 2 years, marginally significant beneficial effects on weight were reported in girls only. No effects were seen for BMI.

In summary, the findings overall for intervention programs for youth in school settings reviewed above are modestly positive. Significant beneficial effects in BMI or other measures of obesity were reported in approximately half of the studies reviewed. The literature is too sparse to allow meaningful consideration of specific component contributors to effects, although the studies involving high physical activity levels seem particularly interesting. Perhaps the most tempering aspect of these findings is the observation that the biggest and most methodologically rigorous of these studies, the CATCH and Know Your Body program studies, were not successful in showing intervention effects on body weight.

Obesity prevention intervention in adults

This review considered obesity prevention studies in adults of two kinds. First are studies in entire communities that, like the majority of the school intervention studies for youth, targeted multiple behavioral risk factors for chronic disease with specific emphasis on diet and physical activity habit changes that would be expected to be beneficial for weight control. Second are a small group of interventions specifically targeting the prevention of weight gain in adults as opposed to weight loss. This review will not cover the large body of literature on obesity treatment in adults, either in clinical settings or in more community settings like worksites. For a comprehensive review of worksite studies on obesity see Hennrikus and Jeffery (36).

Six sizable community studies targeting behavioral risks for obesity have now been published. They include the Minnesota Heart Health Program (37), the Pawtucket Heart Health Program (38), the North Karelia Heart Health Program (39), a national program on the island of Mauritius (40), and two community trials that originated out of Stanford University, the Stanford Three-Cities Study (41) and the Stanford Five-Cities Project (42). All six of the above studies attempted to implement community-wide efforts to reduce cardiovascular risk factors, including reducing the fat content of the typical diet, increasing physical activity, controlling blood pressure, and quitting cigarette smoking. Although not all of these goals, particularly quitting cigarette smoking, are compatible with population weight control, they were expected to have beneficial effects on body weight. Interventions in these studies included mass media exposure to healthy eating and exercise messages, and programs in schools, churches, social organizations, and worksites. Some included population risk factor screening with individualized behavioral prescriptions and others included environmental interventions to promote heart healthy eating choices in grocery stores and restaurants. All of these studies included assessments of obesity outcomes. Evidence from these studies indicated that implementation of the interventions was good in that there was widespread awareness and participation in the intervention activities related to these projects. Outcomes of these studies were also positive with respect to self-reported changes in diet and physical activity and some cardiovascular risk factors, specifically smoking and blood pressure. Results with respect to mean body weight or prevalence of obesity, however, were fairly minimal. Two of the six projects showed significant weight control effects favoring intervention in either a subset of the population or in a restricted time period of the intervention. However, overall, the effectiveness of these large community intervention education trials with respect to body weight was negligible. The three most recent US studies were all conducted during the period of the recent obesity epidemic and in each case the most dramatic effect seen in body weight was rapid increase in mean BMI over time in both treated and untreated communities.

More recently, three studies have specifically looked at methods for promoting weight-gain prevention in adults. Although none of these was truly population oriented, their explicit focus on obesity prevention (as opposed to obesity treatment or multiple risk factor interventions) makes them worthy of note. Two of these three studies were conducted by Jeffery and colleagues at the University of Minnesota; the first, called the Pound of Prevention Study, being a pilot study for the second (43, 44). Individuals were recruited from the community for these studies and randomized to an intervention that consisted primarily of educational materials about weight-gain prevention delivered through monthly newsletters (with or without incentives for readership). Additional optional educational opportunities were also offered at 6-month intervals, including educational classes on weight control and exercise, physical activity and nutrition contests, and a weight control correspondence course. In the pilot version of the Pound of Prevention project, significant treatment effects were observed (i.e. weight loss in the intervention group and no weight change in the control group in the course of 1 year). In the full-scale trial, however, weight gain was observed in treatment as well as control groups and although the intervention groups gained about 10 per cent less weight over 3 years than the control condition, this was not statistically significant.

The final weight-gain specific intervention was one completed in conjunction with the Women's Healthy Lifestyle project, a 5-year, randomized trial testing a method to prevent weight gain and to prevent increase in low-density lipoprotein cholesterol in 575 women going through menopause (45). The approach to weight gain prevention in this study was to counsel women to lose a modest amount of weight as a protection against adverse cardiovascular risk factor changes during menopause. Participants took part in 15 intensive counseling sessions to encourage improved diet and increased physical activity. This was followed by monthly meetings for 3 months, then three meetings over the next 6 months, and finally group mail and telephone contacts every 2–3 months. Significant between-group differences in weight change from baseline to 54 months showed that this lifestyle intervention was effective in preventing menopause-related weight gain. The difference in body weight between the treatment groups in 54 months was about 2.5 kg.

In summary, efforts to date to study ways to prevent weight gain with age in adults, whether with community approaches or more individual level approaches, have not been very successful. Relying almost entirely on individual education strategies, the interventions have been operational successes in the sense of attracting participants and maintaining their participation over time. The effects on body weight in obesity prevalence, however, have been negligible. Interventions targeting weight-gain prevention do not appear to be any more effective than interventions targeting weight loss for achieving long-term change in body weight.

Conclusions

This chapter has reviewed available research on public health interventions for obesity control. Those in youth have been delivered primarily through schools. Those targeting adults have used heterogeneous delivery modes. All have relied heavily on educational messages encouraging greater physical activity and more healthful diet. The overall outcomes of these interventions are thought to be very modestly positive with the strongest results being seen in programs for children with high physical activity requirements. Unfortunately, the sizes of the overall effect seen in these studies are considerably smaller than the rate of increase in population obesity. Clearly, more needs to be done to combat the obesity epidemic. Whether "more" means greater and better-financed educational efforts or whether "more" means other methods, such as altering the population food supply, remains to be seen.

Acknowledgements

This research was supported by the University of Minnesota Obesity Prevention Centre and the National Institute of Diabetes and Digestive and Kidney Diseases (NIDDK) grant DK50456.

References

1. Manson JE, Willett WC, Stampfer MJ, *et al.* (1995). Body weight and mortality among women. *N Engl J Med* **333**, 677–724.
2. World Health Organization (June 1997). *Obesity: preventing and managing the global epidemic.* Report of a WHO Consultation on Obesity, Division of Noncommunicable Diseases. Programme of Nutrition Family and Reproductive Health, Geneva.
3. Lissner L, Barker DJP, Blundell JE, *et al.* (1996). Group report: what are the bio-behavioral determinants of body weight regulation? In: Bouchard C, Bray GA, eds, *Regulation of body weight: biological and behavioral mechanisms*, pp. 159–77. John Wiley and Sons Ltd., New York.
4. Carpenter KM, Hasin DS, Allison DB, Faith MS (2000). Relationships between obesity and DSM-IV major depressive disorder, suicide ideation, and suicide attempts: results from a general population study. *Am J Public Health* **90**, 251–7.
5. Harnack L, Story M, Holy Rock B, Neumark-Sztainer D, Jeffery R, French S (1999). Nutrition beliefs and weight loss practices of Lakota Indian adults. *J Nutr Educ* **31**, 10–5.
6. Cullen KW, Zakeri I (2004). Fruits, vegetables, milk, and sweetened beverages consumption and access to a la carte/snack bar meals at school. *Am J Public Health* **94**, 463–7.
7. Molarius A, Seidell JC, Sans S, Tuomilehto J, Kuulasmaa K, Project WM (2000). Educational level, relative body weight, and changes in their association over 10 years: an international perspective from the WHO MONICA Project. *Am J Public Health* **90**, 1260–8.
8. Swinburn B, Egger G (2002). Preventive strategies against weight gain and obesity. *Obes Rev* **3**, 289–301.
9. Wardle J, Waller J, Jarvis MJ (2002). Sex differences in the association of socioeconomic status with obesity. *Am J Public Health* **92**, 1299–304.
10. Ronk CE, Roche AF, Chumlea WC, Kent R (1982). Longitudinal trends of weight/stature in childhood in relationship to adulthood body fat measures. *Hum Biol* **154**, 751–64.
11. Braddon FEM, Rodgers B, Wadsworth MEJ, Davies JMC (1986). Onset of obesity in a 36 year birth cohort study. *BMJ* **293**, 299–303.
12. Rimm IJ, Rimm AA (1976). Association between juvenile onset obesity and severe adult obesity in 73,532 women. *Am J Public Health* **66**, 479–81.

13. Sobal J, Stunkard AJ (1989). Socioeconomic status and obesity: a review of the literature. *Psychol Bull* **105**, 260–75.

14. Willett WC (1998). Is dietary fat a major determinant of body fat? *Am J Clin Nutr* **67**, 556S–62S.

15. Neumark-Sztainer D, Wall MM, Story M, Perry CL (2003). Correlates of unhealthy weight-control behaviors among adolescents: implications for prevention programs. *Health Psychol* **22**, 88–98.

16. Lahti-Koski M, Pietinen P, Heliovaara M, Vartiainen E (2002). Associations of body mass index and obesity with physical activity, food choices, alcohol intake, and smoking in the 1982–1997 FINRISK studies. *Am J Clin Nutr* **75**, 809–17.

17. Jeffery RW (2002). Public health approaches to the management of obesity. In: Fairburn CG, Brownell KD, eds, *Eating disorders and obesity*, pp. 613–8. Guilford Press, New York.

18. Jeffery RW, McGuire MT, French SA (2002). Prevalence and correlates of large weight gains and losses. *Int J Obes* **26**, 969–72.

19. Field AE, Wing RR, Manson JE, Speigelman DL, Willet WC (2001). Relationship of large weight loss to long-term weight change among young and middle-aged U. S. women. *Int J Obes* **25**, 1113–21.

20. Robinson TN (1999). Reducing children's television viewing to prevent obesity: a randomized controlled trial. *JAMA* **282**, 1561–7.

21. Gortmaker SL, Peterson K, Wiecha J, *et al.* (1999). Reducing obesity via a school-based interdisciplinary intervention among youth. *Arch Pediatr Adolesc Med* **153**, 409–18.

22. Mo-Suwan L, Pongprapai S, Junjana C, Puetpaiboon A (1998). Effects of a controlled trial of a school-based exercise program on the obesity indexes of preschool children. *Am J Clin Nutr* **68**, 1006–11.

23. Donnelly JE, Jacobsen DJ, Whatley JE, *et al.* (1996). Nutrition and physical activity program to attenuate obesity and promote physical and metabolic fitness in elementary school children. *Obes Res* **4**, 229–43.

24. Sallis JF, McKenzie TL, Alcaraz JE, Kolody B, Faucette N, Hovell MF (1997). The effects of a 2-year physical education program (SPARK) on physical activity and fitness in elementary school students. *Am J Public Health* **87**, 1328–34.

25. Dwyer T, Coonan WE, Leitch DR, Hetzel BS, Baghurst RA (1983). An investigation of the effects of daily physical activity on the health of primary school students in South Australia. *Int J Obes* **12**, 308–13.

26. Simonetti D'Arca A, Sanarelli G (1986). Prevention of obesity in elementary and nursery school children. *Public Health* **100**, 166–73.

27. Luepker RV, Perry CL, McKinlay SM, *et al.* (1996). Outcomes of a field trial to improve children's dietary patterns and physical activity. *JAMA* **275**, 768–76.

28. Van Dongen R, Jenner D, Thompson C, *et al.* (1995). A controlled evaluation of a fitness and nutrition intervention program on cardiovascular health in 10- to 12-year-old children. *Prev Med* **24**, 9–22.

29. Resnicow K, Cohn L, Reinhardt J, *et al.* (1992). A three-year evaluation of the Know Your Body program in inner-city schoolchildren. *Health Educ Q* **19**, 463–80.

30. Lionis C, Kafatos A, Vlachonikolis J, Vakaki M, Tzortzi M, Petraki A (1991). The effects of health education intervention program among Cretan adolescents. *Prev Med* **20**, 685–99.

31. Tamir D, Feurstein A, Brunner S, Halfon S, Reshef A, Palti H (1990). Primary prevention of cardiovascular diseases in childhood: Changes in serum total cholesterol, high density lipoprotein, and body mass index after 2 years of intervention in Jerusalem schoolchildren age 7–9 years. *Prev Med* **19**, 22–30.

32. Bush PJ, Zuckerman AE, Theiss PK, *et al.* (1989). Cardiovascular risk factor prevention in black schoolchildren: two-year results of the "Know your Body" program. *Am J Epidemiol* **129**, 466–82.

33. Walter HJ, Hofman A, Vaughn BA, Wyader EL (1988). Modification of risk factors for coronary heart disease: five-year results of a school-based intervention trial. *N Engl J Med* **318**, 1093–100.

34. Alexandrov A, Isakova G, Maslennikova G, *et al.* (1988). Prevention of atherosclerosis among 11-year-old schoolchildren in two Moscow administrative districts. *Health Psychol* **7** (suppl), 247–52.

35. Tell GS, Vellar OD (1987). Noncommunicable disease risk factor intervention in Norwegian adolescents: the Oslo Youth Study. In: Hetzel B, Berenson GS, eds, *Cardiovascular risk factors in childhood: epidemiology and prevention*, pp. 217–318. Elsevier, New York.

36. Hennrikus DJ, Jeffery RW (1996). Worksite intervention for weight control: a review of the literature. *Am J Health Prom* **10**, 471–98.

37. Jeffery RW (1995). Community programs for obesity prevention: the Minnesota Heart Health Program. *Obes Res* **3** (Suppl 2), 283S–8S.

38. Carleton RA, Lasater TM, Assaf AR, *et al.* (1995). The Pawtucket Heart Health Program: community changes in cardiovascular risk factors and projected disease risk. *Am J Public Health* **85**, 777–85.

39. Vartiainen E, Puska P (1987). The North Karelia Youth Project 1978–80: effects of two years of educational intervention on cardiovascular risk factors and health behavior in adolescence. In: Hetzel B, Berenson GS, eds, *Cardiovascular risk factors in childhood: epidemiology and prevention*, pp. 183–202. Elsevier, New York.

40. Dowse GK, Gareeboo H, Alberti KG, *et al.* (1995). Changes in population cholesterol concentrations and other cardiovascular risk factor levels after five years of the Noncommunicable Disease Intervention Programme in Mauritius. *BMJ* **311**, 1255–9.

41. Fortmann SP, Williams PT, Hulley SB, Haskell WL, Farquhar JW (1981). Effect of health education on dietary behavior: the Stanford Three-Community Study. *Am J Clin Nutr* **34**, 2030–8.

42. Taylor CB, Fortmann SP, Flora J (1991). Effect of long-term community health education on body mass index: the Stanford Five-City Project. *Am J Epidemiol* **134**, 235–49.

43. Forster JL, Jeffery RW, Schmid TL, Kramer FM (1988). Preventing weight gain in adults: A pound of prevention. *Health Psychol* **7**, 515–25.

44. Jeffery RW, French SA (1997). Preventing weight gain in adults: design, methods and one year results from the Pound of Prevention Study. *Int J Obes* **21**, 457–64.

45. Simkin-Silverman L, Wing RR, Hansen DH, *et al.* (1995). Prevention of cardiovascular risk factor elevations in healthy premenopausal women. *Prev Med* **24**, 509–17.

Chapter 9

The cost-effectiveness of obesity prevention

Rob Carter and Marj Moodie

Introduction

The purpose of this chapter is to explore the economics of obesity prevention, particularly the available evidence on the cost-effectiveness of interventions and how the economic credentials for obesity prevention might be developed. The chapter begins with a discussion of the contribution that the discipline of economics can offer to an understanding of obesity prevention, explaining the separate but related tasks of description, prediction, and evaluation. Using these concepts, the chapter then explores what is known about the economics of obesity prevention. First, the depth and quality of the available economic literature on obesity is reviewed, and then Australia is used as a case study to illustrate the application of economic methods to describe the disease burden and to evaluate options for change.

Despite the public health significance of obesity, the evidence base on the cost-effectiveness of interventions to address obesity remains patchy and incomplete, particularly for children. It is clear that much remains to be done before a economic credentials for obesity prevention are fully established. Accordingly, a case study is used to illustrate how economic techniques (such as "threshold analysis") can be used to answer important policy questions, such as the "economically warranted" level of investment in obesity prevention, even though important data gaps exist. Finally, given that the economically warranted level of investment is likely to outstrip resources available for obesity prevention, and that important choices therefore need to be made, a suggested approach for prioritizing action in obesity prevention from an economic perspective is outlined.

How can the economics discipline contribute?

The starting point for understanding the contribution that health economics can offer is to appreciate that the discipline carries out three separate but related tasks, that is: "description", "prediction", and "evaluation".

With "description", the task is to measure and report on current activities, health status, resource use, behavior, or system effects. There is naturally a heavy emphasis on empirical data collection and analysis. While economics brings its own techniques to empirical studies, it is often heavily dependent on other disciplines for data input and analysis. Those disciplines include: epidemiology for disease incidence/prevalence data; demography for population trends; clinical medicine for treatment pathways; biostatistics for data analysis; and accounting for cost records. Importantly, description often involves the construction of particular concepts and this process of construction may involve particular assumptions or definitions. In estimating the cost of illness (COI), for example, assumptions are required concerning the elements of illness that represent a "cost". All COI studies will estimate the direct cost of disease management and care, while some will try to estimate the indirect costs of lost production in the broader economy, and may also try to impute a cost to pain and suffering.

With "prediction", the task is to estimate future trends in health status, resource use, risk factors, or system effects. As the research question moves from describing the status quo, to predicting future trends, it becomes increasingly important for assumptions to be clearly specified. Those arguing for the importance of particular diseases, for example, will quite often use disease models based on current practice to predict future "needs". Sometimes this is done without clearly specifying that their predictions are based on assumptions that current practice is acceptable (i.e. efficacious, efficient, affordable, etc.) or that technology and/or societal expectations will not change. The task of prediction focuses attention on the concept of "evidence", as well as the need for uncertainty analysis to support the estimates.

While the tasks of description and prediction have their contentious aspects, it is the third task of "evaluation", with its central role of judging "value-for-money", that is the most debated and often the most misunderstood contribution of economics. Evaluation in economics has distinctive characteristics that separate it from evaluation as practised by other disciplines. Evaluation in economics involves both a comparison of alternatives (one of which is often the "status quo" and the other an option for change) and, importantly, has regard to both their costs and benefits. A prime task in economic evaluation is to address the question: "What difference will the proposed intervention make compared to current practice?" Evaluation often involves both description (e.g. describing current practice and the current health burden) and prediction (e.g. estimating cost and benefit streams through time) but, importantly, involves a judgment (implied or explicit) about the "appropriate" use of resources. The issue of appropriateness is guided by decision rules that relate incremental benefit achieved by the proposed intervention to its incremental cost. These decision rules in turn raise an important issue about how "benefit" is defined – is it just health gain or are there broader dimensions involving acceptability, feasibility, and social justice? The task of economic evaluation is thus intimately linked to the contribution that economics can make to health service planning and priority setting.

The discipline distinguishes between "positive economics" and "normative economics", with the former covering "what is", and the latter "what ought to be."

Positive economics is meant to be as value free as possible and is dominated by the task of description. There is an unavoidable normative judgment that data is worthwhile collecting and that particular definitions are appropriate. Beyond this, positive economics strives to be value free. Normative economics, on the other hand, is quite consciously based on value judgments that underlie suggested change. The failure of some economists to make these values transparent can lead to confusion as to whether pronouncements for change are based upon economic theory or ideology. The reliance on the market by "economic rationalists", for example, embodies the ethical judgment that it is acceptable for access to services to be determined by the consumer's ability and willingness to pay. For many societies, health care is viewed as a "merit good" and governments intervene on social justice grounds to ensure access on the basis of "need", rather than income and preferences. We return to this issue below, when considering how the economic credentials for obesity prevention might be developed.

Description: what is the size of the obesity problem and how much is spent on it?

Overview

Governments, health authorities, research departments and a range of other bodies often seek reliable information on the burden of disease (BOD), both in terms of health status and its resource implications. The uses to which such descriptive information on the BOD can be put vary widely. BOD information is often utilized, for example, in developing measures of public health significance and/or monitoring trends through time. It can be employed to examine the performance of the health-care system and its various components, in planning health service provision, in measuring the potential for health status gains and/or cost offsets, and as an input into economic evaluation and priority setting.

Over and above its mortality and morbidity impacts, disease has important second-order effects on income and production patterns throughout the economy, as well as on resource utilization within the health-care system. COI or disease costing studies are one type of BOD study that describe the relationship between current disease incidence and/or prevalence and the consequent resource implications, particularly for the structure and utilization of health services. It is important to recognize that they are descriptive studies (i.e. describing the status quo), not evaluation studies that compare the status quo with options for change. This distinction stands behind the "best buys" rationale – that resource allocation decisions should be based on the net cost of securing health gains through identified interventions, not simply the size of the problem.

Economists make a distinction in COI studies between the "direct costs" of providing health-care services, "indirect costs" (production gains or losses), and "intangibles" (such as pain and suffering). Direct costs (such as hospitals, medical, and allied health services, pharmaceuticals, etc.) are the least contentious, but there is an important issue related to study perspective. Often studies are dominated by the perspective of third-party funders, and while including some cost impacts on patients (such as insurance copayments), other cost impacts on patients are ignored (such as the value of carer time; travel and waiting time; home modifications, etc.).

Indirect costs focus on lost production in the economy attributable to illness and premature death, but may also include costs impacting outside the health-care sector (such as police and court costs for drug abuse; vehicle damage for alcohol abuse; impact of regulations on industry, etc.). The estimation of production effects has been a contentious issue in the COI literature. This is a reflection of a number of factors, namely the variety of measurement techniques available, the difficult ethical and equity issues involved, and the fact that when measurement is attempted, the resulting estimates often swamp direct costs.

Intangible costs, such as pain and suffering, are by their very nature difficult to value in monetary terms. As a consequence they are not often costed in COI studies and (arguably) are best measured through health status indicators such as the quality adjusted life year (QALY) or disability adjusted life year (DALY).

Review of the economic literature describing the obesity problem

The economic literature on obesity is currently focused on "describing" the size of the problem, rather than "evaluating" interventions for its prevention or management. The mounting concern about obesity is, in part, a response to the large body of research in recent years which has addressed the mortality and morbidity arising from the disease (Chapter 1). A number of epidemiological studies have documented the increased risk of all-cause mortality amongst people who are obese (1–3). Some have confined their attention to measuring the burden of illness arising from obesity as a risk factor for a particular disease such as cardiovascular disease (4, 5), diabetes (6–8), and cancer (9, 10). Other studies have been concerned with the measurement of obesity-related burden of disease for particular geographic jurisdictions (11, 12) and/or demographic groups (13, 14).

Whilst the body of literature which quantifies the obesity-related illness burden is substantial, there is a small but growing literature on the cost burden, including several reviews of COI studies (15–17). The COI studies (Table 9.1) vary in their methodology. As noted by Kortt et al., 1998 (16), they generally measure costs attributable to obesity within a prevalence-based framework. In other words, they measure the annual cost burden stemming from all cases of the disease (new or pre-existing), rather than the lifetime costs of a cohort of new cases using an incidence-based assessment as employed by others (18–20). The preferred approach depends on the purpose of the study and data availability. If the results are to be used for cost control or financial planning, then prevalence-based costs are preferable. If the estimates are to input into evaluation of prevention measures (as a description of current practice), then the incidence-based approach is preferable (as only new cases can be prevented).

Table 9.1 Studies of the cost burden attributable to obesity

Author, country, year	BMI criteria	Prevalence or incidence-based	Comorbidities attributable to obesity considered	Costs attributable to obesity	Costs included
Colditz US, 1992 (21)	≥29	Prevalence	NIDDM, gallbladder disease, CVD, hypertension, cancers	US$39.9 billion (1986) = 5.5% of US health-care expenditure	Includes direct and indirect costs
Sjöström et al. Sweden, 1992 (22)		Prevalence	Dyspnea, angina pectoris, myocardial infarction, hypertension, high blood pressure, diabetes, claudication, stroke, gall bladder disease; back, neck and shoulder pain	7% of total productivity loss in Sweden	Sickness pensions
Wolf and Colditz US, 1994 (23)	≥29	Prevalence	NIDDM, gallbladder disease, CVD, hypertension, cancers, musculoskeletal disorders	US$45.8 billion (1990) = 6.8% of US health-care expenditure	Direct and indirect costs, including excess physician visits, work lost days, restricted activity and bed-days attributable to obesity
Segal et al. Australia, 1994 (24)	≥30	Prevalence	NIDDM, gallstones, CHD, hypertension, breast cancer, colon cancer	AUD$395 million in 1989 = 2% recurrent health expenditure	Direct costs: hospital, medical, general practitioner, specialists, pharmaceuticals, allied health, nursing home costs
Seidell Netherlands, 1995 (25)	≥30	Prevalence	Contacts with general practitioners, medical specialists, hospital; admissions, and medications	1 billion Dutch guilders = 4% of Dutch health-care costs	Direct costs only
Levy et al. France, 1995 (26)	≥27	Prevalence	Hypertension, myocardial infarction, angina pectoris, stroke, venous thrombosis, NIDDM, hyper-lipidemia, gout, osteoarthritis, gallbladder disease, colorectal cancer, breast cancer, genitourinary cancer, hip fracture	11.89 billion French francs = 2% French health-care costs	Includes direct costs (personal and health care, hospital care, physician services, drugs) and indirect costs (lost output)

continued

Table 9.1 (continued) Studies of the cost burden attributable to obesity

Author, country, year	BMI criteria	Prevalence or incidence-based	Comorbidities attributable to obesity considered	Costs attributable to obesity	Costs included
Wolf and Colditz US, 1996 (27)	≥29	Prevalence	NIDDM, CHD, hypertension, gallbladder disease	US$22.6 billion in 1993	Direct costs and indirect morbidity costs (lost productivity), days of restricted activity and days in bed, excess physician visits
Gorsky et al. US, 1996 (18)	≥29	Incidence	NIDDM, CHD, hypertension, gallbladder disease, osteoarthritis	US$53 million in 1990 = excess 25-year costs per 10 000 women (aged 40 years) of BMI ≥29	25-year direct health care and medication costs
Swinburn et al. New Zealand, 1997 (28)	≥30	Prevalence	NIDDM, CHD, hypertension, gallstones, breast cancer, colon cancer	NZ$135 million in 1991 = 2.5% total health-care costs	Hospital (inpatient and outpatient) services, general practitioner consultations, pharmaceuticals, laboratory tests and ambulance services
Wolf and Colditz US, 1998 (29)	≥29	Prevalence	NIDDM, CHD, hypertension, gallbladder disease, endometrial cancer, breast cancer, colon cancer, osteoarthritis	US$51.6 billion in 1995 = 5.7% of overall US health-care spending	Includes direct (personal health care, hospital care, physician services, allied health services, medications) and indirect costs (lost output). Also costs of excess physician visits, work-lost days, restricted activity and bed-days

Study	BMI	Measure	Comorbidities	Cost	Description
Thompson et al. US, 1998 (30)	≥25	Prevalence	NIDDM, CHD, hypertension, hypercholesterolemia, stroke, gallbladder disease, endometrial cancer, knee osteoarthritis	US$7.7 billion in 1996 = 5% of medical care cost burden to US business	Includes obesity-attributable expenditure on selected employee benefits: health, life and disability insurance and paid sick leave by private sector firms
Birmingham et al. Canada, 1999 (31)	≥27	Prevalence	NIDDM, hypertension, stroke, CHD, hyperlipidemia, pulmonary embolism, gallbladder disease, postmenopausal breast cancer, colorectal cancer, endometrial cancer	CAN$1.8 billion in 1997 = 2.4% overall health-care spending in Canada	Includes direct costs on hospital care, physician services, services by other health professionals, drugs, other health care and health research
Colditz US, 1999 (32)	≥30	Prevalence	NIDDM, CHD, hypertension, gallbladder disease, breast cancer, endometrial cancer, colon cancer, osteoarthritis	US$70 billion in 1995 = 7.0% of overall health-care spending in US	Includes direct costs of inactivity and obesity
Oster et al. US, 1999 (20)	≥27.5 ≥32.5 ≥37.5	Incidence	Hypertension, hypercholesterolemia, NIDDM, CHD, stroke	A sustained 10% reduction in body weight would decrease expected lifetime obesity-attributable medical care costs by US$2300–$5300 for men, US$2200–$5200 for women	Includes direct costs (hospital care, physicians, allied health, nursing home care, drugs, laboratory tests, rehabilitation). Varied depending on the comorbidity
Thompson et al. US, 1999 (19)	≥32.5 ≥37.5	Incidence	NIDDM, CHD, hypercholesterolemia, hypertension, stroke	US$8600–$11 200 = excess lifetime costs per person of BMI of 32.5 US$14 500–$17 100 – BMI 37.5	

continued

Table 9.1 (continued) Studies of the cost burden attributable to obesity

Author, country, year	BMI criteria	Prevalence or incidence-based	Comorbidities attributable to obesity considered	Costs attributable to obesity	Costs included
Pereira et al. Portugal, 2000 (33)	≥30	Prevalence	Osteoarthritis, NIDDM, hypertension, cardiovascular disease, gallbladder disease, arthropaties, colon cancer, breast cancer, endometrial cancer, obesity	PTE 46.2 billion in 1996 = 3.5% of health-care spending in Portugal	Hospital costs, ambulatory care, pharmaceuticals
Oster et al. US, 2000 (34)	≥25	Prevalence	NIDDM, CHD, hypertension, hypercholesterolemia, stroke, gallbladder disease, knee osteoarthritis, endometrial cancer	US$346 million in 1996 = medical care cost per million persons in a managed care setting	Medical care costs associated with a hypothetical health plan with one million members aged 35–84 years
Finkelstein et al. US, 2004 (35)		Prevalence	No diseases specified	State level expenditure on obesity ranges from US$87 million in Wyoming to US$7.7 billion in California. Estimated % of annual state medical expenditure ranges from 4% (Arizona) to 6.7% (Alaska)	Medicare and Medicaid obesity-attributable medical expenditures

NIDDM = non-insulin-dependent diabetes mellitus; CVD = cardiovascular disease; CHD = coronary heart disease

It is acknowledged that a table similar to this appears in Thompson and Wolf, 2001 (17), however, the format and content has been changed and recent studies added.

The majority of studies confine the cost burden to the direct costs arising from the current prevalence and treatment of obesity. The methodology used to estimate the cost of comorbidities attributable to obesity varies from a *pro rata* allocation of related costs (21, 36), to more rigorous epidemiological approaches of calculating and applying population attributable fractions (24–26) or the use of regression models (37).

Very few studies take into account the indirect costs of obesity. Colditz, 1992 (21), estimated the costs arising from lost productivity to be $20 billion for the US in 1986, and in a later paper (23), revised this to $23 billion. Sjöström *et al.*, 1992 (22), estimated that obese patients were up to 2.4 times more likely to be absent for reasons of sickness, and up to 2.8 times more likely to be in receipt of a disability pension than normal weight individuals. From these figures, they extrapolated that 7 per cent of the total productivity loss in Sweden was obesity related. Gorstein and Grosse, 1994 (38), outlined some key factors influencing the indirect costs of obesity and methods for their quantification, whilst Seidell,1998 (39), and Lobstein *et al.*, 2004 (40), documented the problems in calculating the costs associated with obesity, including intangible costs pertaining to obese individuals in terms of diminished social functioning and quality of life. The studies generally do not include any allowance for such intangible costs (32).

The range of comorbidities considered also differs between studies. Most studies typically focus on non-insulin-dependent diabetes mellitus, gallbladder disease, cardiovascular disease, hypertension, and some cancers (such as 21, 24, 28). Others (such as 26, 31, 33) included conditions such as stroke, gout, osteoarthritis, and hip fractures. This is indicative of the lack of consensus about "obesity-related" illnesses. COI studies are also hampered by the absence of good data on population attributable fractions specific to particular geographic jurisdictions. Segal *et al.*, 1994 (24), for instance, adapted the estimates employed in the US study of Colditz, 1992 (21), to the Australian situation, whereas Birmingham *et al.*, 1999 (31), developed their own methodology using both data from local sources and the literature to develop estimates for Canada. The wide variation in the proportions of diseases attributable to obesity employed in different studies (e.g. 21, 24, 26, 31) may be as much due to differences in methodology as differences in the prevalence of obesity.

The studies also vary in terms of the BMI cut-off points used to define obesity. Some studies focus solely on the obese category (BMI $\geq 30\,\text{kg/m}^2$), whereas others combine the overweight and obese (BMI $\geq 25\,\text{kg/m}^2$), or assume a cut-off point somewhere in between.

Generally, the studies were performed from a national health system perspective. Table 9.1 shows that the costs attributable to obesity generally represent somewhere between 2 and 8 per cent of total health-care expenditure. It does not always follow that the proportion is linked to the number of comorbidities considered, indicating both differences in measurement methodology and in disease risk estimates.

Some studies assume a narrower perspective, either in terms of geographical juris-diction or target group. A recent US study by Finkelstein *et al.*, 2004 (35), produced estimates of obesity-attributable expenditure by States. An earlier study by Thompson *et al.*, 1998 (30) set out to measure obesity-attributable expenditure on selected employee benefits, including health, life, and disability insurance, and paid sick leave by private sector firms. Gorsky *et al.*, 1996, in their study (18) calculated the 25-year cost burden of US women who remain overweight after 40 years of age. Oster *et al.*, 1999 (20), used cost burden analysis to estimate the lifetime cost savings stemming from a sustained 10 per cent reduction in body weight amongst Americans aged 35 to 64 years. Queseneberry *et al.*, 1998 (41), found there was a significant association between the BMI of patients in a specific medical care program and their direct health service costs (inpatient and outpatient costs, pharmacy, radiology costs, etc.), amounting to about 6 per cent of total health-care costs of that population.

Finally, as noted by Kortt *et al.*, 1998 (16), in their review article, there is a lack of economic studies that attempt explicitly to model the association between medical care utilization and obesity. Some studies (41–43) employed individual-level data to model this relationship, whilst another, Wang and Dietz 2002 (44), used multi-year hospital discharge data to examine the trend of obesity-associated diseases in youth and the related economic costs. Modeling the association between obesity and resource utilization is an important area for further research and provides an example of where the description function of economics is flowing over into the prediction function.

Case study: estimating the BOD and COI for obesity in Australia

Whilst acknowledging the importance of the "best buys" approach, being able to examine how health resources are currently funded and allocated among different users, health services, and diseases can be useful in considering a variety of equity, access, and utilization issues. Of particular interest to those in the health promotion field, for example, is the use of limited resources in the diagnosis, treatment, and man-agement of preventable illness. Planners may wish to have this information to generate options for change, to identify what potential changes in service utilization may follow the achievement of national goals and targets, or to develop broad order estimates of the potential health-care offsets to the cost of prevention activities. To illustrate some of these uses, we will develop COI/BOD information for Australia in the case study set out below. In a later section we will integrate this descriptive information into an evaluation that addresses the question: "What is an economically warranted level of investment in a national obesity prevention program for children?"

The steps involved in undertaking a burden of disease study for overweight and obesity in adults are set out in Box 9.1.

Box 9.1: Steps in developing COI and BOD estimates for obesity

+ **Step One:** identify the diseases that are causally related to overweight and obesity in adults;

+ **Step Two:** identify the prevalence and excess relative risk for overweight/obesity in adults and calculate the population attributable fractions (PAFs);

+ **Step Three:** estimate the total health burden and total health-care expenditure associated with each disease causally related to overweight/obesity in adults;

+ **Step Four:** estimate the share of this health burden and health-care expenditure that is attributable to overweight/obesity using the PAFs from step two.

Step one: identify diseases causally related to overweight/obesity in adults

Diseases for which there is sound evidence of a causal association with overweight and obesity in adults are: type 2 diabetes mellitus (6, 7, 45–47); gallbladder disease (48, 49); coronary heart disease (4, 5, 26, 50, 51); ischemic stroke (52, 53); hypertension (22, 26, 54, 55); hypercholesterolemia (3, 19, 20, 26); bowel cancer (52, 56); breast cancer (women 50–69 years) (9, 57–61); endometrial cancer (62); kidney cancer (63, 64); osteoarthritis (65); and back problems (66, 67).

While there are other diseases mentioned in the obesity literature (such as respiratory disease, cancer of the uterus, gout, depression, and anxiety), the causal evidence is not sufficient to include them in the calculations at this stage. Obesity is also known to increase the risk of surgical complications, increase health-care costs for surgical procedures, and result in poorer than expected outcomes from surgery. Again these effects are difficult to quantify with any precision and are not included in the case study at this stage. Further, there are also substantial health expenditures associated with various interventions aimed at the immediate treatment of obesity as a condition in its own right. These include stomach stapling, liposuction, community-based weight control programs, and weight control management through primary care physicians and other health-care professionals. These expenditures were estimated at $AUD28.7 million in 1989/90 by Segal *et al.* (24). The authors acknowledged this estimate to be conservative, as it included no provision for the private weight reduction programs operating in approximately 600 to 1000 centers in Australia. Again, in this exploratory case study, these direct expenditures on the treatment of obesity/overweight have not been included. At every step there has been a conscious decision to be conservative and provide a "floor estimate" of the burden of disease associated with obesity. This is to ensure that

our "threshold analysis", given below, on the "economically warranted" level of investment in a national obesity prevention program for children is not over-stated.

Step two: identify the prevalence and excess relative risk for overweight/obesity in adults and calculate the population attributable fractions (PAFs)

The epidemiological data on risk factor prevalence, relative risks, and PAFs utilized
in the analysis is summarized in Table 9.2 (for overweight) and Table 9.3 (for obesity).
A number of epidemiological studies have shown that there is an increased risk of
all-cause mortality among people who are overweight/obese (1, 2). The International
Obesity Taskforce (IOTF) undertook a systematic review of studies examining the
relationships between disease and obesity/overweight. The studies identified in that

Table 9.2 Prevalence, relative risks, and population attributable fractions (PAFs) for overweight adults

Disease	Prevalence[a] of overweight		Relative risks[b] for overweight		Population attributable fractions (PAFs)[c]	
	Men	Women	Men	Women	Men	Women
Diabetes	0.483	0.302	1.80	1.80	0.279	0.195
Gallbladder disease	0.483	0.302	1.50	1.50	0.195	0.131
CHD < age 65	0.483	0.302	1.35	1.40	0.145	0.108
CHD > age 65	0.483	0.302	1.00	1.00	0.000	0.000
Stroke (ischemic)	0.483	0.302	1.05	1.10	0.024	0.029
Hypertension	0.483	0.302	1.40	1.40	0.162	0.108
Hypercholesterolemia	0.483	0.302	1.18	1.10	0.080	0.029
Breast cancer (women 50–69)	0.483	0.302	–	1.00	–	0.000
Bowel cancer	0.483	0.302	1.20	1.20	0.088	0.057
Kidney cancer	0.483	0.302	1.00	1.00	0.000	0.000
Endometrial cancer	0.483	0.302	–	1.00	–	0.000
Osteoarthritis	0.483	0.302	1.35	1.35	0.145	0.096
Back problems	0.483	0.302	1.21	1.10	0.092	0.033

[a]The prevalence of overweight in men and women is taken from the 1999–2000 Australian Diabetes, Obesity and Lifestyle Study (AusDiab) (68). "Overweight" is defined as a BMI between 25 and 30 and is specified for the reference year 2000.

[b]For most diseases the relative risks were taken from Table 7.8 in *The burden of disease and injury in Australia* (69). For stroke, age was not split between <65 and >65, and a conservative approach was taken to selection of the relative risks. For hypercholesterolemia, the relative risk was taken from a study by Must *et al.* 1999 (3) as this disease was not included in the Mathers *et al.* study for obesity.

[c]The PAFs are derived using the formulae: PAF = P(rr − 1)/[P(rr − 1) + 1]. The PAFs are calculated in an Excel Spreadsheet.

Table 9.3 Prevalence, relative risks, and population attributable fractions (PAFs) for obese adults

Diseases	Prevalence[a] of obesity in 2000		Relative risks[b] for obesity		Population attributable fractions (PAFs)[c]	
	Men	Women	Men	Women	Men	Women
Diabetes	0.191	0.218	3.20	3.20	0.296	0.324
Gallbladder disease	0.191	0.218	2.25	2.25	0.193	0.214
CHD < age 65	0.191	0.218	1.80	2.00	0.133	0.179
CHD > age 65	0.191	0.218	1.20	1.25	0.037	0.052
Stroke (ischemic)	0.191	0.218	1.15	1.20	0.028	0.042
Hypertension	0.191	0.218	2.35	2.35	0.205	0.227
Hypercholesterolemia	0.191	0.218	1.17	1.10	0.031	0.021
Breast cancer (women 50–69)	0.191	0.218	–	1.30	–	0.062
Bowel cancer	0.191	0.218	1.40	1.40	0.071	0.080
Kidney cancer	0.191	0.218	1.00	1.50	0.000	0.098
Endometrial cancer	0.191	0.218	–	1.75	–	0.141
Osteoarthritis	0.191	0.218	2.40	2.40	0.211	0.234
Back problems	0.191	0.218	1.50	1.25	0.087	0.052

[a]The prevalence of obesity in men and women is taken from the 1999–2000 Australian Diabetes, Obesity and Lifestyle Study (AusDiab) (68). "Obesity" is defined as a BMI >30 and is specified for the reference year 2000.

[b]For most diseases the relative risks were taken from Table 7.8 in *The burden of disease and injury in Australia* (69). For stroke, age was not split between <65 and >65 and a conservative approach was taken to selection of the relative risks. For hypercholesterolemia, the relative risk was taken from a study by Must *et al.* 1999 (3), as this disease was not included in the Mathers *et al.* study for this risk factor.

[c]The PAFs are derived using the formulae: $PAF = P(rr-1)/[P(rr-1)+1]$. The PAFs are calculated in an Excel Spreadsheet.

review were utilized by the Australian BOD study (69) which informs this case study. It is important to note that this Australian BOD study has adopted conservative excess relative risks to adjust for possible confounding by other risk factors, such as physical exercise and the consumption of fruit and vegetables. The relative risks reported in Tables 9.2 and 9.3 are approximately half those which appear in other studies citing obesity-related relative risks (17, 24).

Step three: estimate the total health burden and health-care expenditure for diseases causally related to overweight/obesity in adults

The estimates of health burden and associated health-care expenditure for diseases causally related to overweight/obesity are presented in Table 9.4. The health burden is reported as deaths and as DALYs, using the Australian BOD study (69). The DALY is a useful measure because it can be utilized both for descriptive purposes (as a summary

Table 9.4 Total health burden and total recurrent direct health-care expenditure for adults[a] in selected diseases causally related to overweight/obesity

Diseases	Deaths[b]		DALYs[c]		Health-care expenditure[d] (AUD$M)	
	Men	Women	Men	Women	Men	Women
Diabetes	1616	1479	35792	31694	262.76	296.92
Gallbladder disease	116	120	1357	1882	39.35	39.35
CHD < age 65	4508	1541	76971	29587	841.09	504.89
CHD > age 65	12755	13877	103659	101113		
Stroke (Ischemic)	5216	7623	64330	72248	423.93	524.91
Hypertension	618	1025	4999	8042	503.84	746.73
Hypercholesterolemia	0	0	n/a	n/a	125.51	174.42
Breast cancer (women 50–69)	–	1184	–	23677	–	56.73
Bowel cancer	2674	2299	35511	31440	93.76	93.76
Kidney cancer	510	510	6475	4937	18.42	12.28
Endometrial cancer	–	325	–	6045	–	12.79
Osteoarthritis	25	71	22610	33695	352.15	586.91
Back problems	5	5	4390	3501	384.20	447.11
Totals	28043	30059	356094	347861	3045.00	3496.80

[a]The percentage of these diseases that impact on children and adolescents is negligible and, in this scoping analysis, the estimates have not been adjusted for this refinement.

[b]The deaths are for Australia in the year 1996 and are taken from relevant entries for each disease in Annex Table E in *The burden of disease and injury in Australia* (69). Note, deaths have not been adjusted for demographic change since 1996 and may therefore underestimate the number of deaths in the reference year 2000.

[c]The DALYs are for Australia in the year 1996 and are taken from relevant entries for each disease in Annex Table H in *The burden of disease and injury in Australia* (69). Note DALYs have not been adjusted for demographic change since 1996 and may therefore underestimate the number of DALYs in the reference year 2000.

[d]The estimates of health-care expenditure for each disease are based on the AIHW Disease Costs and Impacts database (DCIS) and associated publications (70–74). The DCIS database provides estimates of disease related health expenditure for the year 1993/94. These estimates were updated to the reference year 2000 using the ratio of recurrent health-care expenditure in 1999/2000 over the recurrent health-care expenditure in 1993/94. Information on recurrent health-care expenditure in 1993/94 and 1999/2000 is taken from the AIHW Health Expenditure Bulletin for 2000/01 (75).

measure of population health), as well as in economic evaluations as the outcome measure (76). Like the QALY, the DALY incorporates both mortality (YLL: years of life lost) and morbidity (YLD: years lived with disability) and facilitates comparisons across different disease types.

The estimates of health-care expenditure for each disease are based on the Disease Costs and Impacts database (DCIS) and associated publications from the Australian Institute of Health and Welfare (AIHW) (70–73). The full methodology for these disease cost estimates is reported in *Disease Costing Methodology used in the Disease Costs and Impact Study* (74). The DCIS database provides estimates of disease-related health expenditure for the reference year 1993/94, including: hospitals, nursing homes, medical services, pharmaceuticals, allied health services, and a range of other minor expenditures. These estimates were updated to our reference year (2000) using the ratio of recurrent health-care expenditure in 1999/2000 over the recurrent health-care expenditure in 1993/94. The estimates thus reflect current levels of health-care expenditure and are reported in current prices for the year 1999/2000. This method assumes that the distribution of health-care expenditures between diseases was approximately the same in 1999/2000 as it was in 1993/94. Information on recurrent health-care expenditure in 1993/94 and 1999/2000 was taken from the health expenditure series published by AIHW (75).

It should also be noted that these disease cost estimates are derived from health sector expenditures based on national accounts methods adopted by the AIHW. This means that certain types of expenditures (such as time costs and carer costs) are not included as recurrent health-care expenditure.

Step four: estimate the share of this health burden and health-care expenditure that is attributable to overweight/obesity in adults

In step four, the PAFs from step two are applied to the health burden and health expenditure estimates (step three) to estimate the share attributable to overweight and obesity. The results are reported in Table 9.5 (health burden) and Table 9.6 (health-care expenditure). The use of BOD/COI data to establish public health significance can be illustrated by reporting the mortality, morbidity, and cost estimates associated with obesity as a percentage of the corresponding "all disease" estimates.

Health-care expenditure attributable to overweight/obesity is estimated as $AUD1686 million in 2000, which, as a percentage of total health-care expenditure, is a little over 3 per cent (Table 9.6). The available literature confirms this to be a conservative estimate. Segal *et al.*, 1994 (24), for example, estimated the cost of obesity alone (i.e. not including overweight) to be 2 per cent of health-care expenditure in Australia in 1989/90, but in this study the relative risks were not adjusted for the impact of other risk factors (such as physical exercise and consumption of fruit and vegetables). Given the upward trend in the prevalence of obesity, however, the percentage would be higher today based on the methods used in that study. Similarly, Hughes *et al.*, 1999 (77), reference overseas studies that suggest a magnitude of between 2 and 8 per cent of health-care expenditure as the cost of treating obesity-related disease. We have confirmed this finding in Table 9.1. As noted above, however, the methods and key assumptions adopted in these studies varied and the criteria used to define obesity have not always been made explicit. Further, it is not always clear whether these obesity-specific studies have used relative risks adjusted for possible confounding with related risk factors.

Table 9.5 Health burden attributable to overweight and obesity for Australian adults

Diseases	Deaths[a] due to overweight		DALYs[b] due to overweight		Deaths due to obesity		DALYs due to obesity	
	Men	Women	Men	Women	Men	Women	Men	Women
Diabetes	450	288	9975	6167	478	479	10 590	10 273
Gallbladder disease	23	16	264	247	21	26	262	403
CHD < age 65	652	166	11 130	3189	598	276	10 202	5296
CHD > age 65	0	0	0	0	469	717	3814	5226
Stroke (ischemic)	123	223	1517	2118	145	318	1792	3018
Hypertension	100	110	809	867	127	233	1025	1829
Hypercholesterolemia	0	0	n/a	n/a	0	0	n/a	n/a
Breast cancer (women 50–69)	–	0	–	0	–	73	–	1466
Bowel cancer	236	131	3128	1791	190	184	2520	2522
Kidney cancer	0	0	0	0	0	50	0	485
Endometrial cancer	–	0	–	0	–	46	–	849
Osteoarthritis	4	7	3270	3221	5	17	4770	7879
Back problems	0	0	404	103	0	0	383	181
TOTAL	1588	941	30 490	17 703	2035	2420	35 358	39 427
% of total deaths/ DALYs in men or women	2.33	1.56	2.29	1.50	2.98	4.00	2.66	3.34

[a]The attributable deaths are derived by multiplying the deaths in Table 9.4 for the relevant diseases by the respective PAFs in Tables 9.2 and 9.3.
[b]The attributable DALYs are derived by multiplying the DALYs in Table 9.4 for the relevant diseases by the respective PAFs in Tables 9.2 and 9.3.

Table 9.6 Health-care expenditure attributable to overweight/obesity for adults

Diseases	Expenditure[a] due to overweight AUD$M (2000)		Expenditure[b] due to obesity AUD$M (2000)		Total expenditure obesity and overweight	
	Men	Women	Men	Women	Men	Women
Diabetes	73.23	57.78	77.74	96.24	150.97	154.02
Gallbladder disease	7.66	5.16	7.58	8.43	15.24	13.59
CHD < age 65	121.63	54.42	111.48	90.37	233.11	144.78
CHD > age 65						
Stroke (ischemic)	10.04	15.39	11.81	21.93	21.80	37.32
Hypertension	81.58	80.48	103.28	169.79	184.86	250.28
Hypercholesterolemia	10.04	5.11	3.95	3.72	13.99	8.83
Breast cancer (women 50–69)	–	0	–	3.51	–	3.51
Bowel cancer	8.26	5.34	6.65	7.52	14.91	12.86
Kidney cancer	–	0	–	1.21	–	1.21
Endometrial cancer	–	0	–	1.80	–	1.80
Osteoarthritis	50.92	56.11	74.30	137.24	125.22	193.35
Back problems	35.38	13.11	33.49	23.11	68.87	36.21
TOTAL	398.69	292.89	430.29	564.87	828.98	857.76
% of total recurrent health expenditure on men or women	0.77	0.56	0.83	1.08	1.59	1.65

[a]The attributable expenditure for overweight was derived by multiplying the health-care expenditure in Table 9.4 for the relevant diseases by the respective PAFs in Tables 9.2 and 9.3. The reference year for the estimates is 2000.

[b]The attributable expenditure for obesity was derived by multiplying the health-care expenditure in Table 9.4 for the relevant diseases by the respective PAFs in Tables 9.2 and 9.3. The reference year for the estimates is 2000.

The DALY and cost data can also be utilized to develop broad order estimates of the potential health benefit and cost offsets of introducing a national obesity prevention program in Australia. The case study is developed below to illustrate this application.

Use and interpretation of descriptive data on direct costs of disease

While such direct cost estimates can certainly be useful to planners and researchers for the variety of purposes mentioned above, it is important that they are not over-interpreted. From an economic perspective, the most important points to note are set out in Box 9.2 below.

Used sensibly and carefully, disease cost estimates (and BOD information in general) can have a role that goes beyond simple description and monitoring. Such information can also be a useful input for evaluation and the priority setting process. It has been

Box 9.2: limitations with cost-of-illness studies

- Existing expenditure on a disease, no matter how large, is not sufficient in itself to justify further expenditure (i.e. description is not evaluation, but may input into evaluation). In other words, it is not so much the size of the disease burden *per se* that should guide resource allocation, but rather the efficiency of specific interventions designed to reduce the disease burden.

- Care should be taken in interpreting direct costs associated with disease treatment as an estimate of financial savings that would result from prevention of disease. Such potential "cost offsets" are not estimates of immediately realizable savings, but rather "opportunity cost" estimates measuring resources devoted to the treatment of preventable disease that could be available for other purposes. Conversion of opportunity cost savings into financial savings involves a number of practical issues (such as workforce restructuring, professional interests, management policies, and public reaction) as well as theoretical issues (such as the mix between "fixed" and "variable" costs and "lumpiness" in the expansion/contraction of capital equipment and assets).

- Underlying COI studies are several conceptual and methodological issues that impact on the estimates produced. The choice of study perspective, for example, has an important impact on inclusion/exclusion criteria for cost categories. Similarly, it is important to appreciate whether a "prevalence-based" or "incidence-based" approach to costing is being employed. Data sources are also important, particularly whether a "top-down" approach (using broad aggregate data sets that are attributed to individual diseases) or a "bottom-up" approach (with specified care pathways based on patient level data) is being used.

argued, for example, that priorities for illness prevention and health promotion should be guided by information that includes the public health significance of health problems; their preventability (efficacy/effectiveness); and the relative cost-effectiveness (efficiency) of specific measures aimed at achieving the potential reductions in the disease burden (78).

Prediction: what future trends are likely with regard to obesity?

With prediction, the task is to estimate future trends in risk factors, disease incidence/prevalence, health status, and resource use. In this chapter, prediction will be illustrated within an evaluation context to help ascertain whether the introduction of a national obesity prevention program is likely to represent value-for-money.

Readers interested in other aspects of prediction associated with obesity are encouraged to visit other chapters in Part 1 of the book.

Evaluation: assessing efficiency in obesity prevention

Review of the economic literature on cost-effectiveness

A full economic evaluation analyses both the costs and outcomes of a chosen intervention with a comparator, usually "current practice", to assess what difference the intervention will make to the disease burden. Thus the change in costs is compared with the anticipated change in outcomes and reported as incremental cost-effectiveness ratios (ICERs). Unfortunately, full economic evaluations of obesity interventions are relatively few and have only started to appear in academic journals over the past few years. It is imperative that future studies of the effectiveness of interventions for both the prevention and treatment of obesity incorporate full economic evaluations so that informed decisions can be made about the allocation of resources to obesity relative to other diseases and to specific interventions for its prevention and management (79). Table 9.7 provides a summary of the available economic evaluation studies, while Box 9.3 provides a brief glossary of key economic appraisal terminology.

Interventions for the prevention of obesity

The only economic evaluation identified of an intervention directed at the prevention of obesity is that by Wang *et al.*, 2003, (80) which assessed the cost-effectiveness of Planet Health, an interdisciplinary school-based intervention. Whilst there are no other obesity prevention interventions to which it can be compared, the authors indicate that the program's cost-effectiveness ratio of US\$4305 per QALY compares favorably with other related interventions. The dearth of economic evaluations of potential preventative interventions has been noted and commented upon in the literature (81).

Interventions for the treatment of obesity

Hughes and McGuire in their 1997 review of economic work in the field of obesity (15) reported only two economic evaluations relating to the treatment of obesity, whereas the recent systematic review by Avenell *et al.*, 2004, (82) identified 15, plus four systematic reviews. The latter review groups the studies by intervention types (pharmacological, seven; surgery, eight; and lifestyle, four) and by study design (cost-utility analysis, six; cost-effectiveness, eight; and cost-minimization, one). We have identified several additional studies, one a cost-utility analysis of a surgical intervention (83) and the other, a cost-effectiveness analysis of a lifestyle intervention (84). Acknowledgement is made of the above two reviews (15, 82) which have been drawn upon in preparing Table 9.7.

Pharmacological interventions. Pharmacological interventions for obesity include Orlistat, Sibutramine, and Metformin. Whilst the systematic review of Orlistat by

Table 9.7 Evaluation studies

Type of intervention	Author	Year	Country	Intervention	Study design	Results
Preventive interventions	Wang et al. (80)	2003	US	School-based intervention designed to increase physical activity, decrease TV viewing, increase fruit and vegetable intake and reduce fat intake	Cost-utility	$US4305 per QALY saved
Treatment interventions **i. Pharmacological** Orlistat	Foxcroft et al. (85)	2000	UK	120 mg of Orlistat three times a day in combination with a hypocaloric diet vs. placebo plus diet	Cost-utility	£45 881 per QALY gained (range £19 452 to £55 391)
	Lamotte et al. (86)	2002	Belgium	2-year treatment with Orlistat with diet vs. placebo with diet in 4 types of obese Type 2 diabetic patients	Cost-effectiveness	ICER (euros per life-year gained): €19 986 if no other conditions €7407 if hypercholesterolemia €7388 if arterial hypertension €3462 if both
	Maetzel et al. (87)	2003	US	1- year treatment with Orlistat plus standard diabetes therapy and weight management strategies vs. standard diabetes therapy and weight management strategies for Type 2 diabetes patients	Cost-effectiveness	$US8327 per event-free life-year gained
Sibutramine	BASF (unpublished) (88)	2000	UK	2 placebo-controlled trials in which Sibutramine was combined with diet and exercise	Cost-utility	Cost/QALY gained through reduction in coronary heart disease alone £42 000; cost/QALY gained through reduction in diabetes

	Author	Year	Country	Intervention	Type of analysis	Results
						incidence alone £77 000; cost/QALY gained through weight loss alone £19 000; combined cost £10 500 per QALY gained
	Warren et al. (89)	2004	UK	Sibutramine vs. diet and lifestyle advice	Cost-utility	Cost/QALY £4780
Metformin	Clarke et al. (90)	2001	UK	Metformin in blood glucose control vs. conventional diet therapy	Cost-effectiveness	71% chance of being cost savings and 95% chance that cost per life year gained < £1600
ii. Surgical	Martin et al. (91)	1995	US	Gastric bypass surgery vs. very low calorie diet in obese persons	Cost-effectiveness	Report average rather than incremental cost effectiveness ratios. Cost per pound lost US$260–US$300 for surgical therapy, and US$65–US$300 for medical therapy
	Chua, Mendiola (92)	1995	US	Laparoscopic vertical banded gastroplasty vs. open gastric bypass	Cost-minimization	Intervention cheaper (US$12 800 compared to US$16 700), shorter hospital stay, but longer operating time
	Sjöström et al. (93)	1995	Sweden	Banding or vertical banded gastroplasty or gastric bypass vs. conventional treatment	Cost-effectiveness	Direct cost of surgery 16.5 million Swedish krona/100 patients over 10 years; patients lost 30–40 kg over 2 years
	Segal et al. (94)	1998	Australia	Gastric bypass surgery for seriously obese	Cost-effectiveness	ICER of AUD$12 300 unless targeted to impaired glucose tolerance patients (AUD$4600)
	Van Gemert et al. (95)	1999	Netherlands	Vertical banded gastroplasty vs. no treatment	Cost-utility	Surgery saved US $3928–$4004 per QALY

continued

Table 9.7 (continued) Evaluation studies

Type of intervention	Author	Year	Country	Intervention	Study design	Results
	Nguyen et al. (96)	2001	US	Laparoscopic vs. open gastric bypass for morbidly obese patients	Cost-utility	ICERS not reported. Costs not significantly different, and laparoscopic procedure produced greater weight loss and improvement in quality of life during recovery period
	Craig and Tseng (83)	2002	US	Gastric bypass surgery for severely obese vs. no treatment	Cost-utility	ICER = US$5000–US$16100 per to QALY for women; US$10000–US$35 600 for men depending on age and initial BMI
iii. Lifestyle	Kaplan et al. (97, 98)	1987 1988	US	4 treatment groups – (i) diet and behavior therapy (ii) exercise and behavior therapy (iii) diet, exercise and behavior therapy (iv) control – education about diabetes	Cost-utility	ICER US$10 870 per well life year. Sensitivity analysis on effectiveness of intervention and duration of benefit produced a range of estimates US$4503–US$18 011
	Johannesson et al. (99)	1992	Sweden	Diet vs. drug treatment (generally atenolol) for hypertension in obese men	Cost-effectiveness	ICER for additional life year saved from diet vs. drug ranged from 46 000 to 205 000 Swedish crowns
	Salkeld et al. (100)	1997	Australia	2 interventions – (i) video plus written self-help materials; (ii) video; control routine care in general practice	Cost-utility	If assumed changes in risk factors were sustained for 2 years, ICER = AUD$4342 per additional QALY amongst high-risk males

Dalton et al. (84)	1997	Australia	GP-led behavioral change program involving weight reduction targeted at diabetes prevention	Cost-effectiveness	ICER = AUD$63 000 per life year saved if implemented as an independent program, or AUD$4000 if piggy-backed onto a CVD intervention
Segal et al. (94)	1997	Australia	Interventions: (i) diet and behavioral therapy for seriously obese (ii) diet and behavioral therapy for women with previous gestational diabetes (iii) group behavioral therapy for overweight and obese men (iv) GP advice for high-risk adults (v) media campaign	Cost-effectiveness	Group behavioral therapy and media campaign – cost savings. Diet, behavioral and GP programs – ICERS of AUD$1000–$2600
Goldfield et al. (101)	2001	US	Group vs. mixed family-based behavioral treatment for childhood obesity	Cost-effectiveness	At 12 months, decrease of 0.0004Z-BMI units per $ in mixed group, decrease of 0.001Z-BMI units per $ in group treatment

ICER: Incremental cost-effectiveness ratio

Box 9.3: Glossary of economic appraisal terminology

Cost–benefit analysis (CBA): An analytic tool for estimating the net social benefit of a program or intervention as the incremental benefit of the program less the incremental cost, with all benefits and costs measured in dollars (102).

Cost-effectiveness analysis (CEA): An analytic tool in which costs and effects of a program and at least one alternative (usually current practice) are calculated and presented in a ratio of incremental cost to incremental effects. Effects are measured as physical health outcomes (such as cancers prevented, women screened, or life years saved), rather than monetary measures as in CBA (based on 102).

Cost-utility analysis (CUA): An analytic tool in which costs and effects of a program and at least one alternative (usually current practice) are calculated and presented in a ratio of incremental cost to incremental effects. Effects are measured as quality adjusted life years, rather than monetary measures as in CBA (based on 102). Quality adjusted life years are a measure of health outcomes that combine both mortality and morbidity impacts. For CUA, the measurement instrument must be a preference-based instrument, rather than a simple descriptive instrument.

Cost-minimization analysis (CMA): An analytic tool used to compare the net costs of programs, where there is sufficient evidence to conclude that the outcomes are equivalent (based on 102).

Threshold analysis: A decision aid that can be undertaken in various ways to assist resource allocation decisions. Usually the critical value(s) of a parameter or parameters central to a decision to invest or disinvest are identified. For example, the decision maker might specify an acceptable level of investment or an acceptable return on investment. The analyst then uses available information to assess which combinations of parameter estimates could cause the threshold to be exceeded or achieved. Alternatively, the threshold values that cause the program to be regarded as too costly or not cost-effective could be defined (103).

Steady-state analysis: A form of economic modeling where the program under analysis is assumed to be fully implemented and running in accordance with its efficacy potential. A representative period is selected (usually 1 year) and the net costs are compared with the net benefits attributable to the program for the representative period.

Incremental cost-effectiveness ratio (ICER): The ratio of the difference in net costs between two alternatives to the difference in net effectiveness between the same two alternatives (based on 102).

Acceptability curve approach: A way of presenting the ICER results which incorporates both the decision rule and the level of uncertainty associated with the available evidence on costs and outcomes. Acceptability curves provide more information on uncertainty, for example, than do confidence intervals (based on 104).

O'Meara *et al.*, 2001(105), identified 14 RCTs investigating its efficacy, there have been only three economic evaluations to date, one of which was a confidential submission by a drugs manufacturer (106). A cost-utility study, conducted by Foxcroft and Milne, 2000 (85), as part of a systematic review, confined itself to the estimated effects of the drug on short-term QALYs, given the absence of data enabling the modeling of long-term benefits.

Several studies have focused on Orlistat for type 2 diabetes patients. The cost-effectiveness study by Lamotte *et al.*, 2002 (86), used Markov modeling to predict the morbidity and mortality over a 10-year period associated with a 2-year Orlistat treatment. Economic evaluations are based on the making of assumptions around parameters subject to uncertainty, and it has been suggested that this study greatly overestimated the cost-effectiveness of Orlistat by using some inappropriate parameter estimates (107). Maetzel *et al.*, 2003 (87), in a simulation of the diabetes-related complications and mortality of a shorter course of the drug (1 year) over a longer timeframe (11 years), used higher rates of complications and lower relative risk reductions, and concluded that Orlistat combined with conventional diabetes and weight management approaches was cost-effective.

A systematic review by O'Meara *et al.*, 2002 (108), identified 16 randomized controlled trials of Sibutramine, but no published economic evaluations. It referred to an unpublished cost-utility analysis undertaken as part of a pharmaceutical company submission (88), but queried aspects of the methodology, including the estimated QALY gains per kilogram of weight loss, suggesting the cost-effectiveness may have been over-stated. However, a recent study published since the systematic review (89) reported better results stemming from the use of Sibutramine combined with diet and lifestyle advice. Another cost-effectiveness study of both Orlistat and Sibutramine as long-term therapies (109) has been recently undertaken in The Czech Republic, but is not available in English.

There is one other economic evaluation of a pharmacological intervention for obesity, namely the use of Metformin in blood glucose control vs. conventional diet therapy for obese type 2 diabetic patients (90). It is the only one of the 15 economic evaluations of obesity treatments to make use of an acceptability curve approach.

Surgical interventions. The systematic review of surgical interventions for the morbidly obese by Clegg *et al.*, 2003 (110), plus the recent broad systematic review of all types of obesity interventions (82), and our own literature search identified a total of seven economic evaluations of surgical interventions. Four focused on gastric bypass (83, 91, 94, 96), two on vertical banded gastroplasty (92, 95), whilst the other considered both these options plus gastric banding (93). The analysis of gastric bypass by Segal *et al.*, 1998 (94) was within a group of interventions used to assess the cost-effectiveness of primary prevention of type 2 diabetes.

Three of the studies are cost-effectiveness studies, three cost-utility, whilst one is essentially a cost-minimization analysis in that it does not report effectiveness outcomes.

The results of the various studies do not lend themselves to comparison given their different settings, the different perspectives adopted by the studies and the consequent variation in the costs and benefits taken into account.

Lifestyle interventions. The 2004 systematic review (82) noted the absence of economic evaluations of diet, exercise, or behavior therapy. That review broadened its search to canvass interventions not necessarily targeted exclusively at obese persons, but to persons for whom obesity is often a serious complication or subsequent disease. It identified five studies targeted at either people with type 2 diabetes (97, 98) or overweight people at risk of the sequelae of obesity (94, 99, 100). We have identified an additional two economic evaluations of lifestyle interventions (84, 101).

The Kaplan and Salkeld studies (97, 98, 100) were cost-utility studies. The former (97, 98) compared three different combinations of diet, exercise, and behavior therapy against a control group receiving diabetes education only. The usefulness of the study results is limited by the small sample size, the short follow-up period, and the failure of the study to track associated health service use apart from medications. The cost-utility study by Salkeld et al., 1997 (100) was better in terms of sample size and costs included, but would have benefited from long-term follow-up, given the uncertainty of the results. It investigated two lifestyle interventions delivered by general practitioners to people with one or more modifiable cardiovascular disease risk factors. The other four studies are cost-effectiveness analyses. Johannesson and Fagerberg, 1992 (99), targeted obese men in a trial of diet vs. drug treatment to control hypertension. The study ran a number of simulations each varying the assumptions about the effect of risk factor changes on the risk of coronary heart disease. The Australian study by Segal et al., 1998 (94) used a Markov approach over a 25-year follow-up period to explore six different interventions for the primary prevention of type 2 diabetes. The interventions were not implemented, but were modeled using assumptions about baseline health states, transition rates, and effectiveness based on the literature and existing databases. Whilst the authors are right in suggesting that the cost offsets downstream may be under-estimated, given their exclusion of costs of diseases other than diabetes which are caused by obesity, the assumption that the effectiveness of the interventions is sustained for the full follow-up period is probably an over-statement. Another Australian study by Dalton et al., 1997 (84), reported that a behavioral change weight-reduction program targeted at diabetes prevention was significantly more cost-effective if piggy-backed onto a cardiovascular disease intervention given the joint risk factors shared by diabetes and cardiovascular disease, the associated cost savings, and improved rates of participation and adherence.

The other cost-effectiveness analysis, Goldfield et al., 2001 (101), concluded that group treatment used in a family-based behavioral therapy intervention for obese children was more cost-effective than mixed treatment. The inclusion of costs incurred by participating families may have further strengthened this conclusion, presuming that the mixed treatment consumed more of family time.

The case study revisited – from description to evaluation

The purpose now in our case study is to scope the economic case for introducing a co-ordinated national program to prevent overweight and obesity in children and adolescents. It is important to note that our analysis is not being undertaken to address technical efficiency issues related to the detailed design and composition of a national obesity prevention program. Rather, the purpose is to address the issue of allocative efficiency; that is, whether investment in obesity prevention is likely to be a "worthwhile" use of limited health funds. The consequence of this focus is that marginal analysis of design issues for each intervention, or the balance between interventions that might make up such an initiative, is not addressed in this section. The focus is rather on broad-based incremental analysis comparing the net additional resource costs of obesity prevention in childhood (as a composite program) with the net additional benefits that such an initiative is estimated to yield. While research on the efficiency of individual interventions is highly desirable and should be undertaken as soon as practicable, a decision on the essential economic merit of targeting obesity in children and adolescents can reasonably be based on the economic analysis set out below.

Overview of method

The assessment of whether overweight/obesity prevention in childhood represents "value-for-money" is based on an economic technique called "threshold analysis" (Box 9.3). For this case study, an acceptable cost-effectiveness ratio of AUD$30 000 per QALY is assumed as the key threshold parameter. While notions of cost-effectiveness are inherently subjective and country specific, cost-effectiveness results equal to or below AUD$30 000 per QALY would be regarded favorably in Australia. This judgment reflects available evidence on the current use of resources in the Australian health sector (111–113).

The next step is to make an informed judgment on the potential efficacy/effectiveness of a nationally co-ordinated obesity prevention program introduced in the Australian context. Based on the information set out in Table 9.7, together with information provided in Parts 2 and 3 of this book, it is assumed that a 1–2 per cent fall per annum in the prevalence of overweight/obesity in children and adolescents could be achieved. "Steady-state analysis" (Box 9.3) is utilized, whereby the costs of running the obesity prevention program for a representative period (1 year) is compared with the corresponding impacts attributed to the program. The COI/BOD information, set out above, is then used to work out the potential health gains and cost offsets from investment in obesity prevention.

It is important to note that health gains and cost offsets associated with lower levels of obesity-related disease will accrue to children and adolescents in the near future (i.e. while they are still young), as well as in the longer term (i.e. as adults) if they maintain healthy weight. In the short-term, childhood overweight/obesity is associated with both physical and psychosocial consequences (114, 115). In the longer term, the greatest risk is the increased likelihood of adult overweight/obesity with its associated health risks. The level and quality of evidence available on relative risks associated with overweight and obesity is stronger for adults than it is for children/adolescents. In this initial scoping exercise, therefore, only the longer-term benefits accruing to adults due to overweight/obesity prevention in their childhood/adolescence are estimated. Clearly, this approach will yield a conservative estimate of the total potential benefits, but it will provide a solid foundation for assessing the economic credentials of investment in the prevention of overweight/obesity in children/adolescents.

The steps involved in our threshold analysis are set out in Box 9.4. The first four steps we have already covered above and are listed in Box 9.1. In this section we will focus on the remaining three steps that take us from description to evaluation.

Box 9.4: Steps in developing our COI/BOD study into an economic evaluation (threshold analysis)

+ **Steps One to Four:** see Box 9.1.
+ **Step Five:** estimate the potential health improvement and health cost offsets associated with possible falls in the prevalence of overweight/obesity in adults (i.e. recalculate the PAFs for different levels of risk factor prevalence);
+ **Step Six:** estimate the link between reductions in the prevalence of childhood overweight/obesity and the consequent reductions in adult overweight/obesity; and
+ **Step Seven:** using these building blocks, estimate the level of investment in a national obesity prevention program that achieves an AUD$30 000 per QALY threshold result.

Step five: estimate the health gains and health cost offsets for adults associated with falls in the prevalence of overweight/obesity in adults

The annual health burden and health-care expenditure attributable to obesity/overweight in adults was calculated for the current prevalence of overweight (see Table 9.2) and obesity (see Table 9.3) in the Australian community. It is possible to estimate the potential impact of reducing BMI levels to normal weight by recalculating the PAFs for anticipated falls in prevalence, keeping the relative risks the same. Table 9.8 summarizes the results assuming uniform falls in the prevalence of overweight/obesity of 1 and 2 per cent. It is clear that substantial health gains and cost offsets are potentially

Table 9.8 Potential health gain and cost offsets due to falls in adult overweight/obesity

Prevalence[a] of overweight/obesity in Australian population	Health-care expenditure[b] on overweight/obesity related diseases AUD$M	DALYs[c] due to overweight/obesity related diseases
Current prevalence	1687	122 986
1% fall in prevalence	1632[d]	118 991[d]
Health gain and cost offset	**55**	**3995**
2% fall in prevalence	1578[d]	114 990[d]
Health gain and cost offset	**109**	**7996**

[a]Taken from Tables 9.2 and 9.3.

[b]Taken from Table 9.6.

[c]Taken from Table 9.5.

[d]Calculated using the Excel spreadsheet. The reference year for the estimates is 2000.

available from achieving small reductions in the prevalence of overweight/obesity, even when very conservative estimates are made of those potential gains.

It is important to recall, as stated above, that cost offset estimates are "opportunity cost" estimates which are only broadly indicative of potential financial savings through additional prevention and/or treatment interventions. Cost offsets are usually calculated by applying the percentage reduction in new cases for the specified diseases to the corresponding reference year disease cost estimates. This calculation, in effect, uses the current average cost of care to compute future offsets. As for the corresponding DALY estimates, this assumes that the current relationship between cost (and health status) and incident cases does not change through time.

Step six: estimate the link between reductions in childhood overweight/obesity and consequent reductions in adult overweight/obesity

The measurement of longer-term benefits from preventing overweight/obesity in childhood also requires evidence on the probability that overweight/obese children become overweight/obese adults. Fortunately, there is published evidence available based on logistic models which fit available cohort data between overweight/obesity in children and adolescents with overweight/obesity in adults (116). These data suggest that there is a strong probability of overweight/obese children becoming overweight/obese adults. Overweight children at age 15, for example, have a 75 per cent chance (males) and a 64 per cent chance (females) of becoming overweight adults at age 35. Overweight young adults at age 20 have an 89 per cent chance (males and females) of becoming overweight adults at age 35. The probability of having a BMI >25 at age 35 increased in this study with childhood/adolescent BMI percentile and with age (116).

Table 9.9 Probabilities of childhood overweight/obesity becoming adult overweight/obesity

Age (years)	Probability[a] of adult overweight (%)		Probability[b] of adult obesity (%)	
	Men	**Women**	**Men**	**Women**
12	63	60	38	50
15	75	64	54	60
20	89	89	98	99

[a]and [b]The probabilities are taken from Guo et al., 2002 (116).

In Table 9.9, representative probabilities from this study are documented for ages 12, 15 and 20, for both males and females. These probabilities were used to estimate the likely reductions in *adult* obesity/overweight resulting from potential reductions in *childhood* overweight/obesity attributable to a national obesity prevention program. These likely reductions in the prevalence of adult overweight/obesity were in turn expressed as potential health gains and cost offsets. Discounting (5 per cent) was used to express these potential gains in present value terms for our reference year (2000). A 30-year time lag was incorporated as a simple approximation of the lag between childhood overweight/obesity and the expression of disease in adulthood. The results are presented in Table 9.10.

Step seven: using these building blocks, estimate the level of investment in a national obesity prevention program that achieves an AUD$30 000 per QALY result

The final step in the threshold analysis is to use the various data presented above to compute the level of investment that would yield a cost-utility ratio of AUD$30 000 per DALY recovered. In making this calculation, the formula set out in Box 9.5 was used.

Solving this formula for a 1 per cent fall in the prevalence of overweight/obesity and a 5 per cent discount rate, yields the following results for the representative ages given in Tables 9.9 and 9.10:

◆ age 12 data: $17.07M + $7.73M cost offset = warranted investment of $24.80M;

◆ age 15 data: $19.32M + $8.70M cost offset = warranted investment of $28.02M;

◆ age 20 data: $24.69M + $11.20M cost offset = warranted investment of $35.89M.

The threshold analysis suggests that an investment of only AUD$25 to 36 million per annum would have an important impact on addressing childhood obesity. If a 2 per cent fall in the prevalence of childhood overweight/obesity was achieved, then the "economically warranted" level of investment would approximately double to AUD$50 to 72 million per annum. Alternatively, a 2 per cent fall in prevalence combined with an investment of AUD$25 to 36 million per annum is likely to achieve a cost-effectiveness ratio of approximately AUD$15 000 per DALY avoided.

Table 9.10 Health gain and cost offsets for adult overweight/obesity due to falls in childhood overweight/obesity

Age	1% fall in childhood prevalence			2% fall in childhood prevalence		
	Adult DALY gain (discounted 5% 30 year lag)	Cost offsets undiscounted AUD$M	Cost offsets discounted 5% with 30 year lag AUD$M	Adult DALY gain (discounted 5% 30 year lag)	Cost offsets undiscounted AUD$M	Cost offsets discounted 5% with 30 year lag AUD$M
Age 12	2459 (569)	33.39	7.73	4922 (1139)	66.79	15.46
Age 15	2784 (644)	37.58	8.70	5575 (1290)	75.28	17.42
Age 20	3556 (823)	48.40	11.20	7117 (1647)	96.80	22.40

The estimates in Table 9.10 are derived using the probabilities for men and women in Table 9.9 and the detailed health gain/cost offset information in the Excel spreadsheet. The reference year for the estimates is 2000.

Box 9.5: Formula for the threshold analysis

[Net Investment in Obesity Program]/[DALYs recovered] = AUD$30 000 per DALY where:

◆ "AUD$30 000 per DALY" is the key threshold parameter of acceptable "value-for-money";

◆ "Net Investment in Obesity Program" is the suggested annual investment minus the present value (5 per cent) of the anticipated annual cost offsets; and

◆ "DALYs recovered" is the present value (5 per cent) of the anticipated annual DALYs recovered.

These results assume a discount rate of 5 per cent per annum and a 30-year time lag before cost offsets and health gains are achieved. If the discount rate were reduced from 5 to 3 per cent, for example, then the warranted investment range would increase to AUD$44 to 64 million per annum for the 1 per cent prevalence fall. If the discount rate were increased to 7 per cent, then the warranted investment would decrease accordingly.

Conclusions from threshold analysis

From an allocative efficiency perspective, there are quite reasonable grounds for concluding that an investment of at least AUD$25 to 36 million per annum in a national obesity prevention program is warranted in Australia and would achieve a major impact on addressing childhood obesity. While the estimates from the threshold analysis set out above are more indicative than definitive, they have been constructed on a conservative set of assumptions that should engender confidence. It is noticeable from the analysis that the probability of adult overweight/obesity increases the longer the delay in addressing overweight/obesity in childhood. This is an important finding from a public health perspective.

The "economically warranted" level of investment will clearly vary as key assumptions in the analysis are varied, particularly the assumptions for: the list of diseases where sufficient causal evidence exists to establish a link with overweight/obesity; the estimates for the health burden and recurrent health-care expenditure associated with those attributable diseases; the relative risk of disease with/without exposure to the risk factors of overweight/obesity (conservative relative risks were adopted in the threshold analysis); the inclusion/exclusion of direct expenditures on treating the risk factor itself and not just the resulting diseases (excluded in the present analysis); the inclusion/exclusion of diseases in childhood/adolescence that are causally related to overweight/obesity (excluded in the present analysis); the appropriate probabilities of remaining overweight/ obese in adulthood, if overweight/obese in childhood/adolescence; the appropriate time lag before diseases manifest in adulthood, given childhood overweight/obesity; and the choice of discount rate.

As all of these assumptions were conservative in the threshold analysis, increased confidence can be placed on the economic credentials for obesity prevention presented here. While a formal sensitivity analysis has not been undertaken, sensible variations are much more likely to increase the minimum level of investment that is "economically warranted" than to reduce it. Adding in estimates for the potential health gain/cost offsets for preventing overweight/obesity-related diseases in childhood, for example, would justify additional investment (particularly as time lags would be minimal). Similarly, inclusion of potential reductions in overweight/obesity treatment programs (such as stomach stapling) would also warrant additional expenditures in childhood interventions.

From evaluation to decision-making on obesity prevention priorities

Before closing this chapter, it is worth considering what guidance health economics can offer if the economically warranted level of investment exceeds the resources made available for obesity prevention. Further, even if funding were considered sufficient, how should the funding be distributed between the various interventions that might make up a national obesity prevention program?

Often such resource allocation choices in health care are driven by historical patterns of expenditure and/or the influence of professional, industrial, and community interest groups. Economic analysis can provide additional information to help decision-makers set funding priorities that will improve the effectiveness and efficiency of health services. The traditional economic approach involves maximizing health gain (however measured) subject to a budget constraint, which implies ranking programs according to their incremental cost-effectiveness ratios (ICERs). This traditional approach, however, is subject to three important difficulties: limitations in economic evaluation methodology; incorporating ethical values, particularly equity principles; and practical constraints arising from the political, institutional, and environmental context in which priority setting takes place (76, 117, 118). These limitations suggest a broader approach to economic analysis than one based purely on the mechanistic application of ICERs.

In Australia, Carter and Vos have developed and trialed an innovative approach to priority setting (termed "ACE", derived from Assessing Cost-Effectiveness) that involves: a standardized economic protocol to overcome methodological confounding; the close involvement of policy-makers and clinicians; and a concept of benefit based on health gain, but including broader factors that impinge on policy decisions (119). Trialed in cancer, heart disease, and mental health, the ACE approach is currently being applied to obesity prevention. The key characteristics of the ACE approach are:

♦ a clear rationale for the selection of options for change (either introducing new initiatives or modifying existing interventions);

- adoption of a two-stage approach to the assessment of benefit, involving both health gain (i.e. cost per DALY saved) and explicit "judgment" aspects which are included as second stage filters ("equity", "strength of evidence", "feasibility", and "acceptability to stakeholders");

- use of an economic protocol specifically developed for each study;

- an evidence-based approach facilitated by a small team of multidisciplinary researchers;

- extensive uncertainty analysis; and

- involvement of stakeholders through a Steering Committee, that both guides and participates in the analysis.

The Steering Committee is the primary mechanism for incorporating the views of stakeholders and ensuring "due process". Its functions include selection of the options for change; defining "benefit" and the associated criteria by which the selected interventions are judged; critically examining the evidence and analyses presented by the research team; and formulating conclusions based on the presented evidence.

The ACE approach recognizes the reality that technical approaches, however rigorous or sophisticated, will never be able to deal with the complexity and contested nature of priority setting. Equally, it recognizes the importance of evidence and that "due process" should utilize the sort of information on efficacy/effectiveness, efficiency, equity, and needs provided by technical analysis. Both technical analysis and due process need to be involved in any approach to priority setting that is seeking strong theoretical foundations and empirical validity.

Summary

Obesity prevention programs in countries with high or increasing incidence and mortality rates are likely to have strong economic credentials. Further work is necessary, however, to explore in more detail the value of the relative components of these campaigns as a way of ensuring that they continue to be cost-effective in the long term.

Economic evaluation can play an important role, along with other disciplines, in aiding planners to make optimal decisions about what type of obesity prevention interventions to undertake, for how long, and at what level of investment. For this to occur, however, it is important for planners and decision-makers to become informed users of what the discipline of health economics has to offer. Much is said in the name of "economic theory" that is founded more on ideology than on economic theory or empirical evidence. Users need to be aware when economics is being used in "positive" or "normative" mode and need to be conscious of the important distinctions between the tasks of description, prediction, and evaluation. It is hoped that the ACE: Obesity study currently underway in Australia will assist policy-makers in this regard by providing sound information on cost-effectiveness, balanced by a concern for due process and explicit value judgments.

References

1. Seidell JC, Verschuren WM, van Leer EM, Kromhout D (1996). Overweight, underweight, and mortality. A prospective study of 48 287 men and women. *Arch Intern Med* **156**, 958–63.

2. Bender R, Trautner C, Spraul M, Berger M (1998). Assessment of excess mortality in obesity. *Am J Epidemiol* **147**, 42–8.

3. Must A, Spadano J, Coakley EH, Field AE, Colditz G, Dietz WH. (1999). The disease burden associated with overweight and obesity. *JAMA* **282**, 1523–9.

4. Manson JE, Colditz GA, Stampfer MJ, *et al.* (1990). A prospective study of obesity and risk of coronary heart disease in women. *N Engl J Med* **322**, 882–9.

5. Rimm EB, Stampfer MJ, Giovannucci E, *et al.* (1995). Body size and fat distribution as predictors of coronary heart disease among middle-aged and older US men. *Am J Epidemiol* **141**, 1117–27.

6. Colditz GA, Willett WC, Rotnitzky A, Manson JE (1995). Weight gain as a risk factor for clinical diabetes mellitus in women. *Ann Int Med* **122**, 481–6.

7. Njolstad I, Arnesen E, Lund-Larsen PG (1998). Sex differences in risk factors for clinical diabetes mellitus in a general population: a 12-year follow-up of the Finnmark Study. *Am J Epidemiol* **147**, 49–58.

8. Mokdad AH, Bowman BA, Ford ES, Vinicor F, Marks JS, Koplan JP (2001). The continuing epidemics of obesity and diabetes in the United States. *JAMA* **286**, 1195–200.

9. Huang Z, Hankinson SE, Colditz GA, *et al.* (1997). Dual effects of weight and weight gain on breast cancer risk. *JAMA* **278**, 1407–11.

10. Giovannucci E, Rimm EB, Chute CG, *et al.* (1994). Obesity and benign prostatic hyperplasia. *Am J of Epidemiol* **140**, 989–1002.

11. Flegal K, Carroll M, Kuczmarski R, Johnson C (1998). Overweight and obesity in the United States: prevalence and trends, 1960–1994. *Int J Obes* **22**, 39–47.

12. Martinez JA, Moreno B, Martinez-Gonzalez MA (2004). Prevalence of obesity in Spain. *Obes Rev* **5**, 171–2.

13. Manson JE, Van Itallie TB (1996). America's obesity epidemic and women's health. *J Women's Health* **5**, 329–34.

14. Lobstein T, Frelut ML (2003). Prevalence of overweight among children in Europe. *Obes Rev* **4**, 195–200.

15. Hughes D, McGuire A (1997). A review of the economic analysis of obesity. *Br Med Bull* **53**, 253–63.

16. Kortt MA, Langley PC, Cox ER (1998). A review of cost-of illness studies on obesity. *Clin Ther* **20**, 772–9.

17. Thompson D, Wolf AM (2001). The medical-care cost burden of obesity. *Obes Rev* **2**, 189–97.

18. Gorsky RD, Shaffer PA, Pamuk E (1996). The 25-year health care costs of women who remain overweight after 40 years of age. *Am J Prev Med* **12**, 338–94.

19. Thompson D, Edelsberg J, Colditz GA, Bird AP, Oster G (1999). Lifetime health and economic consequences of obesity. *Arch Intern Med* **159**, 2177–83.

20. Oster G, Thompson D, Edelsberg J, Bird A, Colditz GA (1999). Lifetime health and economic benefits of weight loss among obese persons. *Amer J Public Health* **89**, 1536–42.

21. Colditz G (1992). Economic costs of obesity. *Amer J Clin Nutr* **55**, 503–7S.

22. Sjöström L, Larsson B, Backman L, *et al.* (1992). Swedish obese subjects (SOS). Recruitment for an intervention study and a selected description of the obese state. *Int J Obes Relat Metab Disord* **16**, 465–79.

23. **Wolf AM, Colditz GA** (1994). The cost of obesity: The US perspective. *Pharmacoeconomics* **5**, 34–7.

24. **Segal L, Carter R, Zimmet P** (1994). The cost of obesity: the Australian perspective. *Pharmacoeconomics* **5** (Suppl), 45–52.

25. **Seidell J** (1995). The impact of obesity on health status: some implications for health care costs. *Int J Obes* **19** (Suppl 6), S13–S16.

26. **Levy E, Levy P, Le Pen C, Basdevant A** (1995). The economic cost of obesity: the French situation. *Int J Obes Relat Metab Disord* **19**, 788–92.

27. **Wolf AM, Colditz GA** (1996). Social and economic effects of body weight in the United States. *Amer J Clin Nutr* **63**, 466–9S.

28. **Swinburn B, Ashton T, Gillespie J, et al.** (1997). Health care costs of obesity in New Zealand. *Int J Obes*, **21**, 891–6.

29. **Wolf AM, Colditz GA** (1998). Current estimates of the economic costs of obesity in the United States. *Obes Res* **6**, 97–106.

30. **Thompson D, Edelsberg J, Kinsey KL, Oster G** (1998). Estimated economic costs of obesity to US business. *Amer J Health Promot* **13**, 120–7.

31. **Birmingham CL, Muller JL, Palepu A, Spinelli JJ, Anis AH** (1999). The cost of obesity in Canada. *Canad Med Assoc J* **160**, 483–8.

32. **Colditz GA** (1999). Economic costs of obesity and inactivity. *Med Sc Sports Exer* **31**, S663–7.

33. **Pereira J, Mateus C, Amaral MH** (2000). Direct costs of obesity in Portugal. *J Interl Society Pharmacoeconomics Outcomes Res* **3**, 64.

34. **Oster G, Edelsberg J, O'Sullivan AK, et al.** (2000). The clinical and economic burden of obesity in a managed care setting. *Am J Manag Care* **6**, 681–9.

35. **Finkelstein EA, Fiedelkorn IC, Wang G** (2004). State-level estimates of annual medical expenditures attributable to obesity. *Obes Res* **12**, 18–24.

36. **West R** (1994). Obesity. Office of Health Economics Monographs on Current Health Issues, no. 112. Office of Health Economics, London.

37. **Hakkinen U** (1991). The production of health and the demand for health care in Finland. *Soc Studies Sci* **33**, 225–37.

38. **Gorstein J, Grosse RN** (1994). The indirect costs of obesity to society. *Pharmacoeconomics*, **5** (Suppl 1), 58–61.

39. **Seidell JC** (1998). Societal and personal costs of obesity. *Exp Clin Endocrinol Diabetes* **106** (Suppl 2), 7–9.

40. **Lobstein T, Baur L, Uauy R** for the IASO International Obesity Task Force (2004). Obesity in children and young people: a crisis in public health. *Obes Rev* **5** (Suppl 1), 4–85.

41. **Quesenberry CP, Caan B, Jacobsen A** (1998). Obesity, health services use, and health care costs among members of a health maintenance organization. *Arch Inter Med* **158**, 466–72.

42. **Heithoff KA, Cuffel BJ, Kennedy S** (1997). The association between body mass and health care expenditures. *Clin Ther* **19**, 811–20.

43. **Burton WN, Chen CY, Schultz AB, Edington DW** (1998). The economic costs associated with body mass index in a workplace. *J Occup Envir Med* **40**, 786–92.

44. **Wang G, Dietz WH** (2002). Economic burden of obesity in youths aged 6 to 17 years: 1979–1999. *Pediatrics* **109**, E81–1.

45. **Colditz GA, Willett WC, Stampfer MJ, et al.** (1990). Weight as a risk factor for clinical diabetes in women. *Am J Epidemiol* **132**, 501–13.

46. **Chan JM, Rimm EB, Colditz GA, Stampfer MJ, Willett WC** (1994). Obesity, fat distribution and weight gain as risk factors for clinical diabetes in men. *Diabetes Care* **17**, 961–9.

47. Carey VJ, Walters EE, Colditz GA (1997). Body fat distribution and risk of non-insulin-dependent diabetes mellitus in women. The Nurses' Health Study. *Am J Epidemiol* **145**, 614–9.

48. Stampfer MJ, Maclure KM, Colditz GA, Manson JE, Willett WC (1992). Risk of symptomatic gallstones in women with severe obesity. *Am J Clin Nutr* **55**, 652–8.

49. Sahi T, Paffenbarger RS Jr, Hsieh CC, Lee IM (1998). Body mass index, cigarette smoking, and other characteristics as predictors of self-reported, physician-diagnosed gallbladder disease in male college alumni. *Am J Epidemiol* **147**, 644–51.

50. Harris TB, Launer LJ, Madans J, Feldman JJ (1997). Cohort study of effect of being overweight and change in weight on risk of coronary heart disease in old age. *BMJ* **314**, 1791–4.

51. Harris HE, Ellison GT, Richter LM, de Wet T, Levin J (1998). Are overweight women at increased risk of obesity following pregnancy? *Brit J Nutr* **79**, 489–94.

52. Garfinkel L (1992). Overweight and cancer. *Ann Intern Med* **103**, 1034–6.

53. Rexrode KM, Hennekens CH, Willett WC, *et al.* (1997). A prospective study of body mass index, weight change, and risk of stroke in women. *JAMA* **277**, 1539–45.

54. Witteman JC, Willett WC, Stampfer MJ, *et al.* (1989). A prospective study of nutritional factors and hypertension among US women. *Circulation* **80**, 1320–7.

55. Ascherio A, Rimm EB, Giovannucci EL, *et al.* (1992). A prospective study of nutritional factors and hypertension among US men. *Circulation* **86**, 1475–84.

56. Lee IM, Paffenbarger RS Jr (1992). Quetelet's index and risk of colon cancer in college alumni. *J Natl Cancer Inst* **84**, 1326–31.

57. Lubin F, Ruder AM, Wax Y, Modan B (1985). Overweight and changes in weight throughout adult life in breast cancer etiology. A case–control study. *Am J Epidemiol* **122**, 579–88.

58. Tretli S (1989). Height and weight in relation to breast cancer morbidity and mortality. A prospective study of 570,000 women in Norway. *Int J Cancer* **44**, 23–30.

59. Sellers TA, Kushi LH, Potter JD, *et al.* (1992). Effect of family history, body-fat distribution, and reproductive factors on the risk of postmenopausal breast cancer. *N Engl J Med* **326**, 1323–9.

60. Mayberry RM (1994). Age-specific patterns of association between breast cancer and risk factors in black women, ages 20 to 39 and 40 to 54. *Ann Epidemiol* **4**, 205–13.

61. Yong LC, Brown CC, Schatzkin A, Schairer C (1996). Prospective study of relative weight and risk of breast cancer: the Breast Cancer Detection Demonstration Project follow-up study, 1979 to 1987–1989. *Am J Epidemiol* **143**, 985–95.

62. Armstrong B (1999). Personal Communication.

63. Moller H, Mellemgaard A, Lindvig K, Olsen JH (1994). Obesity and cancer risk: a Danish record-linkage study. *Eur J Cancer* **30A**, 344–50.

64. Tavani A, La Vecchia C (1997). Epidemiology of renal-cell carcinoma. *J Nephrol* **10**, 93–106.

65. Anderson JJ, Felson DT (1988). Factors associated with osteoarthritis of the knee in the first national Health and Nutrition Examination Survey (HANES I). Evidence for an association with overweight, race, and physical demands of work. *Am J Epidemiol* **128**, 179–89.

66. Rissanen A, Heliovaara M, Knekt P, Reunanen A, Aromaa A, Maatela J (1990). Risk of disability and mortality due to overweight in a Finnish population. *BMJ* **301**, 835–7.

67. Tsai SP, Gilstrap EL, Cowles SR, Waddell LC Jr, Ross CE (1992). Personal and job characteristics of musculoskeletal injuries in an industrial population. *J Occup Med* **34**, 606–12.

68. Dunstan D, Zimmet P, Welborn T (2001). Diabetes and associated disorders in Australia – 2000. The accelerating epidemic. *The Australian Diabetes, Obesity and Lifestyle Study (AusDiab)*. International Diabetes Institute, Melbourne.

69. **Mathers C, Vos T, Stevenson C** (1999). *The burden of disease and injury in Australia.* Australian Institute of Health and Welfare, Canberra.

70. **Mathers C, Penm R, Sanson-Fisher R, Carter R, Stevenson R** (1998). *Health system cost of cancer in Australia, 1993–94.* Australian Institute of Health and Welfare, Canberra.

71. **Mathers C, Penm R** (1999). *Health system cost of cardiovascular disease and diabetes in Australia, 1993–94.* Australian Institute of Health and Welfare, Canberra.

72. **Mathers C, Penm R** (1999). *Health system cost of injury, poisoning and muskuloskeletal disorders in Australia, 1993–94.* Australian Institute of Health and Welfare, Canberra.

73. **Mathers C, Penm R, Stevenson R, Carter, R** (1998). *Health system cost of diseases and injury in Australia, 1993–94.* Australian Institute of Health and Welfare, Canberra.

74. **Mathers C, Stevenson R, Carter R, Penm R** (1998). *Disease costing methodology used in the Disease Cost and Impacts Study, 1993–94.* Australian Institute of Health and Welfare, Canberra.

75. **AIHW** (2002). *Health Expenditure 2000–01.* Australian Institute of Health and Welfare, Canberra.

76. **Carter R** (2001). *The macro economic evaluation model (MEEM): An approach to priority setting in the health sector.* PhD Thesis, Faculty of Business and Economics. Monash University, Melbourne.

77. **Hughes D, McGuire A, Elliot H, *et al.*** (1999). The cost of obesity in the United Kingdom. *J Drug Assess* **2**, 327–96.

78. **Carter R** (1994). Macro approach to economic appraisal in the health sector. *Aust Econ Rec* **106**, 105–12.

79. **Hutton J** (1994). The economics of treating obesity. *Pharmacoeconomics* **5** (Suppl 1), 66–72.

80. **Wang L, Yang Q, Lowry R, Wechsler H** (2003). Economic analysis of a school-based prevention program. *Obes Res* **11**, 1313–24.

81. **Ganz ML** (2003). The economic evaluation of obesity interventions: its time has come. *Obes Res* **11**,1275–7.

82. **Avenell A, Broom J, Brown TJ, Poobalan A, Aucott L, SC Stearns, *et al.*** (2004). Systematic review of the long-term effects and economic consequences of treatments for obesity and implications for health improvements. *Health Technol Assess* **8**, 1–458.

83. **Craig BM, Tseng DS** (2002). Cost-effectiveness of gastric bypass for severe obesity. *Amer J Med* **113**, 491–8.

84. **Dalton A, Carter R, Dunt D** (1997). *The cost-effectiveness of GP led behavioural change involving weight reduction: implications for the prevention of diabetes.* Working Paper 65, Centre for Health Program Evaluation, Melbourne.

85. **Foxcroft DR, Milne R** (2000). Orlistat for the treatment of obesity: rapid review and cost-effectiveness model. *Obes Rev* **1**, 121–6.

86. **Lamotte M, Annemans L, Lefever A, Nechelput M, Masure J** (2002). A health economic model to assess the long-term effects and cost-effectiveness of Orlistat in obese type 2 diabetic patients. *Diabetes Care* **25**, 303–8.

87. **Maetzel A, Ruof J, Covington M, Wolf A** (2003). Economic evaluation of orlistat in overweight and obese patients with type 2 diabetes mellitus. *Pharmacoeconomics* **21**, 501–12.

88. **BASF Pharma/Knoll** (2000). *Cost-utility analysis of sibutramine. Submission to NICE.* Knoll Limited, Nottingham. Unpublished.

89. **Warren E, Brennan A, Akehurst R** (2004). Cost-effectiveness of sibutramine in the treatment of obesity. *Medical Decision Making* **24**, 9–19.

90. **Clarke P, Gray A, Adler A, Stevens R, Raikou M, Cull C, *et al.*** (2001). Cost-effectiveness analysis of intensive blood-glucose control with metformin in overweight patients with Type II diabetes (UKPDS No. 51). *Diabetologia* **44**, 298–304.

91. Martin LF, Tan T-L, Horn JR, Bixler EO, Kauffman GL, Becker DA, *et al.* (1995). Comparison of the costs associated with medical and surgical treatment of obesity. *Surgery* **118**, 599–606.

92. Chua TY, Mendiola RM (1995). Laparoscopic vertical banded gastroplasty: the Milwaukee experience. *Obes Surg* **5**, 77–80.

93. Sjostrom L, Narbro K, Sjostrom D (1995). Costs and benefits when treating obesity. *Inter J Obes Relat Metab Disord* **19** (Suppl 6), S9–12.

94. Segal L, Dalton AC, Richardson J (1998). Cost-effectiveness of the primary prevention of non-insulin dependent diabetes mellitus. *Health Promot Int* **13**, 197–209.

95. van Gemert WG, Adang EM, Kop M, Vos G, Greve JW, Soeters PB (1999). A prospective cost-effectiveness analysis of vertical banded gastroplasty for the treatment of morbid obesity. *Obes Surg* **9**, 484–91.

96. Nguyen NT, Goldman C, Rosenquist CJ, Arango A, Cole CJ, Lee SJ, *et al.* (2001). Laparoscopic versus open gastric bypass: a randomized study of outcomes, quality of life, and costs. *Ann Surg* **234**, 279–89.

97. Kaplan RM, Hartwell SL, Wilson DK, Wallace JP (1987). Effects of diet and exercise interventions on control and quality of life in non-insulin-dependent diabetes mellitus. *J Gen Intern Med* **2**, 220–8.

98. Kaplan RM, Atkins CJ, Wilson DK (1988). The cost-utility of diet and exercise interventions in non-insulin dependent diabetes mellitus. *Health Promot* **2**, 331–40.

99. Johannesson M, Fagerberg B (1992). A health-economic comparison of diet and drug treatment in obese men with mild hypertension. *J Hypertension* **10**, 1063–70.

100. Salkeld G, Phongsavan P, Oldenburg B, *et al.* (1997). The cost-effectiveness of a cardiovascular risk reduction program in general practice. *Health Policy* **41**, 105–19.

101. Goldfield GS, Epstein LH, Kilanowski CK, Paluch RA, Kogut-Bossler B (2001). Cost-effectiveness of group and mixed family-based treatment for childhood obesity. *Inter J Obes* **25**, 1843–49.

102. Gold MR, Siegel JE, Russell LB, Weinstein MC, eds. (1996). *Cost-effectiveness in health and medicine.* Oxford University Press, New York.

103. Drummond MF, O'Brien B, Stoddart G, Torrance GW (1997). *Methods for the economic evaluation of health care programmes.* Oxford Medical Publications, New York.

104. Drummond M, McGuire A (2001). *Economic evaluation in health care: merging theory with practice.* Oxford University Press, Oxford.

105. O'Meara S, Riesma R, Shirran L, Mather L, ter Riet G (2001). A rapid and systematic review of the clinical effectiveness and cost-effectiveness of orlistat in the management of obesity. *Health Technol Assess* **5**, 1–81.

106. Roche Submission for the National Institute for Clinical Excellence (2000). *Xenical (orlistat) NICE submission. Achieving clinical excellence in the treatment of obesity.* Roche, Welwyn Garden City, Herts.

107. Edelsberg J, Weycker D, Oster G (2002). Tenascin-C levels in the vitreous of patients with proliferative diabetic retinopathy (Letters: Comments and Responses). *Diabetes Care* **25**, 1899–900.

108. O'Meara S, Riesma R, Shirran L, Mather L, ter Riet G (2002). The clinical effectiveness and cost-effectiveness of sibutramine in the management of obesity: a technology assessment. *Health Technol Assess* **6**, 1–97.

109. Minarcikova I (2003). Long-term drug therapy of obesity in 2002 – pharmaceconomic aspects. *Ceska a Slovenska Farmacie* **52**, 258–61.

110. Clegg A, Colquitt, Sidhu M, Royle P, Walker A (2003). Clinical and cost effectiveness of surgery for morbid obesity: a systematic review and economic evaluation. *Int J Obes* **27**, 1167–77.

111. **Carter R, Marks R, Hill D** (1999). Could a national skin cancer primary prevention campaign in Australia be worthwhile: an economic perspective? *Health Promot Interl* **14**, 73–82.

112. **George B, Harris A, Mitchell A** (1999). *Cost effectiveness analysis and the consistency of decision making: evidence from pharmaceutical reimbursement in Australia 1991–1996.* Centre for Health Program Evaluation, Melbourne.

113. **Carter R, Scollo M** (2000). Economic evaluation of the National Tobacco Campaign. *Australia's National Tobacco Campaign: evaluation report.* Vol. 2. K. Hassard (ed.). Canberra, Commonwealth of Australia.

114. **Jebb SA, Lambert J** (2000). Overweight and obesity in European children and adolescents. *Eur J Pediatr* **159** (Suppl 1), S2–4.

115. **Wabitsch M** (2000). Overweight and obesity in European children: definition and diagnostic procedures, risk factors and consequences for later health outcome. *Eur J Pediatr* **159** (Suppl 1), S8–13.

116. **Guo SS, Wu W, Chumlea WC, Roche AF** (2002). Predicting overweight and obesity in adulthood from body mass index values in childhood and adolescence. *Am J Clin Nutr* **76**, 653–8.

117. **Hauck KH, Smith PC, Goddard M** (2003). *The economics of priority setting for health care: a literature review.* HNP Discussion Paper. The World Bank, Washington DC.

118. **Carter R** (2001). *Priority setting in health: processes and mechanisms.* Expert paper prepared on invitation from the Commonwealth Secretariat for the 13th Commonwealth Health Ministers Meeting, Christchurch, New Zealand, 25–29 November, 2001.

119. **Haby M, Carter R, Mihalopoulos C, Magnus A, Andrews G, Vos T** (2004). Assessing cost effectiveness (ACE) – mental health: introduction to the study and methods. *ANZJP* **38**, 569–78.

Part 3

Chapter 10

Opportunities to prevent obesity in children within families: an ecological approach

Kirsten Krahnstoever Davison and Karen Campbell

Introduction

Preventing the development of obesity among children is an international priority. This reflects the fact that rates of obesity among children have reached epidemic proportions in developed (1) and developing (2) countries, that obesity during childhood is associated with negative health and psychological outcomes (3), and that obese children tend to become obese adults (4). As outlined in Chapter 1, eating, physical inactivity, and sedentary behaviors (e.g. TV/video viewing, computer usage, video game playing) are established risk factors for the development of obesity among children and adults. Each of these behaviors develops at an early age in the context of the family and show a moderate degree of tracking across time (5). Therefore, it is important to understand the impact that the family has on children's emerging eating and activity behaviors and to use this information to design family-based preventive interventions.

To this end, the link between parenting and children's obesity risk behaviors will be reviewed in this chapter. The evidence reviewed and the structure of this chapter will be guided by Ecological Systems Theory which embodies the premise that human behavior cannot be understood without taking into consideration the context in which a person is embedded (6). In the case of young children, the family provides the key context in which socialization occurs and behavioral patterns emerge. The ecological model was used by Davison and Birch (7) to explain the contribution of child-specific characteristics, the family environment, and community characteristics to the development of obesity among children. This chapter will build on the work of Davison and Birch by presenting a more detailed analysis of the role of parenting and the familial environment on children's emerging obesity risk behaviors, with a particular focus on the ecology of parenting. Specifically, this chapter aims to: review research on the links between parenting and children's eating, physical activity, and sedentary behaviors; examine the context in which parenting occurs and the impact it has on parenting

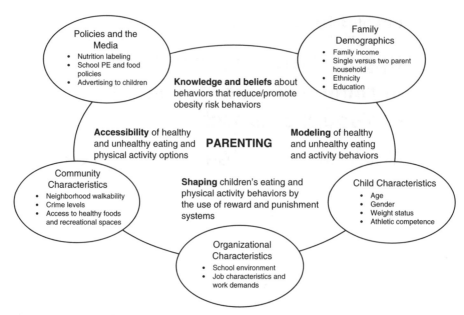

Fig. 10.1 The family ecology and children's eating, physical activity, and sedentary behaviors.

behaviors and family interactions pertaining to obesity risk behaviors; and suggest ways in which parents might directly (i.e. through parenting) or indirectly (i.e. though advocacy efforts to create supportive environments) foster the development of healthful eating and activity behaviors among their children and how practitioners and policy makers can support parents in their efforts.

The ecological model is outlined in Figure 10.1. Four aspects of parenting will be reviewed as they relate to each obesity risk behavior including beliefs and knowledge, modeling, accessibility, and shaping. Beliefs and knowledge refers to the importance that parents assign to a healthy diet and a physically active lifestyle, parents' nutrition knowledge, parents' perceptions of risk among their children, and their belief in their children's competencies. Modeling refers to both vicarious learning through observation and parent and child coparticipation in activities. Accessibility includes the extent to which parents facilitate or impede food access and opportunities to be sedentary or physically active. Finally, shaping describes the manner in which parents mould children's behaviors by pairing a behavior with a positive (e.g. praise) or negative outcome and the use of unhealthy foods and sedentary behaviors (e.g. TV viewing) as rewards. Factors that shape and constrain these parenting practices are reviewed, including: family demographics such as ethnicity, family income, and parent education; child characteristics such as age, gender, and weight status; organizational characteristics such as the school and work environments; community characteristics such as access to safe and clean recreational facilities and healthy foods; and higher order policy and media influences such as nutrition labeling and advertising to children.

Parenting and children's eating, physical activity, and sedentary behaviors

Eating behaviors

Beliefs and knowledge

In a review of the relationships between adult nutrition knowledge and food behaviors, Worsley (8) notes that nutrition knowledge appears to play a small but pivotal role in the adoption of healthier food habits. By way of example, research shows that parents' nutrition knowledge is positively related to healthier dietary behaviors in children. There is also evidence, however, to show that even when parents' nutrition knowledge is high, as reflected in their personal dietary choices, this knowledge many not be reflected in the diet of their children (9). That is, parents may apply different food rules to themselves and their children. One example of this is provided by Gibson *et al.* (10) who report that while mothers' nutrition knowledge was found to be an important predictor of children's fruit intake, it did not predict vegetable or confectionary intake, with these dietary behaviors most strongly linked to other factors, such as mother and child food preferences and mothers' health beliefs. The inconsistency in these findings highlights that parents' nutrition knowledge is but one of the factors impacting on children's eating behavior.

Modeling

The proposition that parental role modeling of eating impacts upon young children's eating is supported by a range of studies. Indirectly, there is evidence to show that dietary habits aggregate within families (e.g. (11)), and that this is likely to reflect the shared environment rather than genetic similarity (12). More specifically, research shows similarities in many aspects of mothers' and daughters' eating, including beverage consumption (13), consumption of fruits and vegetables (10, 14), and fat and micronutrient intakes (15). These findings may reflect a number of factors particular to families, such as children's exposure and accessibility to those fruits and vegetables the family food provider prefers (11, 16), and/or the opportunity to eat with parents at mealtime. Indeed, a number of cross-sectional studies suggest that there is nutritional and social value in sharing family meals. Eating together provides an opportunity for observational learning about food preferences and is associated with children's increased consumption of fruits and vegetables (17), grains and calcium-rich foods (17), and reduced consumption of fried food and soda (16, 17).

In contrast to the body of research that considers observational learning, research regarding the impact of explicit modeling, or parent and child coparticipation in activities such as growing or preparing food, is scant and poorly described. One study showed that children's preferences for vegetables were influenced by growing vegetables at school (18), while no studies have been found which examine the impact of cooking food on food preferences. In both cases however, it seems likely that involvement with an important role model, such as a parent, in the growing and preparation of foods, coupled with increased exposure to the food, is likely to promote preference for that food.

Accessibility

A child cannot learn to prefer a food to which he/she is not exposed. Consistent with this point, research shows that children's consumption of fruits and vegetables increases as the availability and the accessibility in the home increases (17, 19). Practically it seems important, particularly for younger children, that food is not just available but that it is also accessible. For example children are more likely to eat carrots if they are present in the home (i.e. available) and cut up into small pieces and placed in bags in the fridge within children's reach (i.e. accessible) (19).

Shaping

Parents employ a wide range of feeding strategies that are designed to shape children's food intake including restricting foods considered to be "bad", encouraging consumption of foods considered to be "good", and using a preferred food as a reward for the consumption of a less favored food. A growing body of research suggests that such feeding strategies may have negative consequences for children's eating by inadvertently endorsing the foods promoted or restricted. For example a series of studies have shown that restricting access to foods increased preference for and consumption of those foods when they were no longer restricted (20, 21). Further, the restriction of food has been associated with an increase in the contribution of fat to a child's diet (22), and longitudinally with increased eating in the absence of hunger in girls (23). As with restriction, research shows that encouraging a child to "eat up" or "clear your plate" has unintended consequences such as increasing children's energy intake (24), increasing the contribution of fat in the diet (22), increasing the time children spend eating, and increasing the degree of child fatness (25). Similarly, pressure to eat from mothers has been linked with reduced fruit and vegetable consumption among children (14). Finally, there is evidence that using food as a reward may inadvertently promote preferences for the reward food while decreasing preference for the target food. For example offering dessert as a reward for completing meal-time vegetables appears to have the unfortunate effect of increasing the preference for the dessert while further reducing the preference for the vegetables (26).

Physical activity

Beliefs and knowledge

An extensive body of research has examined knowledge, beliefs, and attitudes as predictors of physical activity among adults (e.g. (27)) and children (e.g. (28)). Research, however, has rarely focused on families and assessed associations between parents' beliefs and knowledge and children's activity levels. The research that is available suggests that the value parents assign to physical activity and their belief in their children's physical competencies are indirect predictors of their children's physical activity. Specifically, research shows that parents who assign a higher level of importance to their children being physically active are more likely to support their children's physical activity by, for example, transporting them to sporting events and telling them that physical activity is good for their health (29). Parental support in turn is linked with higher physical activity among their children (29). On a similar note, children's perceptions of the extent to which their parents think they are physically competent and the value their parents assign to being physically fit predict their own perceived physical competency, which in turn predicts their physical activity (30).

Modeling

In general, research shows that active parents tend to have active children (31–33). These associations have been identified using self-report (33) and objective (31, 34) measures of physical activity, and in clinical (i.e. overweight) (32) and non-clinical (33) samples. In addition to vicarious learning, links between parent and child physical activity levels may reflect the fact that parents who are more active themselves are more likely to support their children's physical activity (e.g. provide transportation and watch child perform) (29) and may be more likely to include their children in their physical activities. Research indicates that parents who are active with their children (35) and parents who arrange family outings that include physical activity (36) have children who are more physically active. Research also suggests that fathers are more inclined to explicitly model physical activity, or to be coparticipators, than are mothers (35).

Accessibility

Parents can promote children's access to physical activity in a number of ways. First, parents can create environments that foster physical activity by providing activity-related equipment (e.g. balls, bicycles, basketball hoops, treadmills). Research shows that a greater number of activity-related items in the home is linked with higher levels of physical activity among children (37). Second, parents can enable or facilitate their children's involvement in physical activities. For example, transporting children to a place where they can be active, enrolling them in organized activities, and paying the associated fees have been linked with higher levels of physical activity among children (38). In contrast to what has been noted for modeling, mothers are more likely to facilitate or provide logistic support for children's physical activity than are fathers (35).

Shaping

Few studies have examined parents' use of reward systems specific to children's physical activity. This absence of research may reflect the possibility that parents do not readily use physical activity as a reward for good behavior, nor are they likely to reward children for being physically active; this is in contrast to parents' frequent reports of rewarding children for healthy eating behaviors such as eating their vegetables and their use of food as a reward. The use of less tangible rewards or methods of shaping behavior, however, have been reported. Parents regularly report encouraging their children to be active and parents' reports of encouragement have been linked with higher physical activity among children (39).

Sedentary behaviors

Beliefs and knowledge

Adults, particularly parents, readily identify the amount of time children spend watching TV as a key factor that promotes obesity. In a study of 315 Australian adults, 74 per cent stated that watching too much TV was very or extremely likely to be an important cause of obesity among school-aged children (40). Research comparing parents' concerns about the children's TV viewing time (and use of the internet and video games) and parents' concern about media content, however, clearly indicates that parents are more concerned about overall media content than children's total viewing time (41). Parents' focus on the quality rather than the quantity of viewing time may explain why parental concern about media is not linked with children's total viewing hours (41). A greater focus on media content may reflect the possibility that parents are highly dependent on the care-giving respite provided by TV and justify their children's media use by focusing on what they are watching rather than their viewing time.

Modeling

Sedentary behaviors tend to cluster within families. Children spend significantly more time watching TV when their parents are high volume TV viewers (39, 41). Similarly, children spend more time in sedentary pursuits such as TV/video viewing, using the computer, and reading when their parents are physically inactive (i.e. report no leisure time physically activity) (42). In addition to their independent viewing behaviors, parents can influence children's TV viewing patterns by watching TV with them and using TV viewing as a family recreational activity. While research has examined the impact of parent–child coviewing on children's media literacy, research has rarely examined the impact of parent coviewing on children's total viewing time. Given that parents who coview with their children tend to be high volume viewers (43) and that coviewing is the most frequently shared family activity (44), it is likely that family coviewing increases children's viewing time and consequently their obesity risk.

Accessibility

Opportunities to engage in sedentary behaviors are omnipresent in today's households. Data from a national survey in the US indicate that nearly half of households with children aged 2–17 years have all four media staples including a TV, VCR, video game equipment, and a computer and that the average household has 2.8 TV sets (41). Contrary to what might be expected, however, the number of televisions in the home is not linked with greater TV viewing among children (45). This counterintuitive finding is likely to reflect the fact that low-income families have less media access but report greater TV viewing (41).

In addition to having ready access to sedentary pursuits in the home in general, children are also increasingly likely to have media access in their bedrooms. In the US, approximately 50 per cent of children aged 2–17 years (41) and 40 per cent of preschool children (46) have a TV in their bedroom. In addition, approximately 20 per cent of children have a computer in their bedroom (41). Children with a TV in their bedroom report that they do most of their viewing in their bedroom, out of the purview of parents (41). As a likely consequence of ready access to TV and lack of parental monitoring, children with a TV in their bedroom watch 4.6 hours per week more than children without a TV in their bedroom (46).

The availability (or lack of) a TV in the home or in children's bedroom is an indirect method by which parents can control children's access to sedentary pursuits. Parents can also directly limit children's opportunities to engage in sedentary behaviors. Parents regularly report limiting the types of programs their children watch (47). In contrast, however, just 20 per cent of parents of 3 to 7 year olds (43) and 40 per cent of parents of 8 to 16 year olds (41) limit their children's TV viewing time. Although few parents appear to limit children's total TV viewing time, parents who do instigate such limits have children who watch less television (43).

Shaping

There are few studies that have examined the extent to which parents encourage their children to engage in sedentary behaviors or manipulate access to sedentary behaviors as a means to shape other behaviors. Given that most parents in the US work full time and some families live in unsafe neighborhood environments, it is likely that such activities are indirectly (e.g. by encouraging them to play in their room where there is a TV and a computer), if not directly, encouraged by parents. Indeed, research shows that parents report that TV viewing is a safe distraction for children (45). Similarly, although research has not examined the extent to which parents reward positive behaviors with the "privilege" of watching TV or playing video games or remove such opportunities as a form of punishment, most parents would agree that this form of parenting occurs on a regular basis. As has been shown in the literature on children's eating behaviors (i.e. using unhealthy foods as rewards for particular behaviors) (26), regulating access to sedentary activities as a means to shape children's behavior will likely reinforce the positive valence of sedentary behaviors and further promote children's preferences for such activities. Given that children already watch excessive amounts of TV, watching an average of 2 to 3 hours per day (48), this is clearly an area that warrants investigation.

The ecology of parenting

The design of effective family-based obesity prevention programs needs to combine information on the links between parenting and child behaviors with an understanding of the context in which parenting occurs. Contextual factors that impact on parenting approaches specific to obesity-related behaviors (e.g. child characteristics, family demographics, community and organizational characteristics, and policies) are under-researched. Thus, the following section reviews the available literature on the ecology of parenting and identifies those areas that warrant additional research.

Family demographics

While it is known that rates of obesity, and obesity risk behaviors are disproportionately higher among ethnic minorities (49) and individuals with low levels of education or family income (50), there is little research on the origins of such disparities. Furthermore, very little is known about how parents' cultural beliefs and financial and educational resources permeate the family environment to influence children's obesity risk behaviors.

Although there is little research on the link between cultural beliefs and obesity-related parenting strategies, the idealization of a larger body size among ethnic minorities (51) is likely to translate into differences in parenting approaches. This possibility is highlighted in a qualitative study by Jain and colleagues (52) in which low income, predominantly black, mothers were asked their opinions and beliefs about issues relating to childhood obesity. Results suggested that mothers had a general distrust of growth charts or weight measurements to define a child as being overweight. In addition, mothers did not perceive a child to be obese if he/she had a good appetite and did not exhibit functional limitations. Finally, when mothers were asked about their child feeding practices, they expressed a strong reluctance to deny their children's requests for food and were proud to be able to afford "treats" for their children.

Low maternal education and/or family income have been linked with less healthy diets, lower levels of physical activity, less participation in physical education, and greater participation in sedentary activities (53, 54) among children. While little research has examined how financial and educational limitations translate into differences in parenting practices specific to obesity risk, one can speculate that these associations reflect: increased preference for energy dense food due to low relative costs (55) and decreased preference for fruits and vegetables due to high cost and low perceived quality (56); decreased ability to buy sports equipment and enroll children in organized sports; longer working hours and a greater dependence on TV as a safe activity for children (41); less leisure time to devote to creating a healthy lifestyle for the family; greater use of takeaway or convenience foods (56); lower nutrition knowledge (57); and less social support due to an increased likelihood of single parenthood. Ethnicity, education, and income can also indirectly influence parenting practices as a result of the physical environment in which low socioeconomic families live.

Child characteristics

When considering parenting specific to obesity risk behaviors, a number of child characteristics may influence parenting approaches, or the outcomes of parenting, including characteristics such as children's gender, preferences, competencies, and weight status.

It is generally assumed that parents create different feeding and activity environments for girls and boys. Research, however, does not support this contention (21, 36). Although there are no clear gender differences in family environment exposures, girls and boys appear to respond differently to these environments such that girls are more responsive to the effects of parenting than boys. For example, parents' restriction of access to food is associated with higher snack food intake (when restriction is removed) among girls but not boys (21). In addition, a number of studies have shown that girls benefit more from parents' support of physical activity than boys (58, 59).

Children's preferences and competencies may influence the food and activity environments that parents create. Research shows that parents' food purchase and food preparation decisions are influenced by children's food preferences and requests (60). For example most parents will cease offering a food that has been rejected more than three times (61). On a similar note, children's lack of interest for or enjoyment of physical activity can be a key deterrent in parents' efforts to promote active lifestyles among their children. Conversely, parents are more likely to support children's physical activity when their children are athletic or report high levels of perceived athletic competence (62).

Finally, research shows that parents provide different environments for children based on their risk characteristics, such as being overweight. For example parents are more likely to report monitoring children's dietary intake and restricting their access to food when they are overweight (21). Parents may also take a different approach to encouraging and promoting physical activity among children who are overweight vs. not overweight. Among overweight children there is the risk that interactions specific to physical activity may take on a coercive tone with the enforced goal being weight loss rather than enjoyment and healthful living. Although such efforts by parents may be well-intentioned, they are likely to have the opposite effect to those desired.

Organizational characteristics

A common complaint among parents of school-aged children is that unhealthy foods are readily accessible in schools. Such complaints are warranted given the current status of the school food environment. While standard school lunch menus are highly regulated in the US, à la carte (i.e. canteen) foods and foods available in school shops and vending machines tend not to be regulated. In a recent analysis of 20 middle schools in Minnesota, French and colleagues (63) found that high fat foods were widely available in à la carte areas with chips/crackers and ice cream/frozen desserts being the most widely available food items comprising approximately 20 per cent of à la carte options. In contrast, fruit and vegetable items comprised only 4.5 per cent of the foods available. Furthermore, the majority of schools had multiple soft drink and snack vending machines, which predominantly serve foods and beverages high in sugar or fat. The availability of unhealthy foods in schools has had a negative impact on children's diet quality during the school day (i.e. higher intake of French Fries and soda and lower intake of fruits and vegetables) (64). Foods served at school may also negatively influence the quality of the family diet by way of children's requests for similar foods at home. Thus, many well-intentioned parents may find themselves faced with children who refuse foods that they may have previously eaten. These possibilities have not been examined to date and warrant research attention.

School environments may also foster the development of obesity among children as a result of lack of opportunities for physical activity either during or en route to school, which then transfer into the home. In the US today, for example, only 24 per cent of children walk or bicycle to school at least once a month (65). Low rates of active commuting to school have been linked with lower levels of physical activity among children and higher risks of obesity (66) and likely reflect constraints such as lack of sidewalks and patrolled crossings, as well as the policy of building large satellite schools on cheaper land outside city or town perimeters. In addition to lack of opportunities to be active en route to school, children are inactive during school hours. In 2001, less than half of US children participated in daily physical education (PE) (67). A lack of opportunity for physical activity at school has implications for children's overall levels of physical activity. Children who report no PE at school are less active overall (68). Conversely, schools with adequate space facilities, equipment, and supervision stimulate children to be more active (69). Research also suggests that regular PE helps to establish lifelong patterns of physical activity (70). This continuity in physical activity behaviors may be explained by a link between physical activity at school and in the home. When children are exposed to regular PE at school, and are able to actively commute to school, they are likely to build skills, confidence, and a general appreciation of physical activity (71). As a result, they may be more likely to elicit their parents' support to be active outside of school hours (62). Conversely, when physical activity is not provided or valued in schools, this may translate into reluctant, sedentary children who may reject parents' efforts to encourage them to be active.

The workplace represents a second institution that can have a profound impact on parents' ability to foster and support healthy lifestyles. The vast majority of parents, including mothers of young and school-aged children, now work outside the home (72), working longer hours than ever before (72). The combined demands of work and parenthood mean that parents have less time today to ensure that their children eat well and are physically active. While data showing links between working hours and reliance on convenience foods (which are generally high in fat, sugar, and salt) are not available, it seems likely that increased working hours have contributed to the massive growth in sales of these items. It also seems reasonable to suggest that parents who work longer hours are more likely to use TV and other sedentary activities to engage their children while they attend to competing tasks. Single-parent families are likely to disproportionately experience the negative impact of multiple role demands.

While parents and researchers are well aware of the time limitations experienced by parents, there is virtually no research on this dynamic and, as a result, few validated methods of decreasing or working around such limitations. From the perspective of designing family-based preventive interventions, time demands and role conflicts experienced by parents are likely to be one of the most important barriers to overcome in facilitating parents' ability to create health-promoting family environments.

Community characteristics

Research on the impact of the physical environment on obesity risk is currently the most rapidly growing body of literature in the study of obesity. Findings to date indicate that people are more likely to be physically active if they live in communities in which there are well-maintained sidewalks or footpaths, the streets show a high level of connectivity (in contrast to a series of cul-de-sacs), parks, recreational facilities (e.g. bicycle trails), public transportation, and commercial outlets are accessible, perceived crime rates are low, population density is high, and the environment is perceived as attractive and appealing (73, 74). Similarly, the accessibility of food shops and the quality of food provided will impact on the individual's opportunities to procure foods for a healthy diet.

Access to environments that support healthy behaviors is not uniform across demographic groups. Low-income families are least likely to live in environments that promote physical activity (74). Similarly, low-income families are more likely to live in physical environments that place constraints on their ability to purchase and eat healthful foods. Research from the UK shows that individuals in lower-income groups are more likely to live in neighborhoods with limited access to supermarkets and, consequently, are more likely to use small corner shops to buy many staple items such as bread, milk, fruit, and vegetables (75). This has implications for food purchases because in general, smaller shops sell items at higher costs and in some instances items are of a lower quality (e.g. fresh produce) (75) than in supermarkets. Furthermore, Australian research shows that for lower socioeconomic status families, the purchase and hence consumption of fresh fruits and vegetables is affected by perceptions of poor produce quality (56).

In contrast to the rapidly emerging literature among adults, the impact of community-level characteristics on parenting practices specific to obesity risk behaviors has received much less attention. One exception, however, is a study by Sallis and colleagues (76) which examined factors that influence parents' choice of outdoor play spaces for their young children. Results indicated that safety and the availability of amenities (e.g. toilets, drinking water, lighting, shade, and attractiveness) were the two most important factors influencing parents' decisions. Although that study did not assess the link with children's physical activity, previous research shows that children are most active when they play outdoors (38), thus it is possible that such decision processes mediate the link between community characteristics and young children's obesity-related behaviors.

An additional community-based characteristic that has the potential to influence parenting styles and children's dietary intake is the type and quantity of foods available in fast-food restaurants. The consumption of meals and snacks away from home has increased more than two-thirds in the past two decades in the US, which likely reflects increases in parents' working hours (77). Further, expenditure on the replacement of home cooking (both sit-down meals and take away), continues to increase, with expenditure on raw foods as a proportion of grocery purchases concomitantly declining (78). The reliance on convenience foods and takeout foods has a negative impact on dietary patterns because foods consumed away from home are higher in fat and cholesterol than foods consumed at home (79). The lack of healthy choices for children is particularly noteworthy. A recent report published by the Center for Science in the Public Interest (CSPI) examined children's menus in the top 20 table-service restaurants in the US (80). The analysis revealed that fried chicken, hamburgers, and French fries were offered on the vast majority of menus and that there were few healthy options for children. Furthermore, serving sizes offered in restaurants continue to increase with "super-sizing" being a common practice in the US. This is concerning as research shows that larger portion sizes lead to greater energy intakes in preschoolers, with no compensatory reduction in other food consumed (81). In this context, parents are clearly faced with a dietary conundrum. Much-needed convenience comes at a nutritional price: nutritional quality reduces while energy density and food consumption increases.

Policy and media influences

The final contexts to be considered are the higher order influences of policy and media. Although governments are reluctant to regulate what occurs within families, viewing the family as a private domain, there are a number of polices and guidelines not directed at families that can influence family processes. For example, recommendations for age-appropriate levels of physical activity, TV viewing hours, and dietary intake patterns can be used to inform and educate parents, which in turn may influence parenting strategies. Unfortunately, however, activity, TV, and dietary recommendations are not well known or understood by the general population (82), indicating that health and education practitioners must provide appropriate education (reflecting the guidelines) at all opportunities.

An additional policy that may influence parenting approaches is mandatory nutrition labeling. While nutrition labeling supports consumers in their attempts to achieve dietary change, it appears that nutrition labeling is currently under-utilized by those most at risk of nutrition-related disease. For example, parents in low socioeconomic groups are least likely to use food labels as a source of information regarding diet (83), while in contrast, those with a commitment to dietary change use labels widely (84). Together with consistent nutrition education, food labeling has the potential to support consumers in their purchase of healthy food choices. Clearly however, methods that promote the use of nutrition labeling among nutritionally at-risk groups should be a key research priority.

Similar to policies and national recommendations, the media has the capacity to impact on the eating and activity patterns of a large proportion of the population. It is recognized that television is an effective medium for the sale of food products and that the vast majority of foods advertised to children are high in fat, salt, and/or sugar and low in fiber (85). Across the globe, content analyses of advertising during children's viewing time shows that food advertisements dominate advertising time. The targeting of advertisements for energy-dense foods to children has important implications. Specifically, research suggests that children who watch more television are more likely to request the foods advertised (86), to have a preference for advertised foods (87), and to snack more frequently (88). Further, television viewing is associated with increased consumption of energy (86, 89), increased consumption of high-energy drinks, and decreased vegetable and fruit consumption (90). These findings indicate that the media is a higher order influence that can have a dramatic, and generally negative, influence on children's obesity-related behaviors. The foods that are advertised to children, particularly during child prime-time viewing, are likely to compromise parents' efforts to promote healthy dietary patterns. It is important to acknowledge that television is but one of many mediums used to promote food to children. For example much of young children's sport is sponsored by fast-food chains. Given this, parents would benefit from advice on how they can navigate this pervasive negative information source and minimize its impact on children's obesity-related behaviors.

Implications for parents and practitioners

The information reviewed in this chapter suggests that there are many practical ways in which parents can foster the development of healthful eating and activity behaviors. In this section, we highlight key findings from the literature and extrapolate from these to provide examples of how parents can directly and indirectly foster healthy eating and activity environments for their children, while taking into consideration the context in which parenting takes place (Boxes 10.1 and 10.2). In addition, we outline ways in which policy makers and practitioners can support parents in their efforts (Box 10.3, below).

Parents as role models and children as coparticipators

Given the importance of parents as role models for health behaviors, parents must understand the central role of their own behaviors in their children's risk of obesity. Ideally parents should strive to provide multiple opportunities in which they can directly model health-promoting eating and activity patterns to their children. To achieve this, general themes for parents and for families could include the sharing of family meals, the incorporation of physical activity and food preparation (e.g. food purchase and preparation) into regular family activity, and the displacement of television with other recreational pursuits.

Box 10.1: Examples of parenting strategies that may reduce children's risk of obesity

Eating:

* model healthy eating practices;
* share family meals;
* enable children to participate in selecting, growing, and preparing foods;
* make a wide variety of healthy foods available;
* put healthy foods in places that are easily accessed by children and in forms in which they can be readily eaten (e.g. precut vegetables);
* provide smaller portions of high energy density foods (e.g. soft drinks, cordials, juices, crisps, foods cooked with added fat) and larger portions of low energy density foods (e.g. fruits and vegetables).

Physical activity:

* model a physically active lifestyle;
* incorporate physical activity into family recreation (e.g. hiking, bicycle riding);
* include children in physical activity or exercise routines;
* make activity-related equipment available at home (e.g. balls, bicycles);
* drive or take children to places, such as playgrounds, where they can be active;
* encourage children to play outdoors;
* identify safe play places in the community that children can easily access;
* find activities to do outdoors for all weather conditions.

Sedentary behaviors:

* reduce parents' TV viewing time;
* reduce the family's reliance of on TV as a recreational activity;
* limit children's TV viewing hours to no more than 1–2 hours per day;
* encourage children to adopt selective and circumscribed viewing practices (e.g. select certain programs to watch and then turn TV off);
* remove TV and computers from children's bedrooms.

Increasing children's access to healthy options

In addition to shaping children's behaviors through observational learning, parents also provide more direct forms of influence by controlling children's access to food (types of food and portion sizes) and their opportunities to be physically active or sedentary. Parents can promote active lifestyles in their children by providing resources for physical activity in the home (e.g. balls, bicycles), by encouraging outdoor play, and by removing barriers to physical activity (e.g. driving children to locations where they can be active). With respect to children's sedentary behaviors, parents can reduce children's dependence on media by: placing limits on children's total screen time (i.e. TV, computer, video game); encouraging selective, circumscribed viewing (91); and removing televisions and computers from children's bedrooms.

Supporting and encouraging healthy behaviors

Overt support and encouragement of healthy behaviors is likely to be important in children's adoption of these behaviors, however, parents need to be aware of the emotional tone employed. For example, children are responsive to parents' moral support of their physical activity (e.g. watching them compete in athletic events) and the general feeling that physical activity is valued in the family yet may resent physical activity and consider it a chore when it is regimented or promoted as a method of weight loss. Similarly, emphasis on the consumption of healthy foods as being "good for you" is likely to be ineffective and even counter-productive. Given this, nutrition experts promote the feeding of children in non-coercive environments, where parents provide nutritious food then let children be responsible for their eating, deciding if and how much they will eat. In addition, given children's natural tendency to reject new foods and understanding that repeated exposure can promote food preference, experts support the continued offering of rejected foods (e.g. (92)) and pairing a frequently rejected food with a preferred food (93) as strategies to increase food acceptance over time.

Using advocacy to campaign for the creation of healthy environments

Parents can indirectly influence children's eating and activity environments through efforts to affect change within local and broader environments (Box 10.2). At the most basic level, parents, as consumers, have the capacity to influence supply. For example, parents can advocate for changes to the range of food provided in local shops and restaurants. They can also advocate for safer roads, improved recreational facilities, and policies that promote healthy food and activity environments in their children's schools, child-care centers, and kindergartens. Parents have proved to be powerful advocates for change in issues such as the promotion of soft drinks in schools (94) and the need for safe walking routes to school (95).

How practitioners and policy makers can support parents' efforts to foster healthy lifestyles

While parents can foster the development of healthful eating and activity behaviors among their children, they are likely to be more effective when supported in their parenting through education and the promotion of environments that are supportive of change (Box 10.3). Practitioners and policy makers have an important role to play in

Box 10.2: Examples of how parents can advocate for the creation of environments that support healthy lifestyles

* ask local restaurant to provide healthy options on children's menus;
* request that stores stock healthy alternatives to staple items (e.g. wholemeal breads, low fat milks, good quality fruits and vegetables);
* establish local farmer's markets;
* request that the local municipalities upgrade playgrounds and provide amenities such as water fountains and toilet facilities;
* advocate for schools and day-care centers to make healthy foods widely available and reduce unhealthy food choices; price incentives and cross subsidies may be effective in promoting sales of desired products;
* advocate for schools to remove vending machines, particularly soft-drink machines, from the school premises;
* request that schools provide crossing guards at key intersections around the school;
* put pressure on local transportation councils to include sidewalks/footpaths on all new roads and on existing roads as they are upgraded;
* advocate for the maintenance of existing neighborhood schools (in contrast to closing small local schools and consolidating into one larger school);
* support and encourage safe routes to schools.

Box 10.3: Examples of how policy makers and practitioners can support parents' efforts to foster healthy lifestyles among their children

Health practitioners can:
* provide anticipatory guidance matching obesity prevention messages to receptive moments in parenting, e.g. when making decisions regarding breast or bottle feeding, when considering weaning, when actively managing food conflict, when packing the first snacks and/or lunches, when designing opportunities for play, or when establishing how much television is appropriate;
* provide consistent messages;
* tailor advice to parent circumstances and the contexts in which they live, for example:
  * teach parents about the lower cost of foods in season, the cost effectiveness at certain times of year of buying frozen or canned vegetables and fruit rather

(Continued)

Box 10.3: Examples of how policy makers and practitioners can support parents' efforts to foster healthy lifestyles among their children *(continued)*

than fresh; provide information about local food markets (times of opening, place, bus routes) where profit margins are reduced and fresh produce is more affordable

- understand the impact of cooking skills, access to transport, and the quality of the home kitchen on foods prepared and eaten

- understand the impact of living in a high crime neighborhoods; promote alternatives for play such as involvement in local organizations (e.g. YMCA) where structured activities for children in a safe environment may be available for minimal cost

- in extreme weather conditions promote indoor activities other than TV viewing (e.g. ice skating, playing board games).

Education practitioners can:

◆ promote comprehensive, whole of school approaches to obesity prevention by:

- advocating for school pricing incentives that favor low- over high-energy density foods (63)

- actively promoting low energy density foods to students (19)

- adopting school nutrition policies that promote the use of non-food rewards (100) and the growing of foods (18) and prohibit food advertising at schools (e.g. TV based educational programming (101), sports sponsorship, exclusive marketing contracts to sell food and beverage products, and industry-sponsored educational materials)

- adapting school playgrounds to promote physical activity (e.g. the use of playground markings (102), increased supervision by teachers, increased access to sports equipment)

- promoting active commuting to schools (e.g. mapping of safe routes to school, walk/bicycle to school days, walking school buses, bicycle trains) (103);

◆ consider innovative use of school spaces and curriculum to provide opportunities for food provision and out of school physical activity;

◆ work to be vocal advocates for obesity prevention – use practitioners critical mass;

◆ contribute to national obesity prevention plans.

achieving this support. A range of established services and natural points of contact exist between health and education practitioners and parents. All provide opportunities for anticipatory guidance and continued support for parents in their efforts to create healthy lifestyles for their children. Anticipatory guidance would match obesity prevention messages to receptive moments in parenting such as weaning or packing the first school snacks/lunch. The delivery of consistent messages from multiple practitioners over the course of a child's growth is likely to be powerful in influencing parents in their practice. However, practitioners must, in turn, be well resourced to achieve this goal. Further, practitioners must recognize that for obesity prevention efforts to be maximized, parents need to be supported within their own communities. Therefore, advice to parents should be tailored to their circumstances or the contexts in which they live. In environments in which healthy foods are not readily accessible in stores or are expensive, parents could be advised in very practical ways about the most cost-effective means by which to include such foods in their diets. Similarly, where opportunities for safe play are limited or where sedentary pursuits are considered the safe activity option, practitioners can support parents with appropriately designed advice.

Practitioners also have the potential to impact on the social and political environments in which their clients live. Powerful examples of the capacity to marry individual and community responsibilities when considering child health abound. For example parents' skin cancer prevention efforts are endorsed by school policies which state "No Hat, No Play" (96), the opportunity to increase children's use of bicycle helmets is supported by legislation that makes their use mandatory (97), and legislation in many countries prohibits the promotion of cigarettes to children (98). In all these examples, practitioners have been active in agitating for change.

Health and education practitioners present powerful lobby groups with the capacity to enhance their clients' opportunities to enact health messages. Thus, for example, teachers have the potential to champion comprehensive, whole-of-school approaches to obesity prevention (Box 10.2). Given that time pressures on parents are likely to limit opportunities for food preparation and after school physical activity, approaches to obesity prevention might also include the innovative use of the school space and curriculum to provide opportunities for family food provision (e.g. cooking co-operatives within schools) and children's after-school physical activity. Given that out-of-doors play is predictive of activity in children, the outdoor spaces provided by many schools might be well utilized after school by children of working parents.

Further, through collective interest in and ownership of the need to prevent obesity, practitioners have the capacity to increase the critical mass of interest in this area. In so doing they have the potential to bring large population groups onto the obesity prevention band-wagon. With increased critical mass will come increased capacity to advocate and agitate at the broader political level. The dissent in the US regarding the marketing and sales of soft drinks in schools, and the subsequent changes in legislation to prevent this, provides one important example (94). Finally, as suggested by the

World Health Organization (99), professional organizations and groups can contribute to national obesity prevention plans, promote and document best practice case studies for policy implementation, and increase the consciousness in the non-health sectors of the potential adverse effects of their actions on the ability of people to maintain a healthy weight.

Conclusion

Children's obesity risk are largely defined by their adoption of particular patterns of diet, activity, and sedentary behaviors, many of which are learnt early in life and within the context of their families. As such, parents have a unique role in determining a child's obesity risk. However, this role is undertaken within a contradictory, hostile, and powerfully obesity-promoting environment in which energy dense food is cheap, highly advertised, and readily available, where there are few opportunities to incorporate regular physical activity into our lives, and where sedentariness is actively promoted. In such a milieu, the reality is that parents and families are unlikely to be able to prevent childhood obesity on their own and that parents' ability to shape healthy habits among children requires from us all an understanding of the context in which parents parent and the constraints and limitations under which they operate. Detailed research on the context of parenting, however, is largely non-existent. Addressing this research gap will be a necessary first step to inform successful family-based obesity prevention for children.

References

1. Kromeyer-Hauschild K, Kellner K, Hoyer H (1999). Prevalence of overweight and obesity among school children in Jena (Germany). *Int J Obes* **23**, 1143–50.
2. Stettler N, Bovet P, Shamlaye H, Zemel B, Stallings V, Paccaud F (2002). Prevalence and risk factors for overweight and obesity in children from Seychelles, a country in rapid transition: the importance of early growth. *Int J Obes Rel Met Disord* **26**, 214–9.
3. Dietz WH (1998). Health consequences of obesity in youth: childhood predictors of adult disease. *Pediatrics* **101**, 518–25.
4. Guo SS, Roche AF, Chumlea WC, Gardner JD, Siervogel RM (1994). The predictive value of childhood obesity body mass index values for overweight at age 35. *Am J Clini Nutr* **59**, 810–19.
5. Kelder SH, Perry CL, Klepp KI, Lytle LL (1994). Longitudinal tracking of adolescent smoking, physical activity, and food choice behaviors. *Am J Pub Health* **84**, 1121–6.
6. Bronfenbrenner U, Morris PA (1988). The ecology of human developmental processes. In: Damon W, Eisenberg N, eds. *The handbook of child psychology*, 3rd edn, pp. 993–1027. John Wiley and Sons, New York.
7. Davison KK, Birch LL (2001). Childhood overweight: a contextual model and recommendations for future research. *Obes Rev* **2**, 159–71.
8. Worsley A (2002). Nutrition knowledge and food consumption: can nutrition knowledge change food behaviour? *Asian Pacific Journal of Clinical Nutrition* **11** (Suppl 3), S579–85.
9. St John Alderson T, Ogden J (1999). What do mothers feed their children and why? *Health Edu Res* **14**, 717–27.

10. Gibson EL, Wardle J, Watts CJ (1998). Fruit and vegetable consumption, nutritional knowledge and beliefs in mothers and children. *Appetite* **31**, 205–28.

11. Skinner J, Carruth B, Moran J, *et al.* (1998). Toddlers' food preferences: concordance with family members' preferences. *J Nutr Edu* **30**, 17–22.

12. Rozin P, Millman L (1987). Family environment, not heredity, accounts for family resemblances in food preferences and attitudes: a twin study. *Appetite* **8**, 125–34.

13. Fisher J, Mitchell D, Smiciklas-Wright H, Birch L (2001). Maternal milk consumption predicts the tradeoff between milk and soft drinks in young girls' diets. *J Nutr* **131**, 246–50.

14. Fisher J, Mitchell D, Smiciklas-WH, Birch L (2002). Parental influences on young girls' fruit and vegetable, micronutrient, and fat intakes. *J Am Diet Assoc* **101**, 58–64.

15. Lee Y, Mitchell DC, Smiciklas-Wright H, Birch LL (2001). Diet quality, nutrient intake, weight status, and feeding environments of girls meeting or exceeding recommendations for total dietary fat of the American Academy of Pediatrics. *Pediatrics* **197**, E95.

16. Hannon P, Bowen D, Moinpour C, McLerran D (2003). Correlations in perceived food use between the family food preparer and their spouses and children. *Appetite* **40**, 77–83.

17. Neumark-Sztainer D, Hannan PJ, Story M, Croll J, Perry C (2003). Family meal patterns: associations with sociodemographic characteristics and improved dietary intake among adolescents. *J Am Diet Assoc* **103**, 317–22.

18. Morris J, Zidenberg-Cherr S (2002). Garden-enhanced nutrition curriculum improves fourth-grade school children's knowledge of nutrition and preferences for some vegetables. *J Am Diet Assoc* **102**, 91–3.

19. Hearn M-D, Baranowski T, Baranowski J, Doyle C, Smith M, Lin L-S, *et al.* (1998). Environmental influences on dietary behavior among children: availability and accessibility of fruits and vegetables enable consumption. *J Health Edu* **29**, 26–32.

20. Fisher J, Birch L (1999a). Restricting access to palatable foods affects children's behavioral response, food selection, and intake. *Am Clini Nutr* **69**, 1264–72.

21. Fisher J, Birch L (1999b). Restricting access to foods and children's eating. *Appetite* **32**, 405–19.

22. Zive MM, Frank-Spohrer GC, Sallis JF, McKenzie TL, Elder JP, Berry CC, *et al.* (1998). Determinants of dietary intake in a sample of white and Mexican-American children. *J Am Diet Assoc* **98**, 1282–9.

23. Birch LL, Fisher JO, Davison KK (2003). Learning to overeat: maternal use of restrictive feeding practices promotes girls' eating in the absence of hunger. *Am J Clinic Nutr* **78**, 215–20.

24. Koivisto UK, Fellenius J, Sjoden PO (1994). Relations between parental mealtime practices and children's food intake. *Appetite* **22**, 245–57.

25. Klesges RC, Malott JM, Boschee PF, Weber JM (1986). The effects of parental influences on children's food intake, physical activity, and relative weight. *Int J Eat Disord* **5**, 335–46.

26. Birch LL, Marlin D, Rotter J (1984). Eating as the "means" activity in a contingency: effects on young children's food preference. *Child Dev* **55**, 532–9.

27. Hagger M, Chatzisarantis N, Biddle S (2002). A meta-analytic review of the theories of reasoned action and planned behavior in physical activity: predictive validity and the contribution of additional variables. *Exerc Psychol* **24**, 3–32.

28. Trost S, Pate R, Saunders R, Ward D, Dowda M, Felton G (1997). A prospective study of the determinants of physical activity in rural fifth-grade children. *Prev Med* **26**, 257–63.

29. Trost S, Sallis J, Pate R, Freedson P, Taylor W, Dowda M (2003). Evaluating a model of parental influence on youth physical activity. *Am J Prev Med* **25**, 277–82.

30. Kimiecik JC, Horn TS, Shurin CS (1996). Relationships among children's beliefs, perceptions of their parents' beliefs, and their moderate-to-vigorous physical activity. *Res Q Exerc Sport* **67**, 324–36.

31. Moore L, Lombardi D, White M, Campbell J, Oliveria S, Ellison R (1991). Influence of parents' physical activity levels on activity levels of young children. *J Pediatr* **118**, 215–9.

32. Epstein LH, Paluch RA, Coleman KJ, Vito D, Anderson K (1996). Determinants of physical activity in obese children assessed by accelerometer and self-report. *Med Sci Sports Exerc* **28**, 1157–64.

33. Wold B, Anderson N (1992). Health promotion aspects of family and peer influences on sport participation. *Int J Sports Psychol* **23**, 343–59.

34. Freedson PS, Evenson S (1991). Familial aggregation in physical activity. *Res Q Exerc Sport* **62**, 384–9.

35. Davison K, Cutting T, Birch L (2003). Parents' activity-related parenting practices predict girls' physical activity. *Med Sci Sports Exerc* **35**, 1589–95.

36. Davison K (2004). Activity-related support from parents, peers and siblings and adolescents' physical activity: are there gender differences? *J Phys Activ Health* **1**, 363–76.

37. Dunton GF, Jamner MS, Cooper DM (2003). Assessing the perceived environment among minimally active adolescent girls: validity and relations to physical activity outcomes. *Am J Health Promo* **18**, 70–3.

38. Sallis J, Prochaska J, Taylor W (2000). A review of correlates of physical activity of children and adolescents. *Med Sci Sports Exerc* **32**, 963–75.

39. McGuire MT, Hannan PJ, Neumark-Sztainer D, Cossrow NH, Story M (2002). Parental correlates of physical activity in a racially/ethnically diverse adolescent sample. *J Adolens Health* **30**, 253–61.

40. Hardus PM, van Vuuren CL, Crawford D, Worsley A (2003). Public perceptions of the causes and prevention of obesity among primary school children. *Int J Obes* **27**, 1465–71.

41. Woodard E, Gridina N (2000). *Media in the home 2000: fifth annual survey of parents and children.* Annenberg Public Policy Center of the University of Pennsylvania, Philadelphia.

42. Fogelholm M, Nuutinen O, Pasanen M, Myohanen E, Saatela T (1999). Parent–child relationship of physical activity patterns and obesity. *Int J Obes Rel Met Disord* **23**, 1262–8.

43. St Peters M, Fitch M, Huston A, Wright J, Eakins D (1991). Television and families: what do young children watch with their parents? *Child Dev* **62**, 1409–23.

44. Timmer SG, Eccles J, O'Brien I (1985). How children use their time. In: Juster FT, Stafford FB, eds. *Time, goods and well-being*, pp. 353–82. University of Michigan, Institute for Social Research, Ann Arbor, MI.

45. Taras H, Sallis J, Nader P, Nelson J (1990). Children's television-viewing habits and the family environment. *Am J Dis Children* **144**, 357–9.

46. Dennison B, Erb T, Jenkins P (2002). Television viewing and television in bedroom associated with overweight risk among low-income preschool children. *Pediatrics* **109**, 1028–35.

47. Valerio M, Amodio P, Dal Zio M, Vianello A, Zacchello G (1997). The use of television in 2- to 8-year-old children and the attitude of parents about such use. *Arch Ped Adolens Med* **151**, 22–6.

48. Lawrence F, Wozniak P (1989). Children's television viewing with family members. *Psychol Rep* **65**, 395–400.

49. Crawford P, Story M, Want W, Ritchie L, Sabry Z (2001). Ethnic issues in the epidemiology of childhood obesity. *Pediatric Clinics N Am* **48**, 855–78.

50. Sobal J, Stunkard AJ (1989). Socioeconomic status and obesity: a review of the literature. *Psycho Bull* **105**, 260–75.

51. Stevens J, Alexandrov A, Smirnova S, Deev A, Gershunskaya YB, Davis C (1997). Comparison of attitudes and behaviors related to nutrition, body size, dieting and hunger in Russian, African-American, white-American adolescents. *Obes Res* **5**, 227–36.

52. Jain A, Sherman SN, Chamberlain LA, *et al.* (2001). Why don't low income mothers worry about their preschoolers being overweight. *Pediatrics* **107**, 1138–46.

53. Lowry R, Kann L, Collins JL, Kolbe LJ (1996). The effect of socioeconomic status on chronic disease risk behaviors among US adolescents. *JAMA* **276**, 792–7.

54. Turrell G, Hewitt B, Patterson C, Oldenburg B, Gould T (2002). Socioeconomic differences in food purchasing behaviour and suggested implications for diet-related health promotion. *J Human Nutr Diet* **15**, 355–64.

55. Drewnowski A, Specter S (2004). Poverty and obesity: the role of energy density and energy costs. *Am J Clinical Nutr* **79**, 6–16.

56. Campbell K, Crawford D (2001). Family food environments as determinants of preschool aged children's eating behaviours: implication for obesity prevention policy. *Aust J Nutr Diet* **58**, 19–25.

57. Wardle J, Parmenter K, Waller J (2000). Nutrition knowledge and food intake. *Appetite* **34**, 269–75.

58. Gregson J, Colley A (1986). Concomitants of sport participation in male and female adolescents. *Int J Sports Psychol* **17**, 10–22.

59. Gottlieb N, Chen M (1985). Sociocultural correlates of childhood sporting activities: their implications for heart health. *Soc Sci Med* **21**, 533–9.

60. Stratton P, Bromley K (1999). Families: accounts of the causal processes in food choice. *Appetite* **33**, 89–108.

61. Carruth B, Ziegler P, Gordon A, Barr S (2004). Prevalence of picky eaters among infants and toddlers and their caregivers' decisions about offering a new food. *J Am Diet Assoc* **104** (Suppl 1), S57–64.

62. Davison K, Downs D, Birch L. Parent activity-related support and girls' perceived athletic competence as predictors of girls' physical activity: What comes first? *Soc Sci Med* (submitted).

63. French S, Story M, Fulkerson J, Gerlach A (2003). Food environment in secondary schools: a la carte, vending machine, and food policies and practices. *Am J Pub Health* **93**, 1161–7.

64. Cullen K, Zakeri I (2004). Fruits, vegetables, milk, and sweetened beverages consumption and access to a la carte/snack bar meals at school. *Am J Public Health* **94**, 463–7.

65. Dellinger AM, Staunton CE (2002). Barriers to children walking and biking to school-United States, 1999. *MMWR* **51**, 701–4.

66. Sirard JR, Riner WF, Mciver KL, Russell P (2004). Physical activity and active commuting to school in fifth grade students. *Med Sci Sports Exerc* **36**, S102.

67. Centers for Disease Control and Prevention (2001). Youth risk behavior surveillance – United States 2001. *MMWR* **51**, SS-4.

68. Myers L, Strikmiller PK, Webber LS, Berenson GS (1996). Physical and sedentary activity in school children grades 5–8: the Bogalusa Heart Study. *Med Sci Sports Exerc* **28**, 852–9.

69. Sallis J, Conway T, Prochaska J, McKenzie T, Marshall S, Brown M (2001). The association of school environments with youth physical activity. *Am J Pub Health* **91**, 618–20.

70. Trudeau F, Laurencelle L, Tremblay J, Rajic M, Shepard R (1999). Daily primary school physical education: effects on physical activity during adulthood. *Med Sci Sports Exerc* **31**, 111–17.

71. Pangrazi RP (1995). *Dynamic physical education for elementary school children*, 12th edn. Allyn and Bacon, Needham Heights, MA.

72. US Department of Labor (2002). *Bureau of labor statistics. Employment status of the population by sex, marital status, and presence and age of own children.* US Department of Labor.

73. Saelens BE, Sallis JF, Frank LF (2003). Environmental correlates of walking and cycling: findings from the transportation, urban design, and planning literatures. *Annals Behav Med* **25**, 80–91.

74. Sallis J, Bauman A, Pratt M (1998). Environmental and policy interventions to promote physical activity. *Am J Prev Med* **15**, 379–97.

75. Ellaway A, MacIntyre S (2000). Shopping for food in socially contrasting localities. *Br Food J* **102**, 52–9.

76. Sallis J, McKenzie T, Elder J, Broyles S, Nader P (1997). Factors parents use in selecting play spaces for young children. *Arch Pediatric Adoles Med* **151**, 414–7.

77. Harnack L, Jeffery R, Boutelle K (2000). Temporal trends in energy intake in the United States: an ecologic perspective. *Am J Clinic Nutr* **72**, 1478–84.

78. Bittman M, Meagher G, Matheson G (1998). *The changing boundaries between home and market: Australian trends in outsourcing domestic labour.* Social Policy Research Centre.

79. Lin B, Guthrie J, Frazao E (1999). *Away-from-home foods increasingly important to quality of American Diet.* Agriculture Information Bulletin No. 749. US Department of Agriculture, Economic Research Service, Washington, DC:

80. Hurley J, Liebman B (2004). Kids' cuisine: "What would you like with your fries?" *Nutr Action Healthletter*, March,12–15.

81. Fisher J, Rolls B, Birch L (2003). Children's bite size and intake of an entree are greater with large portions than with age-appropriate or self-selected portions. *Am J Clinic Nutr* **77**, 1164–70.

82. Keenan D, Abu Sabha R, Robinson N (2002). Consumers' understanding of the Dietary Guidelines for Americans: insights into the future. *Health Edu Behav* **29**, 124–35.

83. McArthur L, Chamberlain V, Howard A (2001). Behaviors, attitudes, and knowledge of low-income consumers regarding nutrition labels. *J Health Care Poor Underserved* **12**, 415–28.

84. Kreuter M, Brennan L, Scharff D, Lukwago S (1997). Do nutrition label readers eat healthier diets? Behavioral correlates of adults' use of food labels. *Am J Prev Med* **13**, 277–83.

85. Hill JM, Radimer KL (1997). A content analysis of food advertisements in television for Australian children. *Aust J Nutr Diet* **54**, 174–81.

86. Taras H, Sallis J, Patterson T, *et al.* (1989). Television's influence on children's diet and physical activity. *Dev Behav Pediatrics* **10**, 176–80.

87. Borzekowski DL, Robinson TN (2001). The 30-second effect: an experiment revealing the impact of television commercials on food preferences of preschoolers. *J Am Diet Assoc* **101**, 42–6.

88. Francis LA, Lee Y, Birch LL (2003). Parental weight status and girls' television viewing, snacking, and body mass indexes. *Obes Res* **11**, 143–51.

89. Crespo CJ, Smit E, Troiano RP, Bartlett SJ, Macera CA, Andersen RE (2001). Television watching, energy intake, and obesity in US children: results from the third National Health and Nutrition Examination Survey, 1988–1994. *Arch Pediatric Adoles Med* **155**, 360–5.

90. Matheson D, Killen J, Wang Y, Varady A, Robinson T (2004). Children's food consumption during television viewing. *Am J Clinic Nutr* **79**, 1088–94.

91. Salmon J, Ball K, Crawford D, Booth M, Telford A, Hume C, *et al.* (2005). Reducing sedentary behaviour and increasing physical activity among 10-year old children: overview and process evaluation of the "Switch-Play" intervention. *Health Promo Int* **20**, 7–17.

92. Birch LL, McPhee L, Shoba BC, Pirok E, *et al.* (1987). What kind of exposure reduces children's food neophobia? Looking vs. tasting. *Appetite* **9**, 171–8.

93. Pliner P, Stallberg-White C (2000). "Pass the ketchup, please": familiar flavors increase children's willingness to taste novel foods. *Appetite* **34**, 95–103.

94. Field Research Corporation (2004). A survey of Californians about the problem of childhood obesity. Available from *http://www.calendow.org/news/press_releases/ 2004/03/main.stm.* Accessed on 28 October 2004.

95. Collins DCA, Kearns RA (2001). The safe journeys of an enterprising school: negotiating landscapes of opportunity and risk. *Health and Place* **7**, 293–306.

96. **Giles-Corti B, English D, Costa C, Milne E, Cross D, Johnston R** (2004). Creating SunSmart schools. *Health Edu Res* **19**, 98–109.

97. **Leblanc J, Beattie T, Culligan C** (2002). Effect of legislation on the use of bicycle helmets. *CMAJ* **166**, 592–5.

98. **Chapman S, Wakefield M** (2001). Tobacco control advocacy in Australia: reflections on 30 years of progress. *Health Edu Behav* **28**, 274–89.

99. **Lobstein T, Baur L, Uauy R** (2004). IASO International Obesity TaskForce. Obesity in children and young people: a crisis in public health. *Obes Rev* **5** (Suppl 1), 4–85.

100. **Kubik M, Lytle L, Hannan P, Story M, Perry C** (2002). Food-related beliefs, eating behavior, and classroom food practices of middle school teachers. *J School Health* **72**, 339–45.

101. **Schwartz M, Puhl R** (2003). Childhood obesity: a societal problem to solve. *Obes Rev* **4**, 57–71.

102. **Stratton G** (2000). Promoting children's physical activity in primary school: an intervention study using playground markings. *Ergonomics* **43**, 1538–46.

103. **Staunton C, Hubsmith D, Kallins W** (2003). Promoting safe walking and biking to school: the Marin County success story. *Am J Pub Health* **93**, 1431–4.

Chapter 11

Drawing possible lessons for obesity prevention and control from the tobacco control experience[1]

Shawna L. Mercer, Laura Kettel Khan,
Lawrence W. Green, Abby C. Rosenthal,
Rose Nathan, Corinne G. Husten, and
William H. Dietz

Introduction

While tobacco control experts in many developed countries announce remarkable reductions in tobacco consumption, nutrition and physical activity experts in these same countries bemoan the growing epidemic of obesity. Food and physical activity differ substantially from tobacco in that they are essential to life. Whereas the goal with tobacco control is therefore to eliminate all use, obesity control focuses on reducing some behaviors (excessive and unhealthful food intake) and increasing others (physical activity). Moreover, tobacco control involves preventing use of a single product while controlling food intake requires addressing a variety of products, and engaging in sufficient physical activity may require encouraging a range of activities and dedicating a period of time daily. On the other hand, both tobacco control and obesity control involve influencing complex behaviors. For example, many overweight individuals struggle with similar tendencies to smokers by compulsively ingesting food for gratification even though they have surpassed their nutritional requirements. Both overweight people and smokers are affected by social, economic, and environmental factors, some of which (e.g., sporting event sponsorship, adolescent peer pressure, low taxes, and lack of clean indoor air policies) may encourage smokers to increase their cigarette consumption and others of which (e.g., product placement in stores,

[1] This work began when Shawna Mercer, Lawrence Green, and Rose Nathan were with the Office on Smoking and Health in the Centers for Disease Control and Prevention (CDC) in Atlanta, Georgia. The findings and conclusions in this report are those of the authors and do not necessarily represent the views of CDC.

lack of price subsidies for fresh produce, reduced availability of parks and other green spaces, and neighbourhood crime) may encourage overweight people to consume products in excess of their recommended caloric intake, or to reduce their physical activity level and thereby minimize their energy expenditure. Furthermore, rates, patterns, and causes of relapse are comparable (1,2). Studies have shown patterns of relapse generally involve a steep reduction in adherence or abstinence in the first few weeks after an intervention or quit attempt, approximately 70% of patients relapsing by the end of three months, another 10% relapsing over the next three months, and subsequently a very slow relapse rate (1).

Such similarities suggest that there may be some overlap between elements involved in the control of obesity and the control of tobacco. This review, therefore, builds on and updates our previously published work (3,4,5) in seeking to draw lessons from the successes of the tobacco control experience for the organization of more successful efforts to reduce and prevent obesity.

The evidence from tobacco control of the need for comprehensive approaches

The reduction in tobacco consumption in the United States since 1965 has been declared one of America's ten greatest public health achievements of the twentieth century (6,7). Similar reductions have been achieved in other countries, including Australia, Canada, New Zealand, Singapore, and some northern European countries (8–14). A number of expert groups have recently published reviews aimed at determining what has been responsible for these successes (15–18). Their systematic examination of trends in tobacco consumption, smoking prevalence, attempts to quit, and successful cessation has indicated that no single component of policies and programs can account for all of the significant changes (8,15,16,19). With the possible exception of pricing, the impact of each component of comprehensive tobacco control programs has been shown to be enhanced by the existence of and synergy with other components operating in the same environment (15–18).

Many obesity control programs have targeted behavior change primarily or solely at the level of the individual. Individual-level strategies such as education or counseling have shown themselves to be effective when they can be focused on executing a discrete behavioral change, such as taking medication on a prescribed schedule (20). Both tobacco use and obesity, however, involve not only individual-level factors such as knowledge, attitudes, beliefs and abilities but also complex lifestyle and environmental factors. Thus, smoking cessation counseling alone is unlikely to have a sufficient impact on population-based cessation rates without supportive interventions such as telephone support, system changes (including provider education and provider-reminder systems), community and media initiatives, and increasing the unit price for tobacco products (16,21). Indeed, physician efforts have not been able to single-handedly reduce the broad cultural acceptability of tobacco use and the pressures and cues to smoke in various settings (15).

To the extent that counseling depends on one's commitment to behavior change, its success can be enhanced if the individual receives support at home, work, and from friends, as well as through organizational, community, and broader societal efforts (22–26). Most individuals relapse repeatedly when they try to initiate and maintain complex behavioral changes without sufficient social support in environments that conspire against them (1,27). To date, evidence-based smoking cessation counseling has seen success because it has been reinforced by comprehensive tobacco control efforts that have simultaneously intervened on multiple facets of the environment, thereby reinforcing the counseling (3,16,21).

A framework for successful tobacco and obesity control

A useful framework for identifying and categorizing all of the components necessary for successful tobacco control is provided by the recent Surgeon General's Report entitled *Reducing Tobacco Use* (18). The report discusses five key elements: 1) clinical intervention and management, 2) educational strategies, 3) regulatory efforts, 4) economic approaches, and 5) the combination of all of these into comprehensive programs with synergistic effects (Box 11.1). We use this framework here, as we have previously (5), to describe the importance of each of these elements for tobacco control, and to discuss their application in obesity control. It is essential to note while reading through the next sections of this chapter that although the framework initially presents and discusses the first four elements individually, the greatest gains in tobacco control are achieved by tying these elements together into a comprehensive multi-message, multi-channel approach, built on a foundation of policy-based interventions (3,18,28)—as is discussed in element five.

Box 11.1: Five key elements for successful tobacco control

Five Key Elements[a] for Successful Tobacco Control

1. Clinical Intervention and Management
2. Educational Strategies
3. Regulatory Efforts
4. Economic Approaches
5. Combining all of the Above Elements into Comprehensive Programs

[a]Source: (22)

Clinical intervention and management

Given the large number of current smokers and the significant morbidity and mortality associated with tobacco use, assisting these current smokers to quit and remain abstinent could produce a public health benefit that would be larger (in the short-term) and more quickly achieved than the benefit associated with many other components of a comprehensive tobacco control program (15,29). Physician counseling and associated treatment for smoking cessation has been found to be one of the most clinically significant and cost effective of all disease prevention interventions (30–34). More than 70% of smokers in the United States make one or more visits to a physician each year and the large majority of these smokers would like to quit smoking (35). Some physicians have avoided counseling out of concern that their patients would resent being asked about their personal behaviors. Yet, recent studies have found that physicians who discussed smoking had more satisfied patients than those who did not—even among patients not interested in quitting (36,37). Physician advice to stop smoking has frequently been cited by patients as a reason for why they attempted to quit smoking as well as for their success in quitting (33,38–40). What is unknown and possibly as important as the data on reasons for quitting is the numbers of smokers who use as their excuse or rationale for not quitting that their physician said nothing about it in their recent visits. In any case, the primary care setting is a vastly underused resource for smoking cessation counseling (41).

Recent years have witnessed the production of numerous clinical guidelines for physician-based smoking cessation and treatment (32,33,42–45). One developed by a task force sponsored by the US Public Health Service has been among the most helpful and influential as a result of its delineation of a clear algorithm for assessing and treating tobacco use (33). The algorithm, entitled "the 5 A's for brief intervention, responds to the numerous competing priorities on physicians' time by identifying the essential elements to be covered at each step. The physician is encouraged to: 1) *ask* every patient about tobacco use at every visit; 2) *advise* every tobacco user to quit, using a clear, strong, and personalized manner; 3) *assess* each user's willingness to quit; 4) *assist*, using counseling and pharmacotherapy, all patients willing to make a quit attempt; and 5) *arrange* follow up, preferably within a week of a quit attempt (Figure 11.1).

For patients unwilling to quit, the physician is encouraged to use "the 5 R's to enhance motivation to quit tobacco" (33). This involves having the patient consider the: 1) *relevance* for him or herself personally of quitting, 2) personal *risks* of tobacco use, 3) personal *rewards* of quitting, and 4) personal *roadblocks* to quitting; and 5) having the physician incorporate *repetition* of this motivational intervention into each clinical visit of an unmotivated patient. Finally, never smokers are encouraged to remain abstinent and former smokers are to receive relapse prevention counseling.

These interventions are designed to be very brief, so that physicians could complete all of them in three minutes (33). Many physicians find that of all the patients they see in a given day, a full three minutes of counseling is appropriate for only a very few.

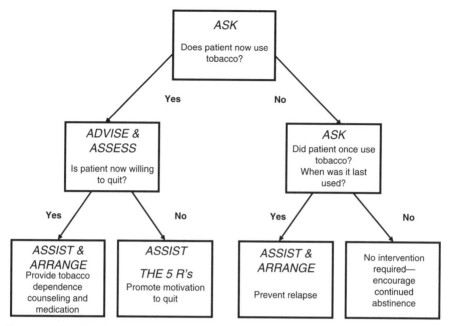

Fig. 11.1 Algorithm for assessing and treating tobacco use. Source: (10); Adapted from (26).

Nonetheless, if physicians carry the sole responsibility for completing all the steps, they are less likely to use the algorithm. Increased adoption and effectiveness result from making structural changes to the health care system that encourage and enable physicians to concentrate on the tasks they are best or uniquely qualified to undertake (33,46,47). Hence, office staff should ask about a patient's smoking status, prompt physicians by providing this information to them right before they begin their visit with the patient, and provide more intensive counseling or arrange referrals to specialized services post visit (3). Physicians can then be freed up to concentrate more intensively on providing smoking cessation and relapse advice and encouragement, assessing readiness to quit, and offering brief assistance through counseling and pharmacotherapy (9,33,46–49).

Receiving advice from a physician to lose weight increases the likelihood that patients will attempt to reduce their weight (50). As with smoking cessation counseling, weight loss counseling is associated with greater benefits when decision-making and goal-setting is shared between the provider and the patient (51). A similar structure of 5 A's has therefore been suggested for obesity counseling: 1) *assess* obesity risk; 2) *ask* about readiness to lose weight; 3) *advise* in designing a weight control program; 4) *assist* in establishing appropriate interventions; and 5) *arrange* for follow up (51). Clinical guidelines have been formulated for obesity management and intervention as they have for smoking cessation (40,52–55). These guidelines have evaluated a variety of approaches that have been used to address obesity and its associated co-morbidities, including counseling about diet and exercise, behavior modification, and pharmacotherapy. The US Preventive Services Task Force (55) recently concluded that there is fair to good evidence of the efficacy of high-intensity counseling—about diet, physical activity or both—together with behavioral interventions—targeting skill development, motivation, and support strategies—in producing modest sustained weight loss, but insufficient evidence to recommend for or against the use of moderate or low intensity counseling together with behavioral interventions. Unlike smoking cessation, however, no programs to date have demonstrated the effectiveness of obesity management in primary care settings. The recent finding that the incidence of type 2 diabetes was reduced through counseling overweight patients about weight and physical activity does suggest that effective interventions may soon be available (56). As is the case for smoking cessation, however, the lack of reimbursement or coverage for obesity prevention and treatment in most countries' medical capitation plans serves as a considerable disincentive for physician's use of such counseling interventions.

Pharmacotherapy to support quitting is recommended for all users of tobacco regardless of amount smoked. In contrast, the relative risks and benefits of pharmacotherapy or surgical treatments for obesity differ by an individual's health status and presence of other co-morbid conditions so that there is no comparable population-based approach for obesity intervention (54,57). As well, while prompts have been found to increase smoking cessation counseling by physicians (16,21), the effect on physician counseling of prompts about the severity of obesity has not been adequately explored. One possible prompt worthy of further exploration in this regard is body mass index (BMI), which the US Preventive Services Task Force concluded is reliable and valid for identifying adults at increased risk for mortality and morbidity due to overweight and obesity (55).

It may be possible for health professionals such as nurses and pharmacists to advise, assess, assist, and motivate less expensively than physicians for both smoking cessation and obesity counseling. Physician-delivered interventions for smoking cessation have been found to be significantly more effective than self-help interventions, but not significantly more effective than non-physician clinicians (33). The relative effectiveness of obesity interventions delivered by physicians versus non-physicians remains unknown.

Educational strategies

Educational interventions and strategies for tobacco control have been delivered principally through school programs, worksites, the mass media, parents, and community programs (18).

School programs

The large majority of smokers start smoking before the age of 18 and many form impressions about tobacco and experiment with it long before they reach high school (58).

While the evidence is inconsistent for the effectiveness of school-based tobacco control interventions when they are implemented alone, school-based interventions have been found to be effective when they are combined with a coordinated mass media campaign and additional community-based educational interventions (16, David P. Hopkins, Personal Communication, July 27, 2005). For example, school-based programs that help youth to identify the social influences that promote tobacco use and teach them skills to resist these influences have led to some reductions in adolescent smoking prevalence (16,58–60). The strength of this effect has been enhanced by other school-based interventions such as comprehensive life skills approaches and enforcement of tobacco-free school policies, as well as community-wide programs with parental and community involvement, mass media campaigns, and restrictions on youth access to tobacco products (10,55,61–64, David P. Hopkins, Personal Communication, July 27, 2005). Linkages with state and local coalitions and counter-marketing programs can also strengthen school-based efforts (58,62). School-based programs often start in the elementary grades and focus on both prevention and cessation of tobacco use (15,58,61,65).

There are considerable complexities and difficulties inherent in establishing and maintaining school-based programs for obesity control just as there are for tobacco control. Nonetheless, because schools provide numerous opportunities for eating and physical activity, and because they are a safe location for physical activity, they are likely places to conduct nutrition and physical activity interventions (66–70). School-based programs that are well-designed and fully implemented have been found to improve physical activity levels and eating behaviors of children and adolescents (71–74). Programs most likely to produce these effects include as key components the implementation of health and physical education curricula that assist students in adopting and maintaining healthful eating behaviors and physically active lifestyles, and that provide health education instruction through tailored activities that address social influences (71,72,75). One such program is the Team Nutrition initiative where the Food and Nutrition Service of the US Department of Agriculture works with state agencies and local school food authorities to educate and motivate children to make healthful food choices and to provide school food service staff with training and technical support (76). Another is Planet Health, an interdisciplinary curriculum aiming to increase physical activity, improve dietary quality, and decrease inactivity through classroom and physical education activities (77).

Advertising, mass media, and counter-marketing

Advertising and promotion of tobacco increase both initiation of tobacco among youth and consumption among adults (58,78,79). Youth are more likely to be influenced by advertising than are adults, youth are highly aware of tobacco advertising, youth exposure to cigarette advertisements that they find appealing is associated with subsequent smoking initiation and maintenance, and youth are more likely to buy the brands of cigarettes that are advertised the most heavily (78–83). Substantial evidence exists that counter-marketing, especially when combined with other program components such as school or community programs, is effective in increasing anti-tobacco attitudes and beliefs and decreasing the initiation and prevalence of tobacco use among both adolescents and adults (48,61,63,84–93). Counter-marketing aims to promote smoking cessation, decrease initiation, and reduce exposure to second-hand tobacco smoke by countering pro-tobacco messages and influences and by increasing pro-health influences and messages that "de-normalize" smoking (15,48,88,94). Counter-marketing can also increase public support for tobacco control and create a climate that is supportive of school, community, and policy efforts (94).

Counter-marketing typically includes media advocacy, press releases, paid advertising, sponsoring of health promotion activities, and replacing tobacco industry promotions and sponsorships of cultural, sports and other events, and it can also include distributing anti-tobacco merchandise, building youth movements against tobacco, and branding of anti-tobacco campaigns ("truth" campaigns, for example) (15,88,94). Effectiveness of counter-marketing has been found to depend on its being of sufficient frequency, duration, and reach (90,94,95). Effectiveness has also been increased by avoiding direct admonitions not to smoke and excessive repetition of individual messages, by using a wide variety of production styles and messages, and by carefully targeting messages for specific audiences (messages eliciting strong emotional responses have greater effect among youth, for example) (15,88,94).

There appears to be a direct relationship between watching television and the prevalence of obesity among children and adolescents (96). Though this relationship may be explained through the displacement of physical activity, a plausible alternative or complementary effect may stem from television's effects on children's food consumption. Televised food advertisements exert a major influence on the dietary intake of children and adults (97–101). A recent study found that more than 60% of the products advertised on Saturday morning television programs for children are food items (102). Additionally, the more television that children and adults watch, the more likely they are to consume the foods they see advertised on television and to consume them inattentively while watching television (96,103,104).

Since the specific mechanisms that account for the effects of television on childhood obesity have not yet been identified, strategies to prevent childhood obesity have focused on reducing television watching. Such interventions have been highly effective in preventing and treating obesity in both school-based and clinical settings (77,96, 103,105–112). The American Academy of Paediatrics has repeatedly released policy statements recommending that parents limit their children's television watching to one to two hours per day (113). Recent reports suggest that television watching may be declining, at least among high school students. The proportion of high school students who reported that they watched television three or more hours on a typical school day has declined significantly from 42.8% in 1999 to 38.2% in 2003 (114).

These figures compare to a 1990 survey that reported children's median television watching was 4.8 hours per day (115). Nonetheless, these findings indicate that many children are still watching substantially more television than is recommended. Furthermore, if displacement of physical activity is responsible for much of the relationship between television viewing and obesity, then it would be troubling if reductions in television watching were associated with increased time spent in front of computer screens and video games.

One of the most ambitious interventions directed at obesity-related behavior has been CDC's VERB campaign, a national youth media campaign first announced in Spring 2002 that engaged kids in promoting healthy activity among kids (116–119). For the first time, substantial financial resources were devoted to an integrated social marketing strategy that used paid media to promote physical activity among children by addressing social norms, presenting physical activity as an opportunity to play and have fun, and partnering with celebrities, athletes, national sports leagues, and recognized children's brands. This campaign explored the factors related to physical activity and assessed the impact of a program designed to address them. After 1 year, 74% of children aged 9-13 surveyed were aware of the VERB campaign, and subgroups of younger children, girls, children whose parents had less than a high school education, children from densely populated urban areas, and children who were low active at baseline engaged in higher physical activity than did children who were unaware of VERB (120).

Regulatory efforts

A growing body of evidence suggests that regulation and its enforcement are critical components of tobacco control programs (16,18,121–128). Regulation has been applied at four levels, all four of which are essential for tobacco control: regulation of the product—to limit the harm of tobacco, a hazardous product; regulation of the industry—to require the industry to function as a responsible corporate citizen; regulation of community, school, and work settings—to ensure safety in public places; and regulation of the individual—to limit opportunities for individuals to harm others or themselves (4).

Regulation of the product can try to ensure that the manufactured tobacco product, like other consumer products, is no more harmful than necessary given the available technology (18). This can include prohibiting constituents that render the product more attractive (such as flavorants) or additives that speed up the neurological effect of nicotine (4,18). It is critical to note, however, that product changes in the form of low tar/low nicotine cigarettes—touted as being associated with reduced risk of disease—have actually been shown to have little, if any, impact on reducing disease risk (129). Instead, use of low tar/low nicotine cigarettes may be at least partially responsible for the increase in lung cancer among long-term smokers who have switched to these cigarettes. It is also important to note that switching to low tar/low nicotine cigarettes may give smokers a false sense of security, given that the cigarettes can be manipulated by the smoker so that the actual amount of tar and nicotine consumed may be the same as, or higher than the brand used previously.

Regulation of the industry has included: ensuring that consumers are informed of the toxic ingredients contained in tobacco products and warned of the dangers of tobacco use; increasing the price of tobacco products through taxation; and restricting or banning tobacco advertising, sponsorships, and promotions. Regulation of community, school, and work settings has included restricting or prohibiting smoking and use of smokeless tobacco in public places. Finally, regulation of individuals has primarily been focused on restricting minors' access to tobacco products (4,18).

Enforcement has received parallel attention because if tobacco control policies are not enforced, the public receives the message that community and government leaders do not consider them to be important (130). Enforcement also enhances the efficacy of tobacco control policies through deterring violators, especially individuals selling tobacco products to children and adolescents (122,125,130). Regulation itself needs to be combined with other program components targeted to changing social norms, as restrictions of products by age or by location of use may simply lead people to adjust where they obtain or use tobacco (15,122,131). Hence, enforcement of minors' access and clean indoor air laws is frequently preceded and accompanied by public information campaigns and employer and retailer education campaigns (18,58,125,132,133).

Most governments around the world now have at least some regulatory provisions for tobacco control, although there is considerable variation in terms of comprehensiveness, stringency, and enforcement (4). Regulation of tobacco products, minors' access laws, and clean indoor air policies to protect the health of non-smokers are the principal areas in which regulation is being developed and enforced in the United States (4,18). The US and Canadian and some other governments support enforcement of minors' access by requiring retailers to verify age (4). Canada has led the world in stringent labeling and disclosure requirements for tobacco products, and a recent telephone survey has suggested that Canada's graphic warning labels have led to some reductions in smoking among adult smokers (4,126). Australia has been particularly active in banning restricting tobacco advertising with a banning on direct cigarette advertising in the mid 1970s and legislation for a general ban in the 1990s, with some exceptions for point of sale advertisements and international sports and cultural event sponsorships (4,134). Many countries, particularly in the Western Pacific region, restrict or ban the sale of tobacco products through vending machines and prohibit the sale of free samples, unpackaged cigarettes, and other promotional tactics aimed at youth (4). South Africa, Poland, and Fiji are particularly noteworthy examples of countries with comprehensive tobacco control regulation (4).

Because of the global nature of the tobacco use epidemic and the considerable variations in tobacco control policies across countries, and in an unprecedented use of its constitutional powers to address health policy, the World Health Organization brought together—from 2000 to 2003—official delegations from more than 150 member states of the World Health Assembly to develop an international legal instrument entitled the Framework Convention on Tobacco Control (FCTC) (135). The FCTC provides a foundation for comprehensive national actions and complementary international actions to control tobacco use and exposure. It addresses regulations in each of the areas discussed in this section, as well as for educational campaigns, clinical interventions, liability and tobacco industry behavior, and supportive and facilitative measures. The FCTC was adopted in May 2003, signed by 168 countries prior to the cut off date of June 29, 2004, has been ratified by 74 countries to the present time, and it will continue to be open indefinitely to countries wishing to become parties to it (136).

Some regulations currently exist or are planned to address the food consumption of large numbers of people (e.g., 137). Most countries permit at least some regulation of marketing to children, but such marketing restrictions are often and easily undermined (138). The European Commission and the UK are proposing to draft regulation of nutrition and health claims while WHO has developed guidelines for the same purpose (138,139).

Two pertinent regulations for obesity control in the US are school lunch programs (an example of regulation of the community, schools and worksites) and food labeling (regulation of the industry) (66). The US National School Lunch Program, for example, is a federally-assisted meal program that operates in more than 97,700 public and non-profit private schools and residential childcare institutions (140,141). It provides nutritionally-balanced, low-cost or free lunches to more than 27 million children each school day. The US Congress expanded the National School Lunch Program in 1998 to reimburse snacks served to children and youth in after-school educational and enrichment programs (142). Regulations stipulate that school lunches must meet the Dietary Guidelines for Americans, so that no more than 30 percent of calories should come from fat, and less than 10 percent from saturated fat. Regulations also indicate that school lunches should provide one-third of the recommended dietary allowances of protein, Vitamin A, Vitamin C, iron, calcium, and calories. Yet, local school food authorities are left to decide what specific foods are served and how they are prepared.

Nutrient labeling has been found to exert a significant effect on consumer purchase behavior (66,143). There is some evidence that consumers act as if they hold "nutrient (or health risk) budgets" (144). When taste and other differences are relatively small, providing nutrient information appears to help consumers to choose between more and less healthful products. If taste and other differences are large, however, nutrient labeling may not reduce the overall consumption of less healthful foods.

In contrast to tobacco, adverse effects of specific dietary practices or foods have not yet been definitively linked to obesity. Therefore, many regulatory strategies that might affect food consumption cannot yet be justified. The identification of these linkages must remain a high priority. In this vein, Yach and his colleagues (138) provide a thorough discussion of how regulation related to a number of the major elements of WHO's FCTC could be applied to diet and nutrition. They maintain, however, that a treaty approach is not appropriate for obesity control because of the inherent differences between controlling a lethal product such as tobacco and controlling obesity, which involves consumption of foods and nutrients from multiple sources as well as physical activity. Nonetheless, it is of note that a commentary accompanying their article suggests that a treaty approach could be warranted (145).

At present, a better case for regulation exists for physical activity. Physical activity has been demonstrated to have beneficial effects on the co-morbidities associated with obesity (68). Additionally, evidence links physical activity in schools to overall physical activity, which in turn has been linked to obesity (66,67,115,146–150). It is therefore disturbing that the proportion of US high school students who report that they participate in daily physical education declined from 42% in 1991 (151) to 29% in 1999 (152). Recent data from the 2003 US Youth Risk Behavior Survey (YRBS) are encouraging since no further reductions were seen in reported daily physical education among high school students (114). Yet, room for regulation is demonstrated by additional data from the 2003 YRBS that indicate 44% of the high school students were not enrolled in any physical education class, and 37% had not participated in sufficient vigorous physical activity during the 7 days prior to the survey (114).

Promising avenues for further research include school-based and school-related policies that focus on improved nutrition and physical activity as obesity prevention strategies (153). Some, for example, are considering transportation policies supportive of active commuting to school (154). Additionally, schools in some communities have refused to sign exclusive contracts with soft drink companies that provide incentives for high sales volumes, given that this encourages students to consume foods of low nutritional value, and schools in other communities have negotiated contracts that require the companies to provide some or exclusively nutritional options (155–157). Currently, data linking soft drink or fast food consumption to obesity are limited, but the criterion of biological plausibility suggests such consumption may increase caloric intake or impair efforts at weight control (158–161). This has led the American Academy of Paediatrics Committee on School Health (162) to release a statement recommending the development of clearly defined, district-wide policies restricting the sale of soft drinks in schools. Moreover, interventions that have reduced the prices of fruit and vegetables in high school and work site cafeterias have increased consumption of fruits and vegetables (163–165). Efforts are underway to determine whether increasing prices of low nutrient foods may also lead to increased fruit and vegetable consumption (166).

Economic approaches

Economic theory postulates that as the price of a product increases, demand for the product will decrease (167). Studies have shown that past consumption levels and perceptions about the costs of current and future consumption are predictors of current consumption of addictive substances such as nicotine (8,18,168). Analyses of the literature suggest that a 10% increase in the price of cigarettes will result in a six to 10% decline in overall consumption in low and middle income countries and a three to five percent decline in high income countries (18). This decline can be attributed to half of the smokers reducing the number of cigarettes they smoke and the other half quitting (18,169). Individuals in low and middle income countries, those of lower socioeconomic status in higher income countries, and adolescents are particularly sensitive to increasing prices, rendering them less likely to smoke at all (8,170). The Guide to Community Preventive Services has concluded that increasing the price of tobacco products is effective both for increasing cessation and for preventing initiation by youth (133). Regulation of tobacco production, importation, and exportation all increase prices and thereby decrease consumption (18). One of the key tobacco control strategies, therefore, and the single most important economic approach to tobacco control, is to lessen the affordability of tobacco by increasing taxes on tobacco products (8,18,138,169). The tax component of the retail price for a pack of cigarettes in countries with comprehensive tobacco control policies is between two thirds and four fifths of the total retail cost (8).

Tobacco taxes can take the form of specific taxes, in which a fixed amount is added to the price of tobacco products, and *ad valorem* taxes (including sales taxes and value-added taxes), which constitute a percentage of the base price and may be added on top of a specific excise tax. Both types of tax are important. With the specific excise tax it is less likely that the tobacco industry will respond by trying to keep low the real amount charged (8). On the other hand, specific excise taxes can decay over time with inflation, necessitating regular requests for tax increases to keep the overall price high.

Studies have found that consumption of fruits and vegetables as well as of low-fat snack choices in schools and worksites can be increased by price reductions or subsidies (97,163,164,166,171,172). Of historical interest is the fact that the introduction into grocery stores in 1973 of soy-ground beef blend resulted almost immediately in adoption of the innovation by approximately one-quarter of ground beef buyers. Fluctuating rates of purchase of ground beef and soy-ground beef and the recovery of ground beef in subsequent months were related almost entirely to the price of ground beef rather than to health motives or social influence (173). Social influence and diffusion or media effects have been found to be secondary to, or coterminous with pricing. Consumption of eggs, butter, and whole milk products has steadily declined—eggs since World War II, butter since the introduction of margarine, and whole milk more recently. Lower or comparable prices of alternative products account for many of the trends, but price effects appear to be augmented by health information about obesity, cardiovascular disease, and other health risks (97,174). A 2002 workshop on "Fruit and Vegetable Environment, Policy, and Pricing' evaluated studies exploring the effect on fruit and vegetable consumption of increasing the price of less nutritious foods, reducing the price of fruits and vegetables, and other strategies such as coupons and point-of-purchase information; although workshop participants identified some promising interventions, they concluded that more research was needed in all settings (166,175–179).

An economic analysis using annual state-based obesity prevalence data from the US Behavioral Risk Factor Surveillance System, along with state-specific data for a variety of other variables, found that the dramatic increases in obesity between 1984 and 1999 were most strongly associated with increases in the number of fast-food and full-service restaurants as well as the increasing cost of cigarettes (180). It was hypothesized that the positive association between the numbers of restaurants and obesity might be related to the increasing proportion of working mothers. They investigators also suggested that when the value of work exceeds the cost of restaurant food, families will choose to buy food rather than to prepare it. Additional economic analyses such as these may identify novel approaches to obesity control.

In the meantime, taxation on food, and possibly also on items related to physical activity, needs to be approached much more carefully because food and physical activity, unlike tobacco, are essential to life. Studies have found, for example, that diets high in fat and sugar can be less expensive than diets high in fruits and vegetables, and that lower socioeconomic status has been associated with higher fat intake and lower intake of fruits and vegetables (181–183). How much the price of processed foods of limited nutritional value would need to increase before seeing corresponding reductions in demand is currently unknown, and it is possible that lower income groups would be the most adversely affected by taxes on these foods (138). How to best use taxation as a tool is therefore not yet clear (97,166,184).

Comprehensive programs

As discussed at the outset of this chapter, individuals make behavioral choices within the complex context of their family and friends, the organizations of which they are a part, their community and culture, the economy and physical environment, and existing and proposed policy and legislation. International experts, therefore, have long called for comprehensive economic, policy, and regulatory interventions to decrease tobacco use, and have increasingly stressed that social environmental and individual level approaches should be mutually supportive (185–190). Comprehensive tobacco programs thus combine tobacco control components into multi-channel, multi-message approaches to tobacco control that simultaneously address many of the factors supporting tobacco use by both individuals and populations (17,18).

Evidence for the efficacy, effectiveness and usefulness of population-based and comprehensive tobacco control efforts has come from a variety of sources (15,18). Much has been learned from the numerous large scale community intervention trials undertaken around the world to prevent cardiovascular disease (10,11,18,191–203). Other information has come from international studies and programs specific to tobacco control including those in Victoria and New South Wales, Australia; India; Ontario and

British Columbia, Canada; US national programs; and US state-based programs including, most notably, those in California, Massachusetts, Florida, Arizona, and Oregon (15,18,85,191,204–217). Of all the jurisdictions employing comprehensive tobacco control—some of which started earlier, and some of which involved even more aggressive efforts on at least some fronts—California has most thoroughly evaluated its efforts over the longest period of time (91,218–222).

CDC's Office on Smoking and Health reviewed all of the above data—from both efficacy and effectiveness trials and from international, national, and state-based programs—in order to synthesize a comprehensive framework to guide the development of comprehensive tobacco control programs. The data collectively suggest that although no one intervention or program to date has included all possible components for which evidence of efficacy or effectiveness has been established, individual tobacco control program components do work together to produce the synergistic effects of a comprehensive program and that changing multiple facets of the social environment reduces individual-level tobacco use as well as the broad cultural acceptability of tobacco use (15,18).

The comprehensive framework integrates four goals within four program components (18,28). The four goals are: 1) prevent initiation of tobacco use, 2) promote quitting by youth and adults, 3) eliminate non-smokers' exposure to environmental tobacco smoke, and 4) eliminate disparities related to tobacco use and its effects on different population groups. The four components provide a structure for including tobacco control elements related to each of the aforementioned clinical intervention and management, educational strategies, regulatory effects, and economic approaches. The components are: 1) community interventions—i.e., programmatic elements that influence the societal organizations, systems and networks in order to promote an environment that encourages and supports individuals to make tobacco-free behavioral changes; 2) counter marketing; 3) program policy and regulation; and 4) surveillance and evaluation—in order to support appropriate evolution and modification in response to changing circumstances and new evidence (18,28). Attention must also be paid to ensuring that comprehensive programs have sound administration and management and that they are accountable and sustainable (15).

Community interventions and programs

Reviews of the evidence by the Community Preventive Services Task Force have found that the effectiveness of individual strategies is enhanced through the infrastructure, support, and community mobilization provided by community interventions (67,133). To support behavior change at the level of the individual, such as smoking prevention and cessation and relapse prevention, community programs need to change knowledge, attitudes, and practices of individual community members, while simultaneously changing the way tobacco products are promoted, made available, sold and used (15,219,223). This requires undertaking initiatives targeted at individuals and also at changing the social environment that promotes tobacco use and accepts exposure to second-hand smoke.

Effective community programs engage people in a wide range of public places including their work sites, schools, places of worship, entertainment venues, and civic organizations, as well as in their homes (15,18,224). Comprehensive programs that operate through multiple community channels foster the development of a synergy that enables social norms undercutting tobacco use to spread through the population more quickly than would otherwise be possible (223). Research has found that even though the effect of community programs on reducing tobacco use may be relatively small overall, this small effect translates into a large public health impact because of the large number of smokers and the substantial morbidity and mortality associated with tobacco use (223,225). The moderate efficacy of community programs is, therefore, more than offset by their considerable reach (15). Additionally, they provide the foundation on which counseling by primary care providers and other individualized tobacco control activities can build.

To meet the four goals for comprehensive tobacco control, community programs have been advised to: a) increase the number of individuals and organizations engaged in planning and implementing education and training programs at the level of the community, b) promote the adoption of public and private tobacco control policies, c) conduct counter-marketing campaigns that educate community members and support local tobacco control policies and initiatives, and d) measure outcomes using surveillance and evaluation (15,22,219). Evidence also shows that community programs need to include initiatives targeted to specific populations. Moreover, involving members of specific populations (for example, youth) in developing and implementing tobacco control interventions for their peers has been shown to strengthen the interventions' effects (88,209,226). Community programs also benefit from implementing local action plans, organizing debates about tobacco in the community, and drawing community leaders into tobacco control activities and advocacy (15,23,227). Finally, sustainability of tobacco use prevention and cessation requires community programs to have sufficient operating funds, resources, organizational support, and educational materials, to be able to support communication campaigns, and to provide adequate education and training.

While numerous broad-based interventions have targeted tobacco, fewer such interventions have been directed at obesity (97). Importantly, the Task Force on Community Preventive Services has concluded that strong evidence exists that physical activity levels can be increased by social support interventions in community settings as well as by combining informational outreach activities with the creation or enhancement of access to places for physical activity (67). School-based obesity prevention and treatment strategies have been envisaged as being among the most promising public health strategies for obesity control. Yet, school-based interventions have not typically been reinforced by community or environmental strategies and they have not had a significant impact on obesity unless they have specifically targeted it as an outcome variable (70,228). It is of note, however, that when interventions to reduce television viewing have been utilized in concert with other strategies, children have shown either reduced rates of weight gain (105) or increased rates of remission of obesity (77,106) compared to control groups. Moreover, a study comparing a home-based and a school-based nutrition program found that the home-based program was associated with changes in parental behavior (including high rates of participation and having more of the encouraged foods in their homes) and in student behavior (including reduced saturated fat, monounsaturated fat, and total fat in their diets) (229). Such studies continue to emphasize the importance of complementing and coordinating school and community efforts in health promotion (62,230).

In contrast to the vigorous advocacy that has been an important component of tobacco control, advocacy to date in the United States around control of obesity has been more limited (97). A number of factors, when taken together, provide a likely explanation. First, obesity has often been viewed as resulting from a lack of self-control, with overweight individuals being held entirely responsible for their status (231). This was also the case earlier in the tobacco control experience, with smokers being blamed entirely for their smoking (18). Moreover, only recently have increases in obesity rates been recognized as of epidemic proportions. The best-known and most visible groups that have advocated for improved nutrition include the American Cancer Society, the American Heart Association, and the Center for Science in the Public Interest. Yet since there is not yet definitive evidence of a causal link between a single type of food or food group and obesity, none of these groups target obesity as their primary focus. Finally, even though physical activity is as important for the energy balance equation as food intake, few constituencies have actively promoted opportunities for physical activity within communities. Organizations such as the National Coalition for the Promotion of Physical Activity and the US National Association for Sport and Physical Education have focused on trying to improve opportunities for physical activity among specific population groups, but a broad public constituency for the promotion of physical activity has not yet been mobilized.

State, province, or county-wide programs and partnership grants: a special case of community interventions and programs

State, province, and county-wide tobacco control programs can provide information, skills, and resources to increase local capacity for implementing strategic, coordinated, and effective tobacco control programs (15,219,227). Resources can include cessation toolkits and materials for mass media campaigns and surveillance. Such jurisdiction-wide programs have also functioned to stimulate and support community action plans, local actions in schools and businesses, and local evaluation efforts (15,232). Moreover, jurisdiction-wide programs have provided local organizations with training and technical assistance on how to implement smoke free policies, reduce minors' access to tobacco, promote media advocacy, and conduct meaningful surveillance and evaluation (15,19,233).

Providing jurisdiction-wide grants to professional, business, and youth groups, as well as to city development and law enforcement organizations has led to increases in group members' knowledge about tobacco use and control and to greater participation of group members in tobacco control efforts. Additionally, the effectiveness of tobacco control efforts among diverse population groups that might not be well reached by government agencies can be increased by providing funding to medical associations and other organizations that interact with these communities, and also by involving the communities themselves in planning and implementation (234,235).

Heightened visibility and support for individual and health system efforts can be provided by state or other governmental-level direction that coordinates efforts and provides a cohesive approach to obesity control. Research has demonstrated that including affected populations in planning and strategy implementation increases participation and helps to ensure relevance. At the same time, one of the lessons from government and foundation funders' insistence on using coalitions is that they must be managed strategically as tools for advocacy and planning, not for micromanagement of programs (236).

One example of a rapidly growing initiative for obesity control at the federal level is the US CDC's State-Based Nutrition and Physical Activity Program to Prevent Obesity and Other Chronic Diseases (237). The purpose of this program is to prevent and control obesity and related chronic diseases by supporting States in their development and implementation of science-based nutrition and physical activity interventions, including population-based strategies such as policy-level change, environmental supports, and social marketing. In 2004-2005, 23 states are being funded at $300,000-$450,000 for capacity-building, including a) gathering data, b) building partnerships, and c) creating state-wide health plans. Five additional states are being funded in 2004-2005 at $800,000 to $1.5 million for basic implementation, including a) developing new interventions, b) evaluating existing interventions, and/or c) supporting complementary state and local efforts to prevent and control obesity and other chronic diseases.

Another example of federal funding and technical support for obesity control is provided by CDC's Steps to a Healthier US cooperative agreement program, launched in 2004. This five year program funds communities to implement coordinated, comprehensive, and evidence-based community-, school-, and work-based prevention and control initiatives for obesity, diabetes, and asthma (116).

Conclusions and comments on future directions

Within the early days of tobacco control research, the actions and inquiries of researchers and health practitioners often tended to be inspired or guided by only one or two of the key elements or intervention modalities important for tobacco control—most typically those interventions that fell within their own discipline (18).

Yet, as described in this chapter, experience has shown that neither single-component interventions nor interventions that are based solely at the level of the individual will be likely to lead to a meaningful reduction in tobacco use at the level of the population (21). Becoming aware of all of the necessary elements for tobacco control and recognizing that these elements work together synergistically enables tobacco control researchers and health practitioners to continue to work within their own particular setting or modality while simultaneously considering how they can influence other settings and contexts in which individuals and populations must negotiate and maintain desired behavior changes. Our goals in preparing this chapter and previous articles, therefore, have been to stimulate parallel consideration of what might be essential elements for obesity control and how might they work together, and to identify existing evidence in this regard, so that obesity researchers might identify future directions for research.

A number of recent documents have attempted to compile the essential elements for obesity control. One compilation, prepared by a working group consisting of key US national, state, and local public health and education professionals, with the assistance of CDC, employed CDC's best practice document for tobacco (15) as a template to begin to formulate guidelines for US state and local health advocates who want to create their own comprehensive obesity control programs (238). For each suggested program component, the document provides a brief rationale, sample activities, and examples of existing US obesity control practices and programs. The working group acknowledges the limitations in the current evidence but provides the document as an important early step that will require modification over time as additional evidence becomes available. CDC has also developed a detailed Resource Guide for Nutrition and Physical Activity Interventions, to help guide the plans and activities of the State-Based Nutrition and Physical Activity Program (239). Additionally, the Task Force on Community Preventive Services is currently undertaking a series of systematic reviews on population-based interventions for obesity control (publication topics available at http://www.thecommunityguide.org/obesity/; accessed 18 July, 2005).

The existing evidence suggests there may be some key differences between comprehensive programs developed to address obesity and tobacco use. For example, some of the reductions in smoking rates have been attributable to changes in social norms about the acceptability of smoking (15,18). With changing social norms came nonsmokers' rights campaigns, which in turn led to stigmatization of smokers through policies prohibiting smoking in public buildings. In contrast, although obese persons have faced stigmatization and discrimination for decades, obesity prevalence has increased rather than diminished. Additionally, whereas increasing the price of a lethal product such as tobacco can be justified for all populations, price measures for high and low nutrient foods need to be considered carefully in order to avoid discriminating against people with lower incomes (138). Finally, there is no equivalent in tobacco control for things such as the small but significant degree of protection from childhood obesity conferred by breastfeeding (66,240).

One of the major emphases of the health promotion field has been to make healthful choices easy choices (137,241,242). This has led to advocacy for tobacco control policies and regulations that modify or control social and physical environments—such as pricing, labeling, and smoke-free environments (18,28). Yet, for both food and physical activity, the current social, physical, and economic conditions in North America as well as in other developed countries seem to make less healthful choices the easier choices (97,137). Finding ways to make more healthful nutritional and physical activity choices the easy choices is one of the challenges ahead.

To determine what has actually been responsible for reductions in tobacco use in real-world communities, researchers and practitioners have had to consider other forms of evidence in addition to randomized clinical trials. In a similar fashion, obesity control experts will need to assess a broad range of influences on eating and physical activity including community, regional, national, and international trends in food marketing. Furthermore, many practitioners, policy makers, and community residents are increasingly determined to become better consumers of research and even to have some control over the research that is done on them or on their behalf, rather than serving solely as objects of research (243). At the same time, most research funding agencies are increasingly concerned with ensuring that the research they fund is actually relevant to and used by its intended beneficiaries. In response, increasing numbers of researchers are utilizing participatory research approaches, in which the intended users and beneficiaries of the research are involved not only subjects of the research, but are engaged in the research process itself—in such things as identifying problems and research questions, designing and conducting the study, and interpreting and applying the study findings in their own community (243).

Participatory approaches will be even more essential for obesity control research than they were for tobacco control. Indeed many food manufacturers, journalists, policy makers, practitioners and lay members of the public may fear that applying lessons learned from tobacco control will lead to attempts to control food and exercise with heavy-handed legal restrictions and environmental controls. Concerns have been expressed that the food industry could be vilified to the same extent as has been the tobacco industry. Yet, since food and physical activity are essential to life, behavior change for obesity control will require more collaborative approaches between researchers, practitioners, governments, and the food industry. Participatory research will be an important means of assuring such cooperation.

References

1. **Brownell KD, Marlatt GA, Lichtenstein ER, Wilson GT** (1986). Understanding and preventing relapse. *Am Psychol* **41**, 765-82.
2. **National Cancer Institute** (1993). *How to help your patients stop smoking: a National Cancer Institute manual for physicians*, NIH Publication No: 93-3064. National Institutes of Health, Washington, DC. [Revised November 1991, Reprinted September 1993].

3. **Green LW, Mercer SL, Rosenthal AC, Dietz WH, Husten CG** (2003). Possible lessons for physician counselling on obesity from the progress in smoking cessation in primary care. In Elmadfa L, Anklam E, Konig JS, eds. *Modern aspects of nutrition: present knowledge and future perspectives,* Vol.56, pp. 191-4. Karger Publishers, Basel, Switzerland.

4. **Green L, Nathan R, Mercer S** (2001). The health of health promotion in public policy: drawing inspiration from the tobacco control movement. *Health Prom J Aus* **12**, 12-8.

5. **Mercer SL, Green LW, Rosenthal AC, Husten CG, Kettel Khan L, Dietz WH** (2003). Possible lessons from the tobacco experience for obesity control. *Am J Clin Nutr* **77** (suppl), 1073S-82S.

6. **Centres for Disease Control and Prevention** (1999). Achievements in public health, 1900-1999: tobacco use—United States, 1900-1999. *MMWR* **48**, 986-93.

7. **Centres for Disease Control and Prevention** (1999). Ten greatest public health achievements— United States, 1900-1999. *MMWR* **48**, 241-3.

8. **Jha P, Chaloupka FJ** (1999). *Curbing the epidemic: governments and the economics of tobacco control.* The International Bank for Reconstruction and Development/The World Bank, Washington, DC.

9. **Solberg LI** (2000). Incentivizing, facilitating, and implementing an office tobacco cessation system. *Tob Control* **9** (suppl), i37-41.

10. **Vartiainen E, Paavola M, McAlister A, Puska P** (1998). Fifteen-year follow-up of smoking prevention effects in the North Karelia youth project. *Am J Public Health* **88**, 81-5.

11. **Vartiainen E, Puska P, Jousilahti P, Korhonen HJ, Tuomilehto J, Nissinen A** (1994). Twenty-year trends in coronary risk factors in North Karelia and in other areas of Finland. *Int J Epidemiol* **23**, 495-504.

12. **World Health Organization** (1997). *Tobacco or health: A global status report.* World Health Organization, Geneva.

13. **Mackay J, Eriksen M** (2002). *The tobacco atlas.* World Health Organization, Geneva.

14. **World Health Organisation, Centres for Disease Control and Prevention, World Bank Group** (2003). *The tobacco country profiles, 2nd ed.* Shafey O, Dolwick S, Guindon GE eds. American Cancer Society, World Health Organisation, and International Union Against Cancer, Atlanta, GA.

15. **Centres for Disease Control and Prevention** (1999). *Best practices for comprehensive tobacco control programs—August 1999.* US Department of Health and Human Services, Centres for Disease Control and Prevention, National Centre for Chronic Disease Prevention and Health Promotion, Office on Smoking and Health. Reprinted, with corrections, Atlanta, GA.

16. **Hopkins DP, Fielding JE, and the Task Force on Community Preventive Services, eds** (2001). The guide to community preventive services: tobacco use prevention and control. Reviews, recommendations and expert commentary. *Am J Prev Med* **20** (suppl), 1-87.

17. **National Cancer Institute** (2000). *Population-based smoking cessation: proceedings of a conference on what works to influence cessation in the general population.* Smoking and tobacco control monograph no. 12, NIH Publication No. 00-4892. US Department of Health and Human Services, National Institutes of Health, National Cancer Institute, Bethesda, MD.

18. **US Department of Health and Human Services** (2000). *Reducing tobacco use: a report of the Surgeon General.* US Department of Health and Human Services, Centres for Disease Control and Prevention, National Centre for Chronic Disease Prevention and Health Promotion, Office of Smoking and Health, Atlanta, GA. Available at http://www.cdc.gov/tobacco/sgr/sgr_2000/ index.htm. Accessed 18 July 2005.

19. **Eriksen MP** (2000). Best practices for comprehensive tobacco control programs: opportunities for managed care organizations. *Tob Control* **9** (suppl), i11-4.

20. Mullen PD, Simons-Morton DG, Ramirez G, Frankowski RF, Green LW, Mains DA (1997). A meta-analysis of trials evaluating patient education and counseling for three groups of preventive health behaviors. *Patient Educ Couns* **32**, 157-73.

21. Hollis JF (2000). Population impact of clinician efforts to reduce tobacco use. In: National Cancer Institute. *Population based smoking cessation: proceedings of a conference on what works to influence cessation in the general population.* Smoking and tobacco control monograph no. 12, pp. 129-154, NIH Publication No. 00-4892. US Department of Health and Human Services, National Institutes of Health, National Cancer Institute, Bethesda, MD.

22. Burns DM (2000). Smoking cessation: recent indications of what's working at a population level. In: National Cancer Institute. *Population based smoking cessation: proceedings of a conference on what works to influence cessation in the general population.* Smoking and tobacco control monograph no. 12, pp. 1-24, NIH Publication No. 00-4892. US Department of Health and Human Services, National Institutes of Health, National Cancer Institute, Bethesda, MD.

23. Carlson CL, Chute P, Dacey S, McAfee TA (2000). Designing tobacco control systems and cessations benefits in managed care: skill-building workshop. *Tob Control* **9** (suppl), i25-9.

24. Green LW (1999). What can we generalize from research on patient education and clinical health promotion to physician counselling on diet? *Eur J Clin Nutr* **53**, (suppl), S9-18.

25. Isham GJ (2000). A proactive health plan: taking action on tobacco control. *Tob Control* **9** (suppl), i15-6.

26. Zhu S, Melcer T, Sun J, Rosbrook B, Pierce JP (2000). Smoking cessation with and without assistance. A population-based analysis. *Am J Prev Med* **18**, 305-11.

27. Marlatt GA, Gordon JR, eds (1985). Relapse prevention: maintenance strategies in the treatment of addictive behaviours. Guilford, New York.

28. Wisotzky M, Albuquerque M, Pechacek TF, Park BZ (2004). The National Tobacco Control Program: Focusing on policy to broaden impact. *Public Health Rep* **119**, 303-10.

29. US Department of Health and Human Services (1990). *The health benefits of smoking cessation: a report of the Surgeon General,* DHHS Publication No (CDC)90-8416. US Department of Health and Human Services, Centres for Disease Control and Prevention, Atlanta, GA. Available at http://profiles.nlm.nih.gov/NN/B/B/C/T/_/nnbbct.pdf. Accessed 18 July 2005.

30. Coffield AB, Maciosek MV, McGinnis JM *et al* (2001). Priorities among recommended clinical preventive services. *Am J Prev Med* **21**, 1-9.

31. Cummings SR, Rubin SM, Oster G (1989). The cost-effectiveness of counselling smokers to quit. *JAMA* **261**, 75-9.

32. Fiore MC, Bailey WC, Cohen SJ *et al* (1996). *Smoking Cessation. Clinical practice guideline no. 18,* AHCPR Publication No. 96-0692. US Department of Health and Human Services, Public Health Service, Agency for Health Care Policy and Research, Rockville, MD.

33. Fiore MC, Bailey WC, Cohen SJ *et al* (2000). *Treating tobacco use and dependence: clinical practice guideline.* US Department of Health and Human Services, Public Health Service, Rockville, MD. Available at www.surgeongeneral.gov/tobacco. Accessed 20 October 2004.

34. Partnership for Prevention (November 2000). *Real reform vs. rhetoric in tobacco prevention.* Priorities in Prevention. Available at http://www.prevent.org/priorities/PinP_1100_Tobacco.pdf. Accessed 18 July 2005.

35. Tomar SL, Husten CG, Manley MW (1996). Do dentists and physicians advise tobacco users to quit? *J Am Dental Assoc* **127**, 259-65.

36. Schaufler HH, Rodriguez T, Milstein A (1996). Health education and patient satisfaction. *J Fam Pract* **42**, 62-8.

37. Solberg LI, Boyle RG, Davidson G, Magnan SJ, Carlson CL (2001). Patient satisfaction and discussion of smoking cessation during clinical visits. *Mayo Clin Proc* **76**, 138-43.

38. **Lancaster T, Stead L, Silagy C, Sowden A** (2000). Effectiveness of interventions to help people stop smoking: findings from the Cochrane Library. *BMJ* **321**, 355-8.

39. **Ockene JK** (1987). Smoking interventions: the expanding role of the physician. *Am J Public Health* **77**, 782-3.

40. **US Preventive Services Task Force** (1996). *Guide to clinical preventive services, 2nd ed.* Williams & Wilkins, Baltimore, MD.

41. **Thorndike AN, Rigotti NA, Stafford RS, Singer DE** (1998). National patterns in the treatment of smokers by physicians. *JAMA* **279**, 604-8.

42. **American Medical Association** (1994). *American Medical Association guidelines for the diagnosis and treatment of nicotine dependence: how to help patients stop smoking.* American Medical Association, Washington, DC.

43. **American Psychiatric Association** (1996). Practice guideline for the treatment of patients with nicotine dependence. *Am J Psychiatry* **153**, 1-31.

44. **British Thoracic Society** (1998). Smoking cessation guidelines and their cost effectiveness. *Thorax* **53** (suppl), S1-38.

45. **Silagy C, Stead LF** (2001). Physician advice for smoking cessation (Cochrane review). In: *The Cochrane Library.* Update Software, 1, Oxford.

46. **Hollis JF, Bills R, Whitlock E, Stevens VJ, Mullooly J, Lichtenstein E** (2000). Implementing tobacco interventions in the real world of managed care. *Tob Control* **9** (suppl), i18-24.

47. **Rigotti NA, Thorndike AN** (2001). Reducing the health burden of tobacco use: what's the doctor's role? *Mayo Clin Proc* **76**, 121-3.

48. **Hopkins DP, Briss PA, Ricard CJ, et al** (2001). Reviews of the evidence regarding interventions to reduce tobacco use and exposure to environmental tobacco smoke. *Am J Prev Med* **20** (suppl), 16-66.

49. **Zhu, S** (2000). Telephone quitlines for smoking cessation. In: National Cancer Institute. *Population based smoking cessation: proceedings of a conference on what works to influence cessation in the general population.* Smoking and tobacco control monograph no. 12, pp. 189-98, NIH Publication No. 00-4892. US Department of Health and Human Services, National Institutes of Health, National Cancer Institute, Bethesda, MD.

50. **Galuska DA, Will JC, Serdula MK, Ford ES** (1999). Are health care professionals advising obese patients to lose weight? *JAMA* **282**, 1576-8.

51. **Serdula MK, Khan LK, Dietz WH** (2003). Weight loss counselling revisited. *JAMA* **89**, 1747-50.

52. **Gandjour A, Westenhofer J, Wirth A, Fuchs C, Lauterbach KW** (2001). Development process of an evidence-based guideline for the treatment of obesity. *Int J Qual Health Care* **13**, 325-32.

53. **McTigue KM, Harris R, Hemphill B et al** (2003). Screening and interventions for obesity in adults: summary of the evidence for the US Preventive Services Task Force. *Ann Intern Med* **139**, 933-49.

54. **National Institutes of Health** (1998). *Clinical guidelines on the identification, evaluation, and treatment of overweight and obesity in adults.* National Institutes of Health, National; Heart Lung Blood Institute, Bethesda, MD.

55. **US Preventive Services Task Force** (2003). Screening for obesity in adults: recommendations and rationale. *Ann Intern Med* **139**, 930-2.

56. **Tuomilehto J, Lindstrom J, Eriksson JG et al** (2001). Prevention of type 2 diabetes mellitus by changes in lifestyle among subjects with impaired glucose tolerance. *N Engl J Med* **344**, 1343-50.

57. **Douketis JD, Macie C, Thabane L, Williamson DF** (2005). Systematic review of long-term weight loss studies in obese adults: clinical significance and applicability to clinical practice. *Intl J Obesity* **2005** July 5 [Epublication ahead of print].

58. **US Department of Health and Human Services** (1994). *Preventing tobacco use among young people: a report of the Surgeon General.* US Department of Health and Human Services,

Public Health Service, Centres for Disease Control and Prevention, National Centre for Disease Prevention and Health Promotion, Office of Smoking and Health, Atlanta, GA. Available at http://www.cdc.gov/tobacco/sgr/sgr_1994/index.htm. Accessed 18 July 2005.

59. **Glynn T** (1989). Essential elements of school-based smoking prevention programs. *J Sch Health* **59**, 181-8.

60. **Rooney BL, Murray DM** (1996). A meta-analysis of smoking prevention programs after adjustment for errors in the unit of analysis. *Health Educ Q* **23**, 48-64.

61. **Flynn BS, Worden JK, Secker-Walker RH** *et al* (1994). Mass media and school interventions for cigarette smoking prevention: effects two years after completion. *Am J Public Health* **84**, 1148-50.

62. **Green LW** (1988). Bridging the gap between community health and school health. *Am J Public Health* **78**, 1149.

63. **Perry CL, Kelder SH, Murray DM, Klepp KI** (1992). Community-wide smoking prevention: long-term outcomes of the Minnesota Heart Health Program and the Class of 1989 study. *Am J Public Health* **82**, 1210-6.

64. **Centres for Disease Control and Prevention** (2001). Effectiveness of school-based programs as a component of a statewide tobacco control initiative—Oregon, 1999-2000. *MMWR* **50**, 663-6.

65. **Lynch BS, Bonnie RJ, eds** (1994). *Growing up tobacco free.* Institute of Medicine, National Academy Press, Washington DC.

66. **Institute of Medicine** (2005). *Preventing childhood obesity: health in the balance.* The National Academies Press, Washington, DC.

67. **Kahn EB, Ramsey LT, Brownson RC** *et al* (2002). The effectiveness of interventions to increase physical activity: a systematic review. *Am J Prev Med* **22** (suppl), 73-107.

68. **US Department of Health and Human Services** (1996). *Physical activity and health: a report of the Surgeon General.* US Department of Health and Human Services, Centres for Disease Control and Prevention, National Centre for Chronic Disease Prevention and Health Promotion, Atlanta, GA. Available at http://www.cdc.gov/nccdphp/sgr/sgr.htm. Accessed 20 October 2004.

69. **US Public Health Service** (1988). *The Surgeon General's report on nutrition and health,* DHHS Publication No (PHS) 88-50210. US Department of Health and Human Services, Public Health Service, Washington, DC.

70. **Wechsler H, Devereaux RS, Davis M, Collins J** (2000). Using the school environment to promote physical activity and healthy eating. *Prev Med* **31** (suppl), S121-37.

71. **Centres for Disease Control and Prevention** (1997). Guidelines for school and community programs to promote lifelong physical activity among young people. *MMWR Recomm Rep* **46** (RR-6), 1-36.

72. **Centres for Disease Control and Prevention** (1996). Guidelines for school health programs to promote lifelong healthy eating. *MMWR Recomm Rep* **45** (RR-9), 1-41.

73. **Contento I, Balch GI, Bronner YL** *et al* (1995). Nutrition education for school-aged children. *J Nutr Educ* **27**, 298-311.

74. **Stone EJ, McKenzie TL, Welk GJ, Booth ML** (1998). Effects of physical activity interventions in youth: review and synthesis. *Am J Prev Med* **15**, 298-315.

75. **French SA, Story M, Fulkerson JA, Hannan P** (2004). An environmental intervention to promote lower-fat food choices in secondary schools: outcomes of the TACOS study. *Am J Public Health* **94**, 1507-12.

76. **US Department of Agriculture, Food and Nutrition Service Online** (2002). *Team Nutrition.* Available at http://www.fns.usda.gov/tn/. Accessed on 18 July 2005.

77. **Gortmaker SL, Peterson K, Wiecha J** *et al* (1999). Reducing obesity via a school-based interdisciplinary intervention among youth: Planet Health. *Arch Pediatr Adolesc Med* **153**, 409-18.

78. **Centres for Disease Control and Prevention** (1994). Changes in brand preference of adolescent smokers—United States, 1989-1993. *MMWR* **43**, 577-81.

79. **Pollay RW, Siddarth S, Siegel M** *et al* (1996). The last straw? Cigarette advertising and realized market shares among youths and adults, 1979-1993. *J Mark* **60**, 1-16.

80. **Arnett JJ, Terhanian G** (1998). Adolescents' responses to cigarette advertisements: links between exposure, liking, and the appeal of smoking. *Tob Control* **7**, 129-33.

81. **Botvin GJ, Goldberg EM, Botvin EM, Dusenbury L** (1993). Smoking behaviour of adolescelts exposed to cigarette advertising. *Public Health Rep* **108**, 217-24.

82. **Feighery E, Borzekowski DLG, Schooler C, Flora J** (1998). Seeing, wanting, owning: the relationship between receptivity to tobacco marketing and smoking susceptibility in young people. *Tob Control* **7**, 123-8.

83. **MacFayden L, Hastings G, MacKintosh AM** (2001). Cross sectional study of young people's awareness and involvement with tobacco marketing. *BMJ* **322**, 513-7.

84. **Centres for Disease Control and Prevention** (1996). Cigarette smoking before and after an excise tax increase and anti-smoking campaign—Massachusetts, 1990-1996. *MMWR* **45**, 966-70.

85. **Centres for Disease Control and Prevention** (1999). Tobacco use among middle and high school students—Florida, 1998 and 1999. *MMWR* **48**, 248-53.

86. **Sparks RE, Green LW** (2000). Mass media in support of smoking cessation. In: National Cancer Institute. *Population based smoking cessation: proceedings of a conference on what works to influence cessation in the general population.* Smoking and tobacco control monograph no. 12, pp. 199-216, NIH Publication No. 00-4892. US Department of Health and Human Services, National Institutes of Health, National Cancer Institute, Bethesda, MD.

87. **Farrelly MC, Davis KC, Haviland L, Messeri P, Heaton CG** (2005). Evidence of a dose-response relationship between "truth" antismoking ads and youth smoking prevalence. *Am J Public Health* **95**, 425-31.

88. **Farrelly MC, Niederdeppe J, Yarsevich J** (2003). Youth tobacco prevention mass media campaigns: Past, present, and future directions. *Tob Control* **12** (suppl), i35-47.

89. **Farrelly MC, Healton CG, Davis KC, Messeri P, Hersey JC. Haviland L** (2002). Getting to the truth: Evaluating national tobacco countermarketing campaigns. *Am J Public Health* **92**, 901-7.

90. **Centres for Disease Control and Prevention** (2004). Effect of ending an antitobacco youth campaign on adolescent susceptibility to cigarette smoking—Minnesota, 2002-2003. *MMWR* **53**, 301-4.

91. **Independent Evaluation Consortium** (1998). *Final report of the independent evaluation of the California Tobacco Control Prevention and Education Program: Wave I data, 1996-1997.* The Gallup Organization, Rockville, MD.

92. **Sly DF, Heald GR, Ray S** (2001). The Florida "truth" anti-tobacco media evaluation: Design, first year results, and implications for planning future state media evaluations. *Tob Control* **10**, 9-15.

93. **Sly DF, Hopkins RS, Trapido E, Ray S** (2001). Influence of a counteradvertising media campaign on initiation of smoking: the Florida "truth" campaign. *Am J Public Health* **91**, 233-8.

94. **Centres for Disease Control and Prevention** (2003). *Designing and implementing an effective tobacco counter-marketing campaign.* U.S. Department of Health and Human Services, Centres for Disease Control and Prevention, National Center for Chronic Disease Prevention and Health Promotion, Office on Smoking and Health, Atlanta, Georgia.

95. **Flay BR** (1987). Mass media and smoking cessation: a critical review. *Am J Public Health* **77**, 153-60.

96. **Dietz WH, Gortmaker SL** (1985). Do we fatten our children at the TV set? Obesity and television viewing in children and adolescents. *Pediatrics* **75**, 807–12.

97. French SA, Story M, Jeffery RW (2001). Environmental influences on eating and physical activity. *Annu Rev Public Health* **22**, 309-35.

98. Hill JO, Peters JC (1998). Environmental contributions to the obesity epidemic. *Science* **280**, 1371-4.

99. Jeffery RW, French SA (1998). Epidemic obesity in the United States: are fast foods and television viewing contributing? *Am J Public Health* **88**, 277-80.

100. Kotz K, Story M (1994). Food advertisements during children's Saturday morning television programming: are they consistent with dietary recommendations? *J Am Diet Assoc* **94**, 1296-300.

101. Kraak V, Pelletier DL (1998). The influence of commercialism on the food purchasing behaviour of children and teenage youth. *Fam Econ Nutr Rev* **11**, 15-24.

102. Gamble M, Cotugna N (1999). A quarter century of TV food advertising targeted at children. *Am J Health Behav* **23**, 261-7.

103. Crespo CJ, Smit E, Troiano RP, Bartlett SJ, Macera CA, Andersen RE (2001). Television watching, energy intake, and obesity in US children. *Arch Pediatric Adoles Med* **155**, 360-5.

104. Maras E (1997). Consumers note what's important in buying snacks. *Autom Merch Oct*, 64-68.

105. Robinson TN (1999). Reducing children's television viewing to prevent obesity: a randomized trial. *JAMA* **282**, 1561-7.

106. Epstein LH, Valoski AM, Vara LS *et al* (1995). Effects of decreasing sedentary behaviour and increasing activity on weight change in obese children. *Health Psychol* **14**, 109–15.

107. Andersen RE, Crespo CJ, Bartlett SJ, Cheskin LJ, Pratt M (1998). Relationship of physical activity and television viewing with body weight and level of fatness among children. *JAMA* **279**, 938-42.

108. Dennison BA, Russo TJ, Burdick PA, Jenkins PL (2004). An intervention to reduce television viewing by preschool children. *Arch Pediat Adol Med* **158**, 170-6.

109. Epstein LH, Paluch RA, Gordy CC, Dorn J (2000). Decreasing sedentary behaviours in treating pediatric obesity. *Arch Pediat Adol Med* **154**, 220-6.

110. Ford B, Tiffany BS, McDonald E, Owens AS, Robinson TN (2002). Primary care intervention to reduce television viewing among African-American children. *Am J Prev Med* **22**, 106-9.

111. Gortmaker SL, Cheung LWY, Peterson KE *et al* (1999). Impact of a school-based interdisciplinary intervention on diet and physical activity among urban primary school children: Eat Well and Keep Moving. *Arch Pediat Adol Med* **153**, 975-83.

112. Robinson TN, Killen JD, Kraemer HC, *et al* (2003). Dance and reducing television viewing to prevent weight gain in African American Girls: The Stanford GEMS Pilot Study. *Ethnicity & Disease* **13** (suppl), 65-77.

113. American Academy of Pediatrics Committee on Public Education (2001). Children, adolescents, and television. *Pediatrics* **107**, 423-6.

114. Centres for Disease Control and Prevention (2004). Youth risk behaviour surveillance—United States, 2003. *MMWR* **53**, 1-96.

115. Gortmaker SL, Must A, Sobol AM, Peterson K, Colditz GA, Dietz WH (1996). Television viewing as a cause of increasing obesity among children in the United States, 1986–1990. *Arch Pediatr Adolesc Med* **150**, 356–62.

116. Gerberding JL, Marks JS (2004). Making America fit and trim—steps big and small. *Am J Public Health* **94**, 1478-9.

117. Bauman A (2004). Commentary on the VERB campaign—perspectives on social marketing to encourage physical activity among youth. *Preventing Chronic Dis* **1**, A02. Available at http://www.cdc.gov/pcd/issues/2004/jul/04_0054.htm. Accessed 18 July 2005.

118. Huhman M, Heitzler C, Wong F (2004). The VERB campaign logic model: a tool for planning and evaluation. *Prev Chronic Dis* [serial online] **1**, A11. Available at http://www.cdc.gov/pcd/issues/2004/jul/04_0033.htm. Accessed 18 July 2005.

119. Wong F, Huhman M, Heitzler C *et al* (2004). VERB—a social marketing campaign to increase physical activity among youth. *Preventing Chronic Dis* **1**, A10. Available at http://www.cdc.gov/pcd/issues/2004/jul/04_0043.htm. Accessed 18 July 2005.

120. Huhman M, Potter LD, Wong FL, Banspach SW, Duke JC, Heitzler CD (2005). Effects of a mass media campaign to increase physical activity among children: year-1 results of the VERB campaign. *Pediatrics* **116**, In Press, August 2005.

121. Brownson RC, Eriksen MP, Davis RM, Warner KE (1997). Environmental tobacco smoke: health effects and policies to reduce exposure. *Annu Rev Public Health* **18**, 163-85.

122. Chaloupka FJ, Pacula RL (1998*). Limiting youth access to tobacco: the early impact of the Synar Amendment on youth smoking.* Paper presented at the Third Biennial Pacific Rim Allied Economic Organizations Conference, Jan 14, 1998, Bangkok, Thailand.

123. Eriksen MP, Gottleib NH (1998). A review of the health impact of smoking control at the workplace. *Am J Health Promot* **13**, 83-104.

124. Fielding R, Chee YY, Choi KM *et al* (2004). Declines in tobacco brand recognition and ever-smoking rates among young children following restrictions on tobacco advertisements in Hong Kong. *J Public Health* **26**, 24-30.

125. Forster JL, Murray DM, Wolfson M, Blaine, TM, Wagenaar, AC, Hennrikus, DJ (1998). The effects of community policies to reduce youth access to tobacco. *Am J Public Health* **88**, 1193-8.

126. Hammond D, Fong GT, McDonald PW, Brown KS, Cameron R (2004). Graphic Canadian cigarette warning labels and adverse outcomes: evidence from Canadian smokers. *Am J Public Health* **94**, 1442-5.

127. Emont SL, Choi WS, Novotny TE, Giovino GA (1993). Clean indoor air legislation, taxation, and smoking behaviour in the United States: an ecological analysis. *Tob Control* **2**, 13-7.

128. Rigotti NA, Pashos CL (1991). No-smoking laws in the United States: an analysis of state and city actions to limit smoking in public places and workplaces. *JAMA* **266**, 3162-7.

129. National Cancer Institute (2001). *Risks associated with smoking cigarettes with low machine-measured yields of tar and nicotine.* Smoking and Tobacco Control Monograph No. 13. US Department of Health and Human Services, National Institutes of Health, National Cancer Institute, Bethesda, MD.

130. Forster J, Wolfson M (1998). Youth access to tobacco: policies and politics. *Annu Rev Public Health* **19**, 203-35.

131. Rigotti NA, DiFranza JR, Chang Y, Tisdale T, Kemp B, Singer DE (1997). The effect of enforcing tobacco-sales laws on adolescents' access to tobacco and smoking behaviour. *N Engl J Med* **337**, 1044-51.

132. Jacobsen PD, Wasserman J, Raube K (1992). *The political evolution of anti-smoking legislation.* RAND Corporation, Santa Monica, CA.

133. Task Force on Community Preventive Services (2005). *The Guide to Community Preventive Services: what works to promote health?* Zaza S, Briss PA, Harris KW, eds. Oxford Press, New York.

134. Chapman S, Wakefield M (2001). Tobacco control advocacy in Australia: Reflections on 30 years of progress. *Health Educ Behav* **28**, 274-89.

135. Taylor A, Bettcher D (2000). WHO Framework Convention on Tobacco Control: a global "good" for public health. *Bull WHO* **78**, 920-9.

136. World Health Organization (2004). Updated status of the WHO Framework Convention on Tobacco Control. Available at http://www.who.int/tobacco/framework/countrylist/en/index.html. Accessed 19 July 2005.

137. UK Department of Health (2004). *Choosing health: making healthier choices easier.* London: The Stationery Office. Available at http://www.dh.gov.uk/PublicationsAndStatistics/Publications/fs/en. Accessed 18 July 2005.

138. **Yach D, Hawkes C, Epping-Jordan JE, Galbraith S** (2004). The World Health Organisation's Framework Convention on Tobacco Control: implications for global epidemics of food-related deaths and disease. *J Public Health Pol* **24**, 274-90.

139. **European Commission** (2005). *Nutrition Policy.* Available at http://europa.eu.int/comm/health/ph_determinants/life_style/nutrition/nutrition_policy_en.htm. Accessed 18 July 2005.

140. **US Department of Agriculture** (1994). *National school lunch program and school breakfast program nutrition objectives for school meals (7CFR 210.220). Fed Regis,* 30218-51.

141. **US Department of Agriculture** (1995). *National School Lunch Program and School Breakfast Program: compliance with the dietary guidelines for Americans and food-based menUSystems.* Food and Consumer Service, Washington, DC.

142. **US Department of Agriculture** (2005). *National School Lunch Program.* Available at http://www.fns.usda.gov/cnd/Lunch/AboutLunch/NSLPFactSheet.htm. Accessed 1 July 2005.

143. **Day S** (2003). US Considers food labels with whole-package data. *New York Times.* November 21, 2003.

144. **Teisl MF, Levy AS** (1997). Does nutrition labelling lead to healthier eating? *J Food Distribution Research* **3**, 19-26.

145. **Daynard RA** (2004). Lessons from tobacco control for the obesity control movement. *J Public Health Pol* **24**, 291-5.

146. **Baranowski R, Thompson WO, Durant RH, Baranowski J, Puhl J** (1993). Observations on physical activity in physical locations: age, gender, ethnicity, and month effects. *Res Q Exerc Sport* **64**, 127-33.

147. **Klesges RC, Eck LH, Hanson CL, Haddock CK, Klesges LM** (1990). Effects of obesity, social interactions, and physical environment on physical activity in preschoolers. *Health Psychol* **9**, 435-9.

148. **Sallis JF, Nader PR, Broyles SL** *et al* (1993). Correlates of physical activity at home in Mexican-American and Anglo-American pre-school children. *Health Psychol* **12**, 390-8.

149. **Datar A, Sturm R** (2004). Physical education in elementary school and body mass index: evidence from the early childhood longitudinal study. *Am J Public Health* **94**, 1501-6.

150. **Neumark-Sztainer D, Story M, Hannan PJ, Rex J** (2003). New Moves: a school-based obesity prevention program for adolescent girls. *Prev Med* **37**, 41-51.

151. **Centres for Disease Control and Prevention** (1992). Participation in school physical education and selected dietary patterns among high school students—United States, 1991. *MMWR* **41**, 597-601, 607.

152. **Kann L, Kinchen SA, Williams BI** *et al* (2000). Youth risk behaviour surveillance—United States, 1999. *MMWR Surveill Summ* **49**, 1-96.

153. **Vereecken CA, Bobelijn K, Maes L** (2005). School food policy at primary and secondary schools in Belgium-Flanders: does it influence young people's food habits? *Eur J Clin Nutr* **59**, 271-7.

154. **Tudor-Locke C, Ainsworth BE, Popkin BM** (2001). Active commuting to school: an overlooked source of childrens' physical activity? *Sports Med* **31**, 309-13.

155. **California Project LEAN** (2002). *Taking the fizz out of soda contracts: A guide to community action.* California Project LEAN, Sacramento, CA.

156. **Erikson D** (2000). School board ditches contract with Coca-Cola; Madison may be the first district in the country to reject such a lucrative vending agreement. *Wisconsin State Journal,* August 29, 2000. Available at www.commercialalert.org/WICoke.htm. Accessed 18 July 2005.

157. **US Department of Agriculture and Centres for Disease Control and Prevention.** *Making it happen! School nutrition success stories.* US Department of Agriculture, Food and Nutrition Service, Washington, DC. Available at http://www.cdc.gov/healthyyouth/nutrition/Making-It-Happen/. Accessed 18 July 2005.

158. **Nestle M** (2000). Soft drink pouring rights. *Public Health Reports* **115**, 308-19.

159. **Anderson PM, Butcher KF** (2005). Reading, writing and raisinets: are school finances contributing to children's obesity? *National Bureau of Economic Research Working Paper No. 11177*, March 2005. Available at http://papers.nber.org/papers/. Accessed 18 July 2005.

160. **Bowman SA, Gortmaker SL, Ebbeling CB, Pereira MA, Ludwig DS** (2004). Effects of fast-food consumption on energy intake and diet quality among children in a national household survey. *Pediatrics* **113**, 112-8.

161. **James J, Thomas P, Cavan D, Kerr D** (2004). Preventing childhood obesity by reducing consumption of carbonated drinks: cluster randomized controlled trial. *BMJ* **328**, 1237-41.

162. **American Academy of Pediatrics Committee on School Health** (2004). Soft drinks in schools. *Pediatrics* **113** (1 Pt 1), 152-4.

163. **French SA, Jeffery RW, Story M** *et al* (2001). Pricing and promotion effects on low-fat vending snack purchases: the CHIPS Study. *Am J Public Health* **91**, 112-7.

164. **French SA, Story M, Jeffery RW** *et al* (1997). Pricing strategy to promote fruit and vegetable purchase in high school cafeterias. *J Am Dietetic Assoc* **97**, 1008-10.

165. **US Department of Agriculture** (2003). *Evaluation of the USDA Fruit and Vegetable Pilot Program: report to Congress, May 2003*. US Department of Agriculture Economic Research Service. Available at http://www.ers.usda.gov/publications/efan03006/. Accessed 18 July 2005.

166. **French SA, Wechsler H** (2004). School-based research and initiatives: fruit and vegetable environment, policy, and pricing workshop. *Prev Med* **39** (suppl), S101-7.

167. **Nicholson W.** *Microeconomic theory: basic principles and extensions, 3ʳᵈ ed.* The Dryden Press, Chicago.

168. **Becker GS, Murphy KM** (1988). A theory of rational addiction. *J Polit Econ* **96**, 675-700.

169. **Sweanor D, Burns DM, Major JM, Anderson CM** (2000). Effect of cost on cessation. In: National Cancer Institute. *Population-based smoking cessation: proceedings of a conference on what works to influence cessation in the general population*. Smoking and tobacco control monograph no. 12, pp. 199-216, NIH Publication No. 00-4892. US Department of Health and Human Services, National Institutes of Health, National Cancer Institute, Bethesda, MD.

170. **Grossman M, Chaloupka, FJ** (1997). Cigarette taxes: the straw to break the camel's back. *Public Health Rep* **112**, 290-7.

171. **French SA, Jeffery RW, Story M, Hannan P, Snyder MP** (1997). A pricing strategy to promote low-fat snack choices through vending machines. *Am J Public Health* **87**, 849-51.

172. **Jeffery RW, French SA, Raether C, Baxter J** (1994). An environmental intervention to increase fruit and salad purchases in a cafeteria. *Prev Med* **23**, 788-92.

173. **Gallimore WW** (1974). Sales of soy-ground beef blends in selected stores. In: *National Food Situation*, pp. 26-9, NFS-147. Economic Research Service, US Department of Agriculture, Washington, DC.

174. **Green LW** (1975). Diffusion and adoption of innovations related to cardiovascular risk behaviour in the public. In: Enelow AJ, Henderson JB, eds. *Applying behavioural science to cardiovascular risk*, pp. p84-108. American Heart Association. Reprinted in *Congressional record, hearings of the Senate Subcommittee on Health*, May 7-8, 1975, pp. 9880-10040. New York.

175. **Glanz K, Yaroch A** (2004). Strategies for increasing fruit and vegetable intake in grocery stores and communities: policy, pricing, and environmental change. *Prev Med* **39** (suppl), S75-80.

176. **McLaughlin EW** (2004). The dynamics of fresh fruit and vegetable pricing in the supermarket channel. *Prev Med* **39** (suppl), S81-7.

177. **Glanz K, Hoelscher D** (2004). Increasing fruit and vegetable intake by changing environments, policy and pricing: restaurant-based research, strategies, and recommendations. *Prev Med* **39** (suppl), S88-93.

178. **Seymour JD, Fenley MA, Yaroch AL, Kettel Khan L, Serdula M** (2004). Fruit and Vegetable Environment, Policy, and Pricing Workshop: introduction to the conference proceedings. *Prev Med* **39** (suppl), S71-4.

179. **Seymour JD, Yaroch AL, Serdula M, Blanck HM, Kettel Khan L** (2004). Impact of nutrition environmental interventions on point-of-purchase behavior in adults: a review. *Prev Med* **39** (suppl), S108-36.

180. **Chou SY, Grossman M, Saffer H** (July 2001). An economic analysis of adult obesity: results from the behavioural risk factor surveillance system. Available at http://www.upenn.edu/ldi/obesity.doc. Accessed 20 October 2004.

181. **Krebs-Smith SM, Cook A, Subar AF, Cleveland L, Friday J, Kahle LL** (1996). Fruit and vegetable intakes of children and adolescents in the United States. *Arch Pediatr Adolesc Med* **150**, 81-6.

182. **Berkey CS, Rockett HR, Field AE** *et al* (2000). Activity, dietary intake, and eight changes in a longitudinal study or preadolescent and adolescent boys and girls. *Pediatrics* **105**, e56.

183. **Drewnowski A, Darmon N, Briend A** (2004). Replacing fats and sweets with vegetables and fruits—a question of cost. *Am J Public Health* **94**, 1555-9.

184. **Jeffery RW** (2001). Public health strategies for obesity treatment and prevention. *Am J Health Behav* **25**, 252-9.

185. **National Cancer Institute** (1991). *ASSIST program guidelines for tobacco-free communities.* National Cancer Institute, Division of Cancer Prevention and Control, Cancer Control Science Program, Public Health Applications Research Branch, Bethesda, MD.

186. **Substance Abuse and Mental Health Services Administration** (1998). *Synar Regulation: report to Congress on FFY 1997 state compliance,* DHHS Publication No (SMA) 98-3183. US Department of Health and Human Services, Substance Abuse and Mental Health Services Administration, Centre for Substance Abuse Prevention, Rockville, MD.

187. **Substance Abuse and Mental Health Services Administration** (1998). *Synar Regulation: report to Congress on FFY 1997 state compliance: summary,* DHHS Publication No (SMA) 98-3185. US Department of Health and Human Services, Substance Abuse and Mental Health Services Administration, Centre for Substance Abuse Prevention, Rockville, MD.

188. **US Department of Health and Human Services** (1999). *Enforcement of tobacco-sales laws: guidance from experience in the field,* DHHS Publication No (SMA) 99-317. US Department of Health and Human Services, Substance Abuse and Mental Health Services Administration, Centre for Substance Abuse Prevention, Rockville, MD.

189. **World Health Organization** (1979). *Controlling the smoking epidemic: report of the WHO expert committee on smoking control.* WHO Technical Report Series No. 636. World Health Organization, Geneva.

190. **World Health Organization** (1998). *Guidelines for controlling and monitoring the tobacco epidemic.* World Health Organization, Geneva.

191. **Tudor-Smith C, Nutbeam D, Moore L, Catford J** (1998). Effects of the Heartbeat Wales program over five years on behavioural risks for cardiovascular disease: quasi-experimental comparison of results from Wales and a matched reference area. *BMJ* **316**, 818-22.

192. **Aravanis C, Corcondilas A, Dontas AS, Lekos D, Keys A** (1970). Coronary heart disease in seven countries. IX. The Greek islands of Crete and Corfu. *Circulation* **41** (suppl), 88-100.

193. **Blackburn H, Taylor HL, Keys A** (1970). Coronary heart disease in seven countries. XVI. The electrocardiogram in prediction of five-year coronary heart disease incidence among men aged forty through fifty-nine. *Circulation* **41** (suppl), 154-61.

194. **Carleton RA, Lasater TM, Assaf AR, Feldman HA, McKinlay S. The Pawtucket Heart Health Program Writing Group** (1995). The Pawtucket Heart Health Program: community changes in cardiovascular risk factors and projected disease risk. *Am J Public Health* **85**, 777-85.

195. Egger G, Fitzgerald W, Frape G *et al* (1983). Results of large scale media anti-smoking campaign in Australia: North Coast "Quit for Life" programme. *BMJ* **287**(6399), 1125-8.

196. Farquhar JW, Maccoby N, Wood PD *et al* (1977). Community education for cardiovascular health. *Lancet* **1**, 1192-5.

197. Farquhar JW, Fortmann SP, Maccoby N *et al* (1985). The Stanford Five-City Project: design and methods. *Am J Epidemiol* **122**, 323-34.

198. Gofin J, Gorin R, Abramson JH, Ban R (1986). Ten-year evaluation of hypertension, overweight, cholesterol, and smoking control: the CHAD program in Jerusalem. *Prev Med* **15**, 304-12.

199. Gutzwiller F, Nater B, Martin J (1985). Community-based primary prevention of cardiovascular disease in Switzerland: methods and results of the National Research Program (NRP 1A). *Prev Med* **14**, 482-91.

200. Murray DM, Hannan PJ, Jacobs DR *et al* (1994). Assessing intervention effects in the Minnesota Heart Health Program. *Am J Epidemiol* **139**, 91-103.

201. Puska P, Nissinen A, Tuomilehto J *et al* (1985). The community-based strategy to prevent coronary heart disease: conclusions from the ten years of the North Karelia project. *Ann Rev Public Health* **6**, 147-93.

202. Steenkamp HJ, Jooste PL, Jordaan PCJ, Swanepoel ASP, Rossouw JE (1991). Changes in smoking during a community-based cardiovascular disease intervention programme: the Coronary Risk Factor Study. *S Afr Med J* **79**, 250-3.

203. Winkleby MA, Feldman HA, Murray DM (1997). Joint analysis of three US community intervention trials for reduction of cardiovascular disease risk. *J Clin Epidemiol* **50**, 645-58.

204. Anantha N, Nandakumar A, Vishwanath N *et al* (1995). Efficacy of an anti-tobacco community education program in India. *Cancer Causes Control* **6**, 119-29.

205. Centres for Disease Control and Prevention (1997). Cigarette smoking before and after an excise-tax increase and anti-smoking campaign—Massachusetts 1990-1996. *MMWR* **45**, 960-70.

206. Centres for Disease Control and Prevention (1999). Decline in cigarette consumption following implementation of a comprehensive tobacco prevention and education program—Oregon, 1996-1998. *MMWR* **48**, 140-3.

207. Centres for Disease Control and Prevention (1999). Tobacco use among middle and high school students—Florida, 1998 and 1999. *MMWR* **48**, 248-53.

208. Centres for Disease Control and Prevention (2001). Tobacco use among adults—Arizona, 1996 and 1999 *MMWR* **50**, 402-6.

209. Connolly G, Robbins H (1998). Designing an effective statewide tobacco program—Massachusetts. *Cancer* **83** (suppl), 2722-7.

210. Dwyer T, Pierce JP, Hannam CD, Burke N (1986). Evaluation of the Sydney "Quit For Life" anti-smoking campaign. Part 2: changes in smoking prevalence. *Med J Austr* **144**, 344-7.

211. Fisher EB Jr (1995). The results of the COMMIT trial [editorial]. *Am J Public Health* **85**, 159-60.

212. Green LW (1997). Commentary: community health promotion: applying the science of evaluation to the initial sprint of a marathon. *Am J Prev Med* **13**, 225-8.

213. Green LW, Richard L (1993). The need to combine health education and health promotion: the case of cardiovascular disease prevention. *Promot Educ.* Dec, Spec No. 11-8.

214. Hill DD (1997). *Quit evaluation studies number 8.* Australian Cancer Centre, Melbourne.

215. Manley MW, Pierce JP, Gilpin EA, Rosbrook B, Berry C, Wun L-M (1997). Impact of the American Stop Smoking Intervention Study on cigarette consumption. *Tob Control* **6** (suppl), S12-S16.

216. Pierce JP, Dwyer T, Frape G, Chapman S, Chamberlain A, Burke N (1986). Evaluation of the Sydney "Quit For Life" anti-smoking campaign. Part 1. Achievement of intermediate goals. *Med J Austr* **144**, 341-4.

217. **Susser M** (1995). The tribulations of trials—intervention in communities [editorial]. *Am J Public Health* **85**, 156-8.

218. **Bal DG, Kizer KW, Felten PG, Mozar HN, Niemeyer D** (1990). Reducing tobacco consumption in California. Development of a statewide anti-tobacco use campaign. *JAMA* **264**, 1570-4.

219. **Fishbein HA, Unger JB, Johnson CA** *et al* (2000). Interaction of population-based approaches for tobacco control. In: National Cancer Institute. *Population-based smoking cessation: proceedings of a conference on what works to influence cessation in the general population.* Smoking and tobacco control monograph no. 12, pp. 223-233, NIH Publication No. 00-4892. US Department of Health and Human Services, National Institutes of Health, National Cancer Institute, Bethesda, MD.

220. **Novotny T** (1995). *Structural evaluation of California's proposition 99-funded tobacco control program.* California Department of Health Services, Tobacco Control Section, Sacramento.

221. **Pierce JP, Gilpin EA, Emery SL** *et al* (1998). Has the California Tobacco Control Program reduced smoking? *JAMA* **280**, 893-9.

222. **Pierce JP, Gilpin EA, Emery SL** *et al* (1998). *Tobacco control in California: who's winning the war? An evaluation of the tobacco control program, 1989-1996.* University of California, San Diego, La Jolla, CA.

223. **Cummings KM** (2000). Community–wide interventions for tobacco control. In: National Cancer Institute. *Population based smoking cessation: proceedings of a conference on what works to influence cessation in the general population.* Smoking and tobacco control monograph no. 12, pp. 1-24, NIH Publication No. 00-4892. US Department of Health and Human Services, National Institutes of Health, National Cancer Institute, Bethesda, MD.

224. **Cummings KM, Sciandra R, Carol J** *et al* (1991). Approaches directed to the social environment. In: National Cancer Institute. *Strategies to control tobacco use in the United States: a blueprint for public health in the 1990's.* Smoking and tobacco control monograph no. 1, pp. 203-65. US Department of Health and Human Services, National Institutes of Health, National Cancer Institute, Washington, DC.

225. **Glantz SA** (1997). After ASSIST, what next? Science. *Tob Control* **6**, 337-9.

226. **Bauer UE, Johnson TM** (2000). Changes in youth cigarette use and intentions: following implementation of a tobacco control program. Findings from the Florida Youth Tobacco Survey, 1990-2000. *JAMA* **284**, 723-8.

227. **Bjornson W** (2000). Strategic partnerships for addressing tobacco use. *Tob Control* **9** (suppl), i67-70.

228. **Resnicow K, Robinson TN** (1997). School-based cardiovascular disease prevention studies: review and synthesis. *Am J Epidemiol* **7** (suppl), S14-31.

229. **Perry CL, Luepker RV, Murray DM** *et al* (1988). Parent involvement with children's health promotion: the Minnesota Home Team. *Am J Public Health* **78**, 1156-60.

230. **Sorensen G, Emmons K, Hunt MK, Johnston D** (1998). Implications of the results of community intervention trials. *Annu Rev Public Health* **19**, 379-416.

231. **Center for Consumer Freedom** (2005). *The onion peels off obesity parody.* The Center for Consumer Freedom, June 16, 2005, Washington, DC.

232. **California Department of Health Services** (1998). A model for change: the California experience in tobacco control. California Department of Health Services, Sacramento, CA.

233. **Mercer SL, MacDonald G, Green LW** (2004). Participatory research and evaluation: from best practices for all states to achievable practices within each state in the context of the Master Settlement Agreement. *Health Promot Pract* **5** (suppl), 167S-178S.

234. **Centres for Disease Control and Prevention** (1998). *Tobacco use among US racial/ethnic minority groups—African Americans, American Indians and Pacific Islanders, and Hispanics: a report of the Surgeon General.* US Department of Health and Human Services, Centres for Disease Control

and Prevention, Atlanta, Georgia. Available at http://www.cdc.gov/tobacco/sgr/sgr_1998/index.htm. Accessed 18 July 2005.

235. **Fisher EB, Auslander WF, Munro JF, Arfken CL, Brownson RC, Owens NW** (1998). Neighbors for a smoke-free north side: evaluation of a community organization approach to promoting cessation among African Americans. *Am J Public Health* **88**, 1658-63.

236. **Green LW** (2000). Caveats on coalitions: in praise of partnerships. *Health Prom Prac* **1**, 64.

237. **Centres for Disease Control and Prevention** (2004). *CDC's state-based nutrition and physical activity program to prevent obesity and other chronic diseases.* Department of Nutrition and Physical Activity, National Centre for Chronic Disease Prevention and Health Promotion, Centres for Disease Control and Prevention. Available at http://www.cdc.gov/nccdphp/dnpa/obesity/state_programs/index.htm. Accessed 18 July 2004.

238. **Nutrition and Physical Activity Work Group** (2002). *Guidelines for comprehensive programs to promote healthy eating and physical activity.* Human Kinetics, Champaign, IL. Available at http://www.humankinetics.com/. Accessed 18 July 2005.

239. **Centres for Disease Control and Prevention** (2004). *Resource guide for nutrition and physical activity interventions to prevent obesity and other chronic diseases.* Nutrition, Physical activity, and Obesity Prevention Program, Centres for Disease Control and Prevention, Department of Health and Human Services. Available at http://www.cdc.gov/nccdphp/dnpa/obesityprevention. htm. Accessed 20 October 2004.

240. **Owen CG, Martin RM, Whincup PH, Smith GD, Cook DG** (2005). Effect of infant feeding on the risk of obesity across the lifecourse: a quantitative review of the published evidence. *Pediatr* **115**, 1367-7.

241. **First International Conference on Health Promotion** (1986). The Ottawa charter for health promotion. *Health Promotion* **1**, i-v.

242. **Milio N** (1976). A framework for prevention: changing health-damaging to health-generating life patterns. *Am J Public Health* **66**, 435-39.

243. **Green LW, Mercer SL** (2001). Can public health researcher and agencies reconcile the push from funding bodies and the pull from communities? *Am J Public Health* **91**, 1926-9.

Chapter 12

The potential for policy initiatives to address the obesity epidemic: a legal perspective from the United States

Ellen J. Fried

Introduction

In 2000, two prominent voices in the fields of public health and nutrition advocacy, Marion Nestle and Michael Jacobson, proposed measures to halt the obesity epidemic through the lens of public health policy (1). *Halting the obesity epidemic: a public health policy approach* chronicled a half century of US government recognition of obesity as a risk factor for chronic health conditions, yet revealed that governmental guidelines regarding diet, activity, and maintenance of healthy weight were both infrequent and, when offered at all, focused primarily on individual behaviors. Worse, the advice was typically banal and by all accounts, ineffective. The authors pointed out:

> Considering the many aspects of American culture that promote obesity, from the proliferation of fast-food outlets to almost universal reliance on automobiles, reversing current trends will require a multifaceted public health policy approach as well as considerable funding. National leadership is needed to ensure the participation of health officials and researchers, educators and legislators, transportation experts and urban planners, and businesses and non-profit groups in formulating a public health campaign with a better chance of success.

Nestle and Jacobson presented policy recommendations aimed at the prevention of excessive weight gain in the areas of education, food labeling and advertising, food assistance programs, health care and training, and transportation and urban development. They argued, as did others who studied the issues, that change must encompass both individual behavior patterns and "environmental barriers to healthy food choices and active lifestyles". The authors acknowledged that such changes are difficult to achieve and concluded "Without such a national commitment and effective new approaches to making the environment more favorable to maintaining healthy weight, we doubt that the current trends can be reversed."

As the world's population of the overweight and obese continues to soar, the critical need for governmental policy initiatives to stop, and ultimately reverse, this raging epidemic grows more imperative still. This chapter examines the current state of regulatory and legislative affairs in the US. This chapter also considers another legal resource, litigation, which has provided a useful arrow in the public health quiver. Legal action has been successful in holding the tobacco industry responsible for the devastating health costs created by its harmful product. The tobacco example, coupled with the alarming escalation of overweight and obesity in the US and the Government's failure to mount a meaningful anti-obesity campaign, has led public health advocates to look to litigation as a means of confronting this epidemic.

To date, litigation based solely on claims that a plaintiff's obesity and related health problems were caused by the consumption of certain foods has not been successful in the US. However, lawsuits that argue consumers have been deceived by dishonest nutrition labels or product health claims have met with greater success; so has a Brazilian lawsuit that argued products harmful to children's health must carry warnings related to over-consumption. Although often viewed as a uniquely American activity, obesity and food-related lawsuits have been initiated in several countries outside the US. It is not surprising that international litigation is based on an American model, in light of the fact that the global obesity epidemic can trace its origins to energy-dense American food products and their relentless promotion. Equally important, the international investment industry has taken a hard look at obesity-related litigation and warned the global financial community that future legal action must be viewed as a potentially serious threat to corporate coffers.

Nestle and Jacobson (1), together with many other public health advocates, have long espoused the view that legislation, regulation, and education are necessary to address the obesity epidemic, heart disease, diabetes, and other diet-induced diseases. Of critical importance, too, is the exercise of responsible personal food and lifestyle choices. Voluntary efforts by the food industry must also play a significant role in improving public health; to date, several food giants, including Kraft, McDonald's and Frito-Lay, have improved the nutritional profile of various products. Some commentators cite the movement by industry towards more healthful food choices as proof that lawsuits are unnecessary; the food industry has gone one step further and has been working feverishly to promote legislation that bans litigation against it related to obesity. Others cite the same industry progress, but argue it has been precisely the threat of costly litigation, coupled with a change in public sentiment, that has prodded the industry to take long overdue action. Only time will tell whether litigation will make a significant difference in stemming obesity in the US, and ultimately, around the world.

The potential for regulation to address the obesity epidemic

Soon after the publication of *Halting the Obesity Epidemic* (1), Dr David Satcher issued *The Surgeon General's Call to Action to Prevent and Decrease Overweight and Obesity* (2), described by the US Department of Health and Human Services (HHS) as the "inaugural event in the development of a national action plan to combat overweight and obesity". It was likely the first time much of the public read in their local newspapers about the dire condition of America's waistline or heard the warning that obesity could soon be responsible for as much preventable disease and death as cigarette smoking (3). It also signaled the need for a shift away from the attitude that responsibility for confronting obesity be placed solely on individuals. The Surgeon General emphasized "people tend to think of overweight and obesity as strictly a personal matter, but there is much that communities can and should do to address these problems" and recognized that "the social, environmental, and behavioral factors responsible for the epidemic of overweight and obesity are firmly entrenched in our society." He also warned, "Identifying and dislodging these factors will require deliberate, persistent action and a degree of patience".

Growing public awareness is a critical step in confronting any epidemic; implementation of meaningful regulations depends on a public both versed in the issues and clamoring for government action. Articles detailing the enormity of the crisis started to spill out beyond the pages of academic and scientific journals. Recent figures measuring media coverage of the obesity epidemic reflect an increase from 593 stories per year in 2000 to 4560 stories in 2003. President Bush introduced the *Healthier US* initiative in June 2002 (4). With an overarching goal of improved personal health and fitness, the program urges Americans to incorporate daily activity and a nutritious diet into their lives. The US HHS next introduced *Steps to a Healthier US* (5). It is based on the concept that the obesity epidemic can be successfully confronted when people implement small lifestyle changes that result in health benefits. An explosion of governmental programs have followed; a detailed outline of "education, communications and outreach, intervention, diet and nutrition, physical activity and fitness, disease surveillance, research, clinical preventive services and therapeutics, and policy and web-based tools that target a wide and varied population range" was recently presented to Congress (6). Indeed, such a roadmap is necessary to comprehend it all.

Critics of the federal government's actions have pointed to the inability of the current programs to be truly effective in combating obesity; many call for studies that, in turn, have recommended actions that are not being undertaken, focus on personal responsibility and individual action rather than societal or environmental issues of obesity, and espouse a voluntary, self-regulatory approach for the food industry that, to date, has been woefully insufficient.

Jacobson has criticized many of the HHS initiatives as "merely rearranging the deck chairs on the Titanic"(7). He has emphasized the need for the government to develop programs such as: voluntary labeling for foods, based on a symbol similar to the Swedish "key" program that allows consumers to readily identify healthy foods; requiring nutrition information on menu boards and other points of sale; reducing the amount of saturated and trans fats in foods; sponsoring mass-media campaigns to encourage the consumption of more fruits, vegetables, and whole grains, and less meat, cheese, and soft drink; offering only healthy meals at schools; barring junk-food advertisements on children's television; and imposing small taxes on unhealthful foods and using those funds for health-related programs. Nestle (8) echoes the criticism and the need for action, and points out that powerful food industry lobbies continue to oppose regulations that would result in reduced consumption of their products or limitations on their marketing techniques.

The influence of industry is gleaned readily from statements by the current Surgeon General, who has explained strategies to confront obesity such as "the government was hoping to partner with the food industry rather than pursue regulatory changes, which could effect advertising" (9). This attitude undercuts the potential effectiveness of otherwise commendable action plans. For example, the US Food and Drug Administration's (FDA) Obesity Working Group (OBG) produced a comprehensive report on combating obesity. However, with regard to food labeling, the OWG is hoping that "encouragement" will be enough to get the food industry to act (10). The exhaustive report issued by the Institute of Medicine's Committee on the Prevention of Obesity in Children and Youth recognizes the need for immediate nationwide action and reinforced the earliest pronouncements of Surgeon General Sachter: "We recognize that several of our recommendations challenge entrenched aspects of American life and business, but if we are not willing to make some fundamental shifts in our attitudes and actions, obesity's toll on our nation's health and well-being will only worsen". It contains many suggestions for action that advocates have long recommended, such as requiring that more nutrition information is available at restaurants and more physical activity in schools, along with stricter nutritional standards. However, it, too, suggests that the critical area of marketing foods to children be primarily industry self-regulated (11).

In view of the conflicts of interest tying the hands of federal regulators, advocates expect that meaningful action will be taken on the state and local level, where the pressures of industry influence are not so keenly felt. This would be reflected in statewide regulation of school foods and local school district bans on the sale of junk foods in school vending machines. Yet even small localities are subjected to budgetary barriers and entrenched attitudes regarding parental responsibility and freedom of choice that may hinder progress. However, it is at the local level that some change has taken root.

Ultimately, the effect of regulatory action taken by the US will extend beyond national boundaries; its participation in multinational trade agreements and the General Agreement on Tariffs and Trade/World Trade Organization (GATT/WTO) ensures that regulation of food-related industries would have a global impact. While regulatory action is critical to reduce the environments that foster obesity, to date, there have been far more words than action.

The potential for legislation to address the obesity epidemic

Another barometer of public awareness of the obesity epidemic is the escalating activity of legislators. Proposed legislation has focused upon a wide range of issues including nutritional education and diet, increased physical activity, and altering the built environment to facilitate activity. And, as is true of many nations around the globe, there is often a long road between the introduction and implementation of legislation; currently in the US, proposed bills far outnumber enacted laws.

In contrast to the paucity of pending legislation regarding, and even public awareness of, an obesity epidemic when *Halting the Obesity Epidemic* (1) first appeared, so many state legislatures, and to a lesser degree federal lawmakers, have begun to grapple with the issue that tracking services have been created to maintain a coherent and easily accessible database. The Centers for Disease Control (CDC) offers a service that both culls and tracks the progress of federal and state legislation; it conveniently provides links directly to the text of the bills, as well as state and federal government websites (12, 13). Federal legislation can also be accessed at Thomas, the Library of Congress website (14).

Federal Congressional representatives and Senators responsible for domestic and international policies are subjected to the competing interests of industry and private citizens, as well as American and foreign agricultural interests. This conflict has stalled the creation of legislative initiatives to combat the obesity public health crisis. Nevertheless, the number of proposed bills has increased in the last 5 years. In 1999, there was a lone bill introduced into the House of Representatives that specifically targeted obesity prevention and reduction. The stated purpose of the *Lifelong Improvements in Food and Exercise (LIFE) Act* was to "provide a national program to conduct and support activities toward the goal of significantly reducing the number of cases of overweight and obesity among individuals in the US". This was to be achieved through training health professionals and the public regarding the health consequences of obesity and to develop intervention strategies at worksites and in community settings. Congress never voted on the bill.

In contrast, the CDC's federal obesity-related legislation compilation, which spans the 2003 legislative year (updated through August 2004 as of this writing), lists a combined total of 13 bills, amendments, and Congressional resolutions that address "obesity prevention". With titles such as the *Healthy Lifestyles and Prevention (HeLP) American Act of 2004* and *IMPACT Act (Improved Nutrition and Physical Activity Act)*, the legislation purports to have a common goal, yet illustrates divergent views on how to achieve it. (*The Commonsense Consumption Act,* known as the "Cheeseburger Bill" is also included; it represents a significant legislative effort, albeit not to prevent obesity but rather to prevent lawsuits against the food industry).

The countervailing forces in the American effort to confront obesity have aligned themselves according to seemingly simple opposing philosophies; personal responsibility vs.

public health initiatives. The former regards one's lifestyle, including food consumption, physical activity, and overall health to be solely a matter of personal choice and, therefore, of personal responsibility. This concept is almost uniformly espoused by food industry sources that argue more exercise and eating in moderation will result in a healthy weight. Since there are no bad foods, just bad diets, there is no need to regulate the advertising of any product. Proponents oppose legislation related to food labeling or banning advertising to children as over-reaching governmental attempts to regulate the personal matter of consumption and a usurping of parental authority. Legislation supporting this view stresses the re-establishment of physical activity in all settings.

The public health approach supports legislation based on the concept that environmental factors that foster over-consumption and under-activity must be altered to encourage healthful eating and to allow individuals to make truly meaningful choices. Proposed legislation incorporates societal changes beyond those that can be made by the individual, such as restricting advertising to children, altering the built environment, and establishing nutritional guidelines that foster healthy eating more than they protect industry.

State legislative proposals have become so prolific that the National Conference of State Legislatures has also developed a tracking service to follow them. It, too, allows direct access to state legislative websites (15). Summaries provided on the site assists those not familiar with regulatory or law-making rituals to make sense of legislative prose. In addition, a recently established publication, whose sole focus is obesity-policy-related news, has also developed a tracking service; although the service is available only to paid subscribers, the publication regularly reports on state and federal legislative activities (16). A mid-year analysis of state legislation for 2004 revealed that over 110 obesity-related bills had already been introduced, making it likely that the number of bills at the end of 2004 would surpass the previous year's total of 120. Schools were the primary focus, with the majority of bills directed to school nutrition and mandatory physical activities. Legislation mandating insurance coverage for obesity-related surgeries were also popular. The report concluded, "obesity continues to be one of the hottest political issues in the country" (17).

Despite the proliferation of bills, when researchers at the University of Baltimore "graded" the legislatures for their effectiveness in taking significant steps to combat obesity not one State received an 'A' and only one state, Arkansas, received a 'B'. The researchers explained that ten states received a 'C' for taking some steps to deal with obesity issues, sixteen states received a 'D' for "ill-conceived" efforts at encouraging healthier lifestyles, and a whopping 23 states received an 'F' for taking no action at all (18).

Since successfully passing a law was the criterion for receiving the top grade, it is clear that legislation is not currently providing the necessary guidance or tools to combat obesity.

Litigation approaches to the obesity epidemic

As discussed in previous sections, progress in stemming and ultimately reversing the obesity epidemic must be addressed through legislative and regulatory action.

However, both of these avenues have their limitations, especially in venues that are fraught with political and industry opposition. Clearly, pressures exerted by myriad interest groups can, and do, interfere with the implementation of objective public health goals and often shape and distort the information made available to the public that affects personal choices. This leaves a third method for public health advocates to consider – litigation (19).

While legislative and regulatory action is influenced by public opinion, it remains a function of government. The government can also initiate litigation; regulatory agencies often have the power to initiate lawsuits against those who are charged with violating the laws and regulations the agency is required to enforce. Litigation can also be a private enforcement tool and in the US has been employed by individuals to achieve benefits that extend beyond the individual plaintiff to the population as a whole. Both individual, and more often class action, lawsuits have served to increase public awareness of safety issues, protect consumers from harmful products, and force industry to modify or cease harmful practices. Indeed, tobacco litigation, which has been ongoing for more than 40 years, was the catalyst for the recent gains made in combating that entrenched public health menace.

Initially, tobacco litigation was considered frivolous and derided as an attempt by smokers to shift the health consequences of their personal choice onto cigarette companies. Nevertheless, despite extraordinary opposition from a powerful industry, litigation was ultimately successful and paved the road for subsequent legislation and regulations that restrict cigarette advertising, impose significant taxes, educate the public about the dangers of smoking, and limit public venues in which smokers can subject others to second-hand smoke. International travelers to the US are often surprised to discover the extent of public prohibitions against smoking in New York City, which has some of the strictest non-smoking regulations in the country.

There are obvious distinctions between tobacco and food, the former is harmful in any quantity while the latter is necessary for survival. However, the success of tobacco litigation was not based upon the direct harm caused by smoking, but rather upon the exposed duplicity of tobacco manufacturers. It is for this reason that tobacco litigation is often described as the model upon which obesity-litigated will be styled (see, for example, 20). Professor Richard Daynard, a prominent figure in tobacco litigation who is now focusing on obesity related litigation, explains:

> ...cases against food manufacturers are likely to be based on evidence that manufactures misrepresented nutritional properties of products, took advantage of the credulity of children to sell them high calorie density products that helped launch them on a career of unhealthy eating, marketed addictive high calorie soda to teenagers in their own school buildings, or otherwise violated consumer protections laws that prohibit "unfair or deceptive acts or practices in commerce"(21).

Not surprisingly, the concept of employing litigation as a tool to combat the obesity public health crisis was initially greeted with the same ridicule that was heaped upon tobacco lawsuits. Undaunted, those who advocate the use of litigation and other legal strategies to combat the obesity crisis seek many of the same goals as those achieved in tobacco litigation, for example forcing the industry to admit the dangers inherent in their current production and advertising practices, and, in the case of food, to help develop strategies that enable and encourage all citizens to maintain a healthy diet and weight. One group, the Public Health Advocacy Institute's Obesity Task Force, a joint effort of "practitioners, academics, and activists from both public health and law" explains its mission in part as: "Informed and timely legal remedies are essential components of comprehensive efforts to control severe population-impacting public health problems. The newly identified obesity epidemic, especially as it impacts children and young adults, represents a clear case in which legal remedies may prove necessary"(22). Attorneys and commentators agree that litigation will initially focus on the most vulnerable segment of the population: children.

The *Surgeon General's Call to Action* includes alarming information about the rise in childhood obesity. Current debate about the responsibility borne by the food industry is not the first time that a spotlight has been trained on the food industry's aggressive tactics aimed at children. Nor is the use of litigation to ban or more carefully regulate those activities an entirely novel concept. In 1977, a California advocacy group sued the large cereal manufacturer General Foods, its advertising agency, and a supermarket that carried its products for undermining children's health by promoting cereals high in sugar content (up to 50 per cent by weight) on children's television shows, in magazines, and on cereal boxes. The plaintiffs argued that the products were more like candy than cereal and were fraudulently marketed in a way that led children to believe that eating the cereals would enhance their physical prowess or give them magical powers (23). The California Supreme Court preliminarily rejected the companies' defense that parents bore the sole and ultimate responsibility as purchasers of cereals because the advertisements directly targeted children. The issue, never directly decided by the court because the case was settled before trial (General Foods provided a $2 million fund to establish a non-profit organization that continues to educate children about good nutrition), remains central to contemporary arguments over personal vs. corporate responsibility.

The concept of "Big Food" litigation, crafted along the line of "Big Tobacco" litigation, did not come as a complete surprise to those who read the business and finance sections of the nation's newspapers. In what now seems like prescient musings in 1995, columnists decried the attempt by "Big Government" to intrude on citizens' private lives and wondered if after the states had collected large sums of money from the tobacco companies,

> ... will government go after the fast food chains and their greasy hamburger? High fat content and cholesterol cause heart attacks among Medicaid recipients and other people. Should hamburger makers be sued? What about the cattle ranchers who provide the beef or those who produce the food the cows eat?...Tobacco today. Alcohol and hamburgers tomorrow (24).

Tobacco litigation continues to have its detractors and the arguments against food litigation are similar; what one chooses to eat is a voluntary act, just as one chooses to smoke. Indeed, the "freedom to choose" is strenuously championed by opponents of societal remedies to the obesity epidemic; adults must be free to smoke and, in the case of food, must be free to eat, both to survive and for pleasure. In the food context, the freedom of choice concept has even been heavily marketed to children and enormous amounts of money are spent by the food industry to create and maintain children's lifelong brand loyalties[1]. Many opponents of litigation continue to warn of the perpetuation of a victim mentality that favors casting blame on others. Many people refuse to acknowledge that attempts by industry to manipulate choice or the flow of information have any effect on them. Thus, even after documents that came to light during the tobacco litigation revealed that tobacco company executives had been lying about the addictive and lethal nature of their product, opponents of the master litigation settlement (in which states would recoup the monetary losses that represented their share of government supported Medicaid costs to treat tobacco-related illnesses) began to warn of the likelihood of *more* government intervention into private matters. That control, the argument continued, would follow on the heels of successful, yet meritless, litigation by unscrupulous lawyers.

As predicted, commentators began to speculate whether food companies could be sued for causing a public health crisis by their over-feeding of the public with unhealthful foods. One financial journalist pondered the connection between cigarettes and guns, and then continued the line to cheeseburgers, reasoning that all three could kill or cause serious bodily harm (28). The author questioned whether the judicial system would be the appropriate forum to tackle social problems given oft-criticized awards of large attorneys' fees attendant to class action litigation. But after he examined the conflicting interests that would no doubt hamper regulatory remedial action he concluded "it shouldn't be surprising if the courts try". The year was 1999 and obesity litigation was still not mainstream thought[2]. Thus, it was not surprising that Nestle and Jacobson did not include litigation as a potential solution to the looming obesity crisis when *Halting the Obesity Epidemic* (1) was published in 2000. Many public health professionals did not consider litigation a viable or preferred solution; that remains true today, although their ranks are shrinking. Even *Food Politics*, Nestle's seminal book describing the relationship between the food industry and the obesity crisis, did not discuss litigation as a tool to be used by public health advocates in combating the problem (25). (She does, however, describe the litigation tactics used by large food

---

[1] For an in-depth analysis of industry efforts aimed at children see (25–27). As succinctly stated by Linn "Burger King, and other corporations who market to children, also benefit from introducing children early on to the idea that they are and should be free to have control over their choices in the marketplace" (25, p. 181).

[2] In a subsequent article Akst focuses on obesity issues and potential cures for social ills, including American's expanding waistline (29).

companies to intimidate its critics – a typical pattern for the food, and previously the tobacco, industry when accused of wrongdoing in a lawsuit, is to defend by attacking the case as "frivolous" and entirely lacking in merit.) Moreover, it appeared that the government had been tracking the sharp increase in obesity, as had various researchers, and that federal, state, and community efforts might soon be marshaled to combat the problem.

As public awareness of the obesity crisis grew, so did the interest in litigation as a tool to facilitate change. And, as the crisis continued unabated and neither legislators nor regulators, despite earlier expectations to the contrary, seem poised to act in a meaningful way to halt its advance, public health advocates began to ponder whether they should, indeed, "give the courts a try". Veterans of the "tobacco wars" were well aware that the strategies and techniques of tobacco litigation could not be applied to food without significant adjustment. The medical complications of smoking are more easily linked to specific disease than long-term overconsumption of different foods. As with tobacco, plaintiffs would have to prove wrongdoing by the defendants, perhaps for "unfair and deceptive" trade practices. Advocates argued:

> Litigation is a new front in the battle to control obesity. While experience with tobacco litigation can help make some predictions, key differences between smoking and obesity will surely affect how the battle will play out. In the absence of proof that particular food industry practices cause obesity, suits seeking compensation for obesity-related injury are unlike to succeed, while suits seeking to protect consumers from unfair or deceptive food marketing techniques are more likely to succeed. Food industry documents analyzed during such lawsuits will likely reveal whether these marketing techniques were intended to deceive or manipulate consumers. This information will play a major role in determining the outcome of food litigation (30).

A widely publicized test of this theory came when "During the summer of 2002, while most Americans blamed themselves for being overweight or obese, at least three people attempted to shift this blame onto fast-food corporations" (31)[3]. *Pelman vs. McDonald's*, popularly dubbed "the McDonald's" or "fat" lawsuit, was brought on behalf of two teenage girls by their parents, who sued the fast-food giant for the alleged

---

[3] This note (31) also describes a case brought by an overweight police officer who sought increased retirement benefits to cover medical costs; he argued that the nature of police work caused him to develop heart disease and that irregular work hours "cause police officers to eat so-called junk food or 'fast foods' high in cholesterol and fat content, contributing to his obesity." The court rejected these medical theories presented by the officer's physician, and instead found that the "testimony as to the singular effects of irregular working hours, 'fast foods', and the inherent stress of police work upon petitioner's obesity, smoking habit, high cholesterol and hypertension was tentative at best". The court also ruled that fast food eaten by the officer was merely one possible contributing factor to his obesity. In other words, too many variables could have contributed to the plaintiff's health problems, making it impossible to single out just one culprit such as fast foods. The dismissal of the case was not surprising; the ability to prove a casual connection between the consumption of fast food and ill health continues to pose a challenge to plaintiffs. The date the case was brought, however, certainly comes as a surprise to most – it was 1982.

health-related consequences of a steady diet of McDonalds's fare[4]. The case was initiated in federal district court in New York, but quickly burst beyond the courthouse doors; the news of its existence traveled around the globe, much like fast food restaurants and obesity.

The judge dismissed the case with leave to replead, in other words, he informed the parties of his views and made suggestions to the plaintiffs about how to best restate their legal arguments. Although most of the popular press ridiculed the suit and applauded its initial dismissal in court, those who actually read the 60 plus page opinion quickly realized that while the teenagers' claims might be difficult to prove, the judge did not consider them frivolous. Supporters were encouraged by the court's serious consideration of the argument that the teenagers' consumption of fast food bore a causal relationship to their weight-related health conditions, while detractors argued the judge should not have permitted the plaintiffs yet another day in court. Ultimately, the court dismissed the amended complaint; neither public health advocates nor trial attorneys were optimistic about the potential for a successful appeal. Most commentators decried the proceedings as a publicity stunt by undisciplined overeaters and greedy trial lawyers.

Nevertheless, the media, delighted by the frenzied debate set off by the case, created the impression that a maelstrom of lawsuits was imminent. This had a three-fold effect. First, it appeared to cement public opinion in opposition to what had been branded "fat" lawsuits, regardless of the claims actually made in the pleadings. Second, it created a groundswell of federal and state legislation that prohibits litigation based on obesity claims. Third, the fear of additional litigation is credited as the catalyst for many changes recently instituted by the food industry. These include statements of intent by Kraft Foods to reformulate products by eliminating trans fats and reducing calories, Coca-Cola's efforts to distance itself from advertising to children, Frito-Lay's labeling baked snacks as "good for you", and a whole host of announcements and actions around the world that are intended to create healthier foods. Since many of the companies involved are multinational, their efforts at revamping products to have a more healthful nutritional profile have a global impact.

The effect of the specter, if not the reality, of lawsuits was noted in Nestle's recent *Science* editorial that explores the political ironies of a world simultaneously beset by issues of obesity and chronic under-nutrition. The author blames the US crisis in large part on the "notorious conflict" of interests under which the US Department of Agriculture (USDA) operates – simultaneously urging Americans to maintain a healthy weight (eat less) while promoting US agricultural interests (eat more). She opined:

> If campaigns to promote more healthful eating are not in the best interest of industry, and government agencies are caught in conflicts of interest, how can any society address its obesity

---

[4] The plaintiffs in *Pelman* are often subjects of harsh criticism. For a window into the daily lives of these teenagers and their consumption of fast food, see (32) According to the movie *Supersize Me* (33), everyday consumption of McDonald's food may prove more dangerous to one's health than even previously thought.

epidemic? The leadership vacuum in the US leaves much room for litigation against the obesity-promoting practices of food companies. Whatever their legal merits, the current lawsuits engage the food industry's rapt attention and encourage scrutiny of their current products and practices (8).

And while litigation may be viewed from a global perspective as a public health tool most frequently employed, or at least threatened, in the US that may be changing. Indeed, the significant potential financial effects upon the international food industry from perceived litigation risks are already being measured.

In March and April of 2003, two international financial institutions, UBS Warburg's Global Equity Research and JP Morgan's European Equity Research departments each issued research reports exploring the impact of the obesity epidemic for investors (34, 35). Both reports highlighted the World Health Organization (WHO) report *Diet, Nutrition and the Prevention of Chronic Diseases* (36) as a major factor in their deliberations. JP Morgan dubbed the report "a time bomb for the food industry" and cautioned investors not to underestimate the potential threat to food industry interests posed by both regulation and litigation. UBS summarized its research findings:

> The recent increase in media focus on the growth of non-communicable diseases has attracted the interest of the mainstream investment community. For the first time, these investors are beginning to explore the links between diet and health concerns and the value of traded stocks. The rationale behind the report is evident: "There is a clear *long term risk* to producers of fast foods, soft drinks, confectionery and snacks that anti-obesity measures will curb their ability to grow revenues in the future". It assumes that the challenge of change will be hardest for companies whose brands are associated most strongly with 'demonized' foods. *It goes on to suggest that the most vulnerable stocks are Coca-Cola, PepsiCo, Cadbury Schweppes, Tate and Lyle, McDonalds and Diageo.* Further, they will become more frequently reported on in the media, and in turn become the focus of risk management and insurance issues (italics in original) (35).

UBS concluded its report with an analysis of the *Pelman* case (32) and a warning; elements of the case were not frivolous, despite McDonald's arguments to the contrary and the lawsuit was likely to be just the "first of many different legal approaches".

JP Morgan's equally detailed analysis concluded with an admonition to the food industry to transform itself for the dual purposes of avoiding overly restrictive regulations ("a total ban of advertising of food and beverages to children on TV could have a negative impact on volumes and profitability") and to take advantage of the growth potential in "healthy segments" of the industry. JP Morgan joined UBS in warning its clients: "litigation risks and their impact on sector sentiment should not be underestimated". The researchers recognized, too, the potential negative impact of even a perceived risk of litigation.

JP Morgan predicted future lawsuits focused on deceptive marketing practices initiated by "well capitalized law firms with a wealth of expertise in tort action lawsuits (in tobacco and asbestos)… target[ing] the deep pockets of the food companies". The report did distinguish, however, between the relatively low monetary damages often awarded by European Courts and the much larger US monetary awards that represent a greater direct financial risk. However, the report was clear that damage to "current equity market valuations in the food sector" could result simply from the initiation of lawsuits and the potential revelation of embarrassing documents. Companies most exposed to "obesity risk" damage were ranked upon the percentage of their portfolios of "not so healthy" and "better than" plus "healthy" foods. Hershey topped the list with 95 per cent of "not so healthy" food, followed by Cadbury, Coca-Cola, PepsiCo, and Kraft as companies whose "not so healthy" products exceeded 50 per cent of total product line.

Corporate executives are keenly aware of the sting of huge monetary settlements and subsequent regulatory restrictions; Altria, parent of Philip Morris (no stranger to the costs of tobacco litigation) and Kraft, presumably prefers to avoid obesity litigation altogether. Despite drastically lower monetary damages sought by European litigants, the negative publicity generated by the suits could certainly have an adverse effect upon corporate image and product sales. And, although still limited in number, lawsuits filed outside the US have already generated significant world-wide public comment.

In Germany, a judge suffering with diabetes sued Coca-Cola on the theory that his habit of drinking two Cokes a day for many years was partly responsible for his weight gain and onset of diabetes (37)[5]. Hans-Josef Brinkmann asserted that Coca-Cola should be held liable for money damages (a modest amount by American lawsuit standards) because it failed to warn consumers that the high sugar content in its beverage could lead to disease. Brinkmann also sued Masterfoods, manufacturers of internationally marketed Mars Bars, Snickers, and Milky Way candies on the same theory – the confections should be labeled to warn consumers of the possible health risks associated with consumption of these products. The BBC reported Brinkmann's sentiment that "...it's about the whole fast-food business and to what extent the manufacturer can deny responsibility for any liability connected with their product" (39).

Characteristically, Coca-Cola's spokesman stated that the company was "taking a relaxed view of the whole thing". Masterfoods' echoed that approach and expressed confidence that research has not established a link between the consumption of sugary foods and the development of diabetes. Although taking place in a German courtroom, the plaintiff's claims and corporate defenses echo those argued in the US in the *Pelman* case. Brinkmann's case differs in that a hearing was held, in Essen (Coke's home in Germany), in which the court received testimony. Ultimately, Brinkmann's claims were rejected on two grounds – the foods are in compliance with regulations and consumers are well aware of the consequences of consuming sugar, obviating the need for a warning label.

Litigation against Coca-Cola by consumers extends beyond the Americas and Europe to Asia. In South Korea, a man sued Coca-Cola claiming that his 30-year, one to

---

[5]   Articles reporting on this lawsuit appeared in several countries including Spain (38), India, and the UK. In the United States, mention of the lawsuit appeared most often on websites and blogs where it was subjected to ridicule and branded lawsuit abuse.

three bottles a day Coca-Cola habit had resulted in the loss of 15 of his teeth. Plaintiff Lee added that had "he tried to quit drinking Coke, but was unable due to a serious addiction to the soft drink". Lee also initiated a second suit against Coke that sought to force the company to place labels on cans and bottles warning of the potential damage to teeth. Lee lost both cases. In rejecting the claims, the Court found that Lee was unable to prove that his dental problems were caused just by Coke and that poor dental hygiene and other causes contributed to the loss of his teeth (40).

Just what constitutes common knowledge about the nutritional value of certain foods, their over-consumption, and its consequences will no doubt be a matter for debate, especially in light of the continued growth of "normal" portion sizes. Lawsuits should question the validity of the much-repeated refrain that everyone knows fast-food (or sugary soft drinks) is bad for their waistline and their overall health. Despite the judicial reliance on these concepts so far, it was flatly rejected by the UBS Warburg report, which pointed out that consumers actually know either very little or are misinformed about processed foods[6]. Nor do children have "common knowledge" about what they are consuming, since most of their nutrition information comes from commercial, rather than educational, sources. UBS concluded:

> It is widely and blithely asserted that consumers know exactly what they're eating and what the consequences of so doing are. This is unlikely – the experts cannot even agree on the role fat and carbohydrates play in weight gain; the true, gruesome consequences of obesity are unlikely to be widely known since this is a modern epidemic, and the delicate nature of human metabolism (just a small, but consistent excess of calories will lead to overweight and ultimately obesity) is almost certainly underestimated.

One court in Brazil has agreed with this reasoning, at least as far as children and sugary soft drinks are concerned. A public interest attorney in Sao Paulo sued Pepsi and Coca-Cola; together these brands account for 66 per cent of Brazilian soft drink sales. The lawsuits were based on Brazilian consumer protection law and supported by research linking obesity and related health risks to children's consumption of sugary, sweetened drinks. In a decision that applies to all of Brazil, Pepsi was required to place warnings on its soft drinks and in advertisements that excessive consumption could damage health. Restrictions were also placed on the sale of sugary soft drinks in schools and other venues, and on advertisements aimed at children. The case against Coca-Cola, heard by a different judge, was dismissed. Both cases have been appealed (42).

As the concept of litigation as a public health tool gained ground and the press continued to write about the purported imminent filing of multiple lawsuits, the National Restaurant Association began a campaign to ban obesity-related lawsuits. The food industry has used the threat of litigation and concomitant risk of losing investor

[6] A survey of nutritionists revealed that few of these food professionals were able to accurately guess the fat and calorie content of typical restaurant servers. Moreover, the nutritional content of many restaurant meals would probably shock judges and consumers alike (41).

confidence to persuade business-oriented federal and state lawmakers to propose legislation that grants immunity to food processors and restaurant chains against lawsuits that allege the consumption of certain foods leads to obesity and related health consequences. The federal *Personal Responsibility in Consumption Act*, dubbed the cheeseburger bill, passed easily in the House of Representatives, however the Senate failed to vote on its version of the bill before the end of the 2004 Congressional session (43).

As of March 2005, fifteen State legislatures have passed 'obesity' lawsuit bans; all of the bills are premised on the dual arguments that individuals, not society or the food industry, are solely responsible for what they choose to eat and that multiple obesity lawsuits threaten the food industry with bankruptcy. One governor refused to sign the bill passed by the State legislature; in another state, counsel to the legislature warned that the bill violated the state constitution because it would prevent an injured person from accessing the courts to redress a grievance.

As the food industry fights to immunize itself from liability and legislators fail to take meaningful steps to halt the obesity epidemic, prominent public health advocates are weighing the positive effects and relevance of litigation. Professor Walter Willet has declared that while lawsuits may be the least desirable option, they may nevertheless be the default, in light of the government's failure to act (44). Although not a proponent of obesity lawsuits, Nestle recognizes their influence on food industry decisions toward more healthful options (8). Professor Kelly Brownell, a distinguished researcher and author in the field whose work appears in this volume, now supports litigation that targets misleading and deceptive food claims as a necessary tool to foster changes in the toxic food environment that envelops the globe (45). Jacobson has gone further and become an outspoken supporter of litigation; he has written and spoken widely of lawsuits as a "powerful engine for change" (46).

This shift in the recognition of litigation as a serious component in the fight against obesity is reflected in the tenor of newspaper reporting, the observations of the business community. Public opinion remains strongly opposed to lawsuits. Newspaper reports with derisive headlines lampooning lawsuits as frivolous have diminished; serious consideration of litigation issues feature attorneys rather than food industry spokespeople (47). The Harvard Business Review, a teaching tool of Harvard Business School and a bellwether of the corporate climate, featured a case study in which a manufacturer of baked goods faced potential litigation because its products contain trans fats (48). The CDC Public Health Law News recently recognized obesity litigation as a new area in public health law and added that "the fate of such cases has big implications for our society's approach to obesity as a public health problem" (49).

In January 2005, the potential significance of obesity litigation was underscored when an appellate Court reinstated the *Pelman* case and directed the lower Court to allow discovery on the plaintiffs' claim that McDonald's has deceptively advertized its foods as healthy and wholesome. This ruling, in turn, has created another round of investment house considerations, introduction of even more state legislation to ban obesity-related lawsuits and the re-introduction of federal legislation to do the same. The increased Replication representation in the Senate is expected to result in the federal cheeseburger bill's passage in 2005 (50).

Pollsters have described public eating habits as contradictory. Poll results often cite the public's general belief in personal responsibility at the core of dietary choices, yet at the same time public opinion tends to favor less targeting of children with junk food advertisements, smaller portion sizes, and readily available nutrition information at restaurant chains. Industry sources trumpet the statistic that 89 per cent of consumers "strongly disagree that lawsuits should be allowed against fast food chains". Perhaps of even greater significance, is the finding that 54 per cent of those polled "believe that the individual, and not the corporation, is solely responsible for healthy eating". That leaves a sizable 46 per cent of respondents casting a critical eye on corporate responsibility for obesity. The jury is out as to whether that will translate into support for litigation as a means to tackle the obesity epidemic (51, 52).

Conclusions

The obesity epidemic in the US shows no signs of significant abatements; nor do global statistics seem any more encouraging. Although there have been a flurry of programs initiated in the US aimed at combating obesity, both their effectiveness and longevity remain open questions. The same is currently true of proposed legislation. Litigation, the last choice of many public health advocates, has already proven to be an effective catalyst for change. The potential and combined power of all three will undoubtedly be required to meaningfully transform the social environment that has created the obesity epidemic.

Acknowledgement

The author gratefully acknowledges the assistance of Dr Nestle (Paulette Goddard Professor of Nutrition, Food Studies, and Public Health and Director of Public Health Initiatives at the Steinhardt School of Education, New York University) and Dr Jacobson (Executive Director, Center for Science in the Public Interest, Washington, DC) in the preparation of this article. She has had the privilege of working with both Dr Nestle and Dr Jacobson in academic and consultant roles, respectively.

References

1. Nestle M, Jacobson M (2000). Halting the obesity epidemic: a public health policy approach. *Public Health Reports* 115, 12–24.

2. US Dept of Health and Human Services (2001). *The Surgeon General's call to action to prevent and decrease overweight and obesity.* US Department of Health and Human Services, Public Health Service, Office of the Surgeon General, Rockville, MD. Available at www.surgeongeneral.gov/topics/obesity. Accessed 9 March 2005.

3. Centers for Disease Control (2004). *Physical inactivity and poor nutrition catching up to tobacco as actual cause of death,* 9 March 2004. Available at www.cdc.gov/od/oc/media/pressrel/fs040309.htm. Accessed 9 March 2005.

4. **Bush G** (2002). Radio address by the President to the Nation. *Healthier US initiative.* Available at http://www.whitehouse.gov/news/releases/2002/06/20020622.html. Accessed 9 March 2005.

5. US Dept of Health and Human Services (2003). *Steps to a healthier US initiative.* Available at http://www.healthierus.gov/steps/index.html. Accessed 9 March 2005.

6. **Crawford L** (2004). *Statement before the Committee on Government Reform,* 3 June 2004. Available at www.fda.gov/ola/2004/obesity0603.html. Accessed 9 March 2005.

7. **Jacobson MF** (2004). *CSPI responds to FDA Obesity Report,* Statement of Michael F Jacobson, March 12, 2004. CSPI Newsroom. Available at http://www.cspinet.org/new/200403121.html. Accessed 9 March 2005.

8. **Nestle M** (2003). The ironic politics of obesity. *Science* **299,** 781.

9. **Atkinson C** (2004). *Surgeon General calls obesity the "terror within": wants ad agencies to help Government 'sell health',* 16 April 2004. Available at www.adage.com/news.cms?newsId=40300. Accessed 9 March 2005.

10. **Obesity Working Group** (2004). *Calories count,* 12 March 2004. Food and Drug Administration. Available at http://www.cfsan.fda.gov/~dms/owg-toc.html. Accessed 9 March 2005.

11. **Committee on the Prevention of Obesity in Children and Youth** (2004). *Preventing childhood obesity: health in the balance,* 30 September 2004. Institute of Medicine of The National Academies. Available at http://www.iom.edu/view.asp?id=22596. Accessed 9 March 2005.

12. **Centers for Disease Control.** *CDC public health law program public health legal preparedness materials. Federal obesity-related legislation.* Available at www.phppo.cdc.gov/od/phlp/Federal_obesity.asp. Accessed 9 March 2005.

13. **Centers for Disease Control.** *CDC public health law program public health legal preparedness materials. State obesity-related legislation (2000–2003).* Available at www.phppo.cdc.gov/od/phlp/statesobesity.asp. Accessed 9 March 2005.

14. **Thomas.** Legislative information on the internet. http://thomas.loc.gov/. Accessed 9 March 2005.

15. National Council of State Legislatures, Health Promotion Program. *State Legislation and Statute Database.* Available at http://www.ncsl.org/programs/health/phdatabase.htm. Accessed 9 March 2005.

16. **Agra Informa, Inc.** *Obesity Policy Report.* Available at http://www.obesitypolicy.com/ (available only to paid subscribers). Accessed 9 March 2005.

17. **Anonymous** (2004). States introduce near-record number of obesity bills. In: *Obesity Policy Report,* Vol. 2, No 7. Available at http://www.obesitypolicy.com/. (available only to paid subscribers). Accessed 9 March 2005.

18. **Cotton A, Stanton KR, Acs ZJ.** *Obesity research.* University of Baltimore. Available at http://www.ubalt.edu/experts/obesity/index.html. Accessed 9 March 2005.

19. **Fried E** (2004). Consumer litigation: a strategy to fight "fat" whose time has come. *The Consumer Advocate* **10,** 1, 3–4, 18–19, 27–28.

20. **Parloff R** (2003). Is fat the next tobacco? January 21. *Fortune Magazine.* **147,** 50–54.

21. **Daynard R, Howard P, Wilking C** (2004). Private enforcement: litigation as a tool to prevent obesity. *J Public Health Policy* **25,** 65.

22. **The Public Health Advocacy Institute.** *PHAI: Projects Obesity.* Available at www.phaionline.org. Accessed 9 March 2005.

23. *Committee on Children's Television, Inc. v. General Foods Corp.* 673 P2d, 660 (Cal.1983)

24. **Thomas C** (1995). A bad lawsuit. *New Orleans Times-Picayune,* Feb. 22, p. B7.

25. **Nestle M** (2002). *Food politics: how the food industry influences nutrition and health.* University of California Press, Berkeley.

26. **Linn S** (2004). *Consuming kids: the hostile takeover of childhood.* The New Press, New York.

27. **Brownell K, Horgen K** (2004). *Food fight: the insides story of the food industry, America's obesity crisis, and what we can do about it.* McGraw Hill, New York.

28. **Akst D** (1999). Challenging that cheeseburger. *New York Times,* Nov. 7, Section 3, at 4.

29. **Akst D** (2003). Finding fault for the fat with two-thirds of Americans now overweight, the obesity crisis is ripe for the courts. And there's plenty of blame to go around. *Boston Globe,* Dec. 7, (Magazine), at 15.

30. **Daynard R, Hash L, Robbins A** (2002). Food litigation: lessons from the tobacco wars. *Medical Student JAMA* **288**, 2179.

31. **Rogers J** (2003). Living on the fat of the land: how to have your burger and sue it too. *Washington University Law Quarterly* **81**, 859, 860.

32. **Shell E** (2003). All-American addiction. Is fast food the next big tobacco? *Seed Magazine* **7**, 58–67, 99–106.

33. **Spurlock M** (2004). *Supersize Me. A film of epic proportions.* Available at www.supersizeme.com. Accessed 9 March 2005.

34. **Streets** (2003). *Obesity update,* 4 March 2003. UBS Warburg. Available at http://www.iblf.org/csr/csrwebassist.nsf/550d4b46b29f68a6852568660081f938/80256adc002b820480256c5b00468409/$FILE/ATTF19G8/investhe.pdf. [A previous report *Absolute risk of obesity – food and drink companies not so defensive?* is also available at this site.] Accessed 9 March 2005.

35. **Langlois A, Adam V, Powell A** (2003). *Food manufacturing. Obesity: the big issue.* JP Morgan, European Equity Research, London, Geneva.

36. World Health Organization (2003). *Diet, nutrition and the prevention of chronic diseases.* World Health Organization.

37. **Anonymous** (2001). Diabetic judge sues Coca-cola over sugar warnings, Sept. 11, 2001. Available at www.ananova.com/news/story/sm_395625.html. Accessed 9 March 2005.

38. **Anonymous** (2001). Unjuez diabetico denuncia a Coca-Cola y Mars por no alerter de riesogog para la salud de sus productos. Available at www.diabetesjuvenil.com/documentos_html/dj_articulo_diario.asp?noticialD=9. Accessed 9 March 2005.

39. BBC News UK edition (2002). *Snack attack,* 2 October 2002. Available at http://news.bbc.co.uk/1/hi/business/3087041.stm. Accessed 9 March 2005.

40. **UPI** (2004). *South Korean man's Coke suit unsuccessful,* 30 August 2004. Available at washington-times.com/upi-breaking/20040828–042121–9969r.htm. Accessed 9 March 2005.

41. **Jacobson M, Hurley J** (1992). *Restaurant confidential.* Workmen Publishing, New York. See also, Wootan M. (2003). Anyone's guess. The need for nutritional labeling at fast-food and other chain restaurants. http://cspinet.org/new/pdf/anyone_s_guess_final_web.pdf. Accessed 9 March 2005.

42. **Anonymous** (2004). *Pais, escolas e governo se unem no combate à obesidade infantil.* Available at http://www.jbonline.terra.com.br/papel/cadernos/vida/2004/02/13/jorvda20040213002.htm. Accessed 9 March 2005.

43. H.R. 339 and S. 1428 (*Commonsense Consumption Act*).

44. **Reuters** (2004). *Are lawsuits the way to fight obesity?* 7 May 2004. Available at msnbc.msn.com/id/4924422. Accessed 9 March 2005.

45. **Brownell K, Horgen K** (2004). *Food fight: the inside story of the food industry, America's obesity crisis, and what we can do about it.* McGraw-Hill, New York.

46. **Jacobson M** (2004). Tipping the Scales. Recipe for reducing American obesity lists labels, legislation, and litigation. *Legal Times,* 31 March, 34.

47. **Zernike K** (2004). Lawyers shift focus from big tobacco to big food. *New York Times* 9 April, A15.

48. **Gerson B** (2004). Taking the cake. *Harvard Business Review* **82**, 29–34, 36–39.

49. *CDC Public Health Law News.* Available at http://www.phppo.cdc.gov/od/phlp/Weeklynews.asp.

50. **Grant J** (2005). Food groups get a taste of fear. *Financial Times*, 24 February, 13.

51. **Anonymous** (2004). *The weight debate: contradictory consumer eating habits challenge food industry.* Available at www.deloitte.com/dtt/cda/doc/content/us_cb_weightdebate.pdf. Accessed 9 March 2005.

52. **Saad L** (2003). *Public balks at obesity lawsuits.* Available at http://www.gallup.com/poll/releases/pr030721.asp?version=pGallupPollAnalyses-PublicBalks. Accessed 9 March 2005.

Chapter 13

The potential of food regulation as a policy instrument for obesity prevention in developing countries

Mark Lawrence

Introduction

The prevalence of obesity and its non-communicable disease (NCD) complications is increasing rapidly in many developing countries (1–8). Tragically, hunger, malnutrition, and food insecurity persist in developing countries. The coexistence of the acute diseases associated with undernutrition and NCDs associated with overnutrition has been described as the 'double-burden' of disease (9). The immediate cause of obesity is a dietary and physical activity behavior pattern resulting in energy intake exceeding energy expenditure. The underlying etiology of obesity is multifaceted, being embedded in environmental determinants rather than an individual's behavior or genetic make up. The rise in the prevalence of obesity in developing countries is one indicator of the so-called 'nutrition transition' which itself is attributed to changes in socioeconomic, demographic, and political circumstances (10). The nutrition transition is characterized by shifts in food consumption patterns away from diets based on traditional indigenous foods towards diets comprising increasing amounts of high fat and energy dense, imported foods (11).

In response to increasing obesity prevalence, governments are now exploring options for obesity prevention programs. The state has available a diversity of instruments to achieve food and nutrition policy objectives. Food regulation is a relatively strong policy instrument that can be used to influence the composition, availability, and accessibility of food products (12). There are other policy instruments, such as nutrition education approaches, and these are important for promoting behavior change for individuals. The value of food regulation is that it can act across the food and nutrition system to help create a supportive environment for behavior change. In the context of the nutrition transition in developing countries, food regulatory approaches are especially relevant for obesity prevention as they can help to protect the domestic food environment against potentially harmful impacts of global food trade.

Many food regulatory approaches have ramifications beyond national boundaries and may have a bearing on a county's involvement in global food trade. In 1995, the World Trade Organization (WTO) was established as the international organization to deal with the rules of trade between Member nations. Central to the work of the WTO is its role in administering the WTO agreements. Members of the WTO are obliged to abide by the rules and provisions documented in the WTO agreements. It is important to understand obligations and commitments contained within the WTO agreements, since international trading obligations can impact upon national food regulation and the conditions for the production, availability, and security of domestic food supplies.

This chapter presents an analysis of the potential of food regulation as a policy instrument for obesity prevention in developing countries. Following a review of the scope of food regulation, an assessment of the feasibility of different food regulatory approaches, from the perspective of working within the rules and provisions of the WTO agreements, is provided. The activities that need to be undertaken to justify the implementation of food regulatory approaches are described. These approaches are illustrated through the case study of Tonga. Finally, the chapter discusses the challenges in developing and implementing food regulatory approaches and makes suggestions towards advancing the case for incorporating food regulatory approaches as integral components within a broad obesity prevention policy framework.

What is the scope of food regulation to help prevent obesity in developing countries?

Food regulation is receiving considerable attention as an integral component of food and nutrition policy activities. For example, according to the World Health Organization's (WHO) Global Strategy on Diet, Physical Activity, and Health, food regulatory approaches can provide structural changes to complement nutrition education initiatives and thereby help make healthier food choices easier choices (13). Food regulation can be used to support obesity prevention programs by intervening at various stages across the food and nutrition system, ranging from setting food production standards to placing controls on food marketing and advertising. Among developing countries, a major contributing factor to obesity is the shift in food availability and accessibility being facilitated by international trade liberalization. Whereas food trade liberalization offers developing countries opportunities to expand their food exports to wider markets, often in practice it has resulted in the increased importation of foods with poor nutritional quality and the inappropriate export of nutritious foods. For example, throughout the island countries of the pacific, cheap fatty meats such as mutton flaps are being imported and displacing local fish as a dietary staple (Figures 13.1 and 13.2). This change in food availability and accessibility is reducing food preparation skills and food security, and creating food dependence (14).

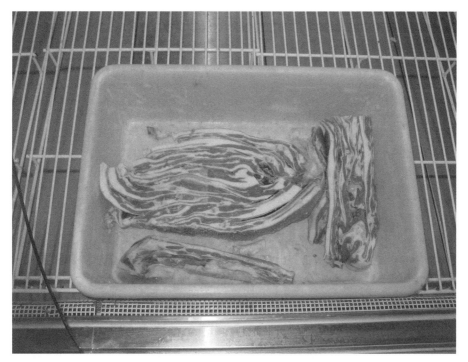

Fig. 13.1 Imported mutton flap.

In 2002, a South Pacific Consultation was held in Fiji to prepare recommendations for the 2002 Commonwealth Finance Ministers Meeting later that year. It was noted (15):

> With globalization, and international trade being seen as the engine of development, most of the efforts of the Pacific Agriculture Ministries are directed at production for trade and export at the cost of home production, which is vital for sustainable livelihoods for the poor. We recommend tariffs to protect local industries and that governments examine the quality of food exports, for example imported mutton flaps, which only cause debilitating lifestyle-related diseases in Pacific Islanders ... there are indications of strong resistance by exporting countries, using WTO rules, to any moves by the Pacific Island Countries to ban or restrict imports of mutton flaps, which provide lucrative income to Australia and New Zealand for products which might well be un-sellable otherwise.

This section presents an overview of the scope of food regulation as a policy instrument within a broad policy framework for obesity prevention in developing countries. The focus is on those food regulatory approaches that have the greatest potential to moderate the problematic aspects of food trade liberalization on domestic food supplies, food consumption patterns, and ultimately obesity. Such food regulatory approaches can serve the dual policy objectives of obesity prevention and food security protection, and therefore help tackle the double burden of disease (16). The three main

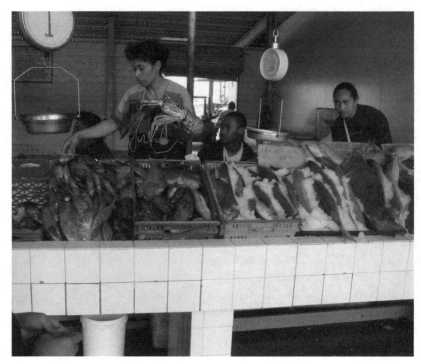

Fig. 13.2 Fish market with locally caught fish.

groupings of regulatory approaches that are described in this section are: restrictions on the supply of fatty foods; pricing controls on foods; and mandating labeling requirements for foods. These three regulatory approaches are complementary, and not 'either/or' policy instruments within a broader policy framework to prevent obesity. Included with the description of these regulatory approaches are examples drawn from international activities where available.

Restrictions on the supply of fatty foods

The purpose of placing restrictions on the supply of fatty foods is to prevent or to reduce the availability of those foods in the marketplace that are deemed to contribute significantly to high-fat intakes among the population. There are three forms of regulatory approach that can restrict the supply of fatty foods. These regulatory approaches are: bans on the import of specific foods; prohibitions on the domestic sale of specific foods; and composition standards for the fat content of specific foods.

Bans on the import of specific foods

An import ban refers to the imposition of a ban to prevent the importation of specific foods. Currently there are no examples of this form of regulatory approach being used in the context of obesity prevention.

Prohibitions on the domestic sale of specific foods

Prohibitions on the domestic sale of specific foods can be introduced to stop the supply of fatty foods. For example, on 8 December 1999, the Fijian Cabinet decided that the meat derived from the belly of sheep (lamb flaps) be prohibited from sale by issue of an order (17) under the provisions of the Fair Trading Decree 1992.

Composition standards for the fat content of specific foods

Composition standards that set maximum fat content levels for specific foods prohibit the supply of those foods that exceed the fat content levels in the marketplace. For example, in Ghana, regulations have been introduced that prohibit the importation of meat with fat content by weight higher than 25 per cent for beef, 42 per cent for pork, 15 per cent for poultry, and 35 per cent for mutton (18). These regulations have effectively halted US exports to Ghana of turkey tails, which typically contain at least 30 per cent fat. Previously, the US had been shipping approximately 1400 metric tonnes of poultry, mostly turkey tails, annually to Ghana. These regulations have also had an impact on US poultry exports to Nigeria, since Ghana was used as a transhipment point for products ultimately destined for the Nigerian market.

Pricing controls on fatty foods

The purposes of pricing controls are to influence the accessibility and availability of certain food products in the marketplace and thereby create an environment likely to influence buying patterns in accordance with dietary messages directed towards obesity prevention. There are three main forms of regulatory approach that can affect pricing controls on fatty foods: tariffs or custom duties on imported fatty foods; domestic taxes; and subsidies on the production, processing, and sale of local foods.

Tariffs or custom duties on imported fatty foods

The imposition of tariffs or custom duties on imported fatty foods would have the effect of increasing the price of the food in the marketplace and making it less accessible to consumers. A differential tariff on imported foods could be based on the fat content of the food products. Currently there are no examples of this form of regulatory approach being used for obesity prevention.

Domestic taxes

The imposition of differential domestic taxes, either as a wholesale sales tax or a retail tax, with the tax level based on public health policy objectives, would have the effect of manipulating the price of both imported and local food products against fat content levels. This regulatory approach would influence the accessibility of different foods to consumers in accord with the food's fat content. In addition to influencing the accessibility of fatty foods, this regulatory approach could be designed to raise funds to support: the administration of the food regulatory system; complementary nutrition education programs; and/or subsidies on the production, processing, and sale of local foods within a broader obesity prevention policy framework.

In their review of policies regarding taxes on less nutritious foods in the US, Jacobson and Brownell identified 19 states and cities that levy taxes at the wholesale or retail level (19). These taxes apply to soft drinks, candy, chewing gum, or snack foods such as potato chips, and may be levied in terms of a fixed tax per volume of product or as a percentage of sale price. Generally the taxes are small. For example, in Arkansas a tax of two cents is levied on the sale of a 12-oz (360 ml) can of soft drink and in California a 7.25 per cent sales tax is levied on soft drinks. It is estimated that these special taxes generate approximately $US 1 billion in revenue annually across the US (19). It is not known whether the special taxes have had a significant affect on the sales and consumption of the targeted, less-nutritious foods. In most jurisdictions the tax revenues go into general treasury and have not been used for public health interventions such as nutrition education or subsidizing the price of more nutritious foods.

Subsidies on the production, processing, and sale of local foods

The implementation of domestic subsidies or other concessions has the direct effect of providing supports for local food industries and the indirect effect of contributing to the improved availability and accessibility of local foods and overall food security. In 1975, Norway became the first industrialized country to adopt a comprehensive food and nutrition policy. The policy incorporated farm subsidies that have had the effect of stabilizing milk and milk product production, based on economic and fiscal priorities and consistent with nutrition policy objectives (20). Milk subsidies to farmers, paid through dairy co-operatives, preferentially favored protein content relative to the fat content of milk with the effect of creating an economic disincentive for farmers if they produced too much milk and an economic incentive for consumers to demand low fat milk.

Labeling requirements for fatty foods

The purposes of labeling requirements are to inform consumers of the fat content of foods and thereby influence negatively the demand for fatty foods. Food labeling standards can complement food composition standards to inform the consumer about the levels of nutrients in a food product and relevant health-related information, and can be an integral component of nutrition education programs to support national nutrition policy (21). There are three forms of regulatory approaches that can effect the labeling requirements for fatty foods. These regulatory approaches are: nutrition claims; warning statements; and nutrition information panels.

Nutrition claims

Nutrition claims can provide information to consumers about the fat content of food products and also can serve as an incentive to food manufacturers to formulate their products in accordance with public health policy objectives. For example the Codex

Guidelines for Use of Nutrition Claims can act as an adjunct to nutrition education activities intended to promote low fat diets. The preamble to the Codex Guidelines states that (22):

Nutrition claims should be consistent with national nutrition policy and support that policy. Only nutrition claims that support national nutrition policy should be allowed.

These Codex Guidelines define a nutrition claim as meaning:

any representation which states, suggests or implies that a food has particular nutritional properties including but not limited to the energy value and to the content of protein, fat and carbohydrates, as well as the content of vitamins and minerals.

Within the context of the Codex Guidelines, the percentage fat statements on a food label are voluntary unless a nutrition claim is made. The most relevant aspect of the Codex Guidelines for informing consumers of the fat content of a food product is the nutrient content claim. According to the Codex Guidelines a nutrient content claim "is a nutrition claim that describes the level of a nutrient contained in a food". The Codex *Guidelines for Use of Nutrition Claims* and the *Table of Conditions for Nutrient Contents* indicate the conditions for making "low fat", "fat free", "low saturated fat", "saturated fat free", "low cholesterol" and "cholesterol free" nutrient content claims.

Warning statements

Warning statements on food labels can alert consumers to the public health risks associated with the consumption of a specific food. They serve as an educational tool to assist in health protection within the context of a broader obesity prevention program. For example "This is a high-fat food. A dietary pattern that is based on the excessive consumption of high fat foods can contribute to an inappropriate dietary fat and energy intake and cause obesity."

Provision to use warning statements has been included in the *Fiji Food Safety Act 2003* (23). Consideration is being given to introducing a regulation that requires the fat content of meats to be included on a label in a manner that alerts the consumer of health risks associated with the consumption of animal fats. The section was included in the Act to help control the consumption of imported of fatty meats such as mutton flaps.

Nutrition information panels

The nutrition information panel on a food product can provide the consumer with information about the quantity of various nutrients, including fat, in a food product. For example, in Australia and New Zealand, *Food Standard 1.2.8* sets out the nutrition information requirements in relation to food that is required to be labeled under the *Australia New Zealand Food Standards Code* (24). This Standard prescribes when nutritional information must be provided, and the manner in which such information is provided. Nutrition information panels are mandatory on most foods. Among the prescribed declarations is the average quantity, expressed in grams, of protein, fat, saturated fat, carbohydrate, and sugars, in a serving of the food and in a unit quantity of the food.

What are the WTO agreements?

The food regulatory approaches outlined in the previous section must be considered within the context of the trade commitments of national governments. Global food trade is being managed within international agreements and in particular the Word Trade Organization (WTO) Agreements. Members of the WTO are obliged to abide by the rules and provisions in the WTO Agreements that set the framework for international trade liberalization. The fundamental WTO principle is non-discrimination. Non-discrimination involves two components: most-favored nation, whereby countries cannot discriminate between their trading partners; and national treatment, whereby imported and locally-produced goods that are otherwise similar are required to be treated equally, in terms of competitive opportunities in the importing country's marketplace.

There are three WTO agreements that are of particular relevance to Member countries in their food control programs and food-related public health measures: the *Agreement on Agriculture*: the *Agreement on the Application of Sanitary and Phytosanitary Measures* (SPS); and the *Agreement on Technical Barriers to Trade* (TBT).

Agreement on agriculture

The primary focus of the *Agreement on Agriculture* is to further a fair and market-oriented agricultural trading system through substantial and progressive reductions in market-distorting agricultural supports and protection. This is done under the Agreement through individual, binding commitments made by each WTO Member to reduce tariffs, taxes, and subsidies. The *Agreement on Agriculture* specifically recognizes the special needs of developing countries[1]. The final clause in the Preamble to the Agreement notes (25):

> that commitments under the reform programme should be made in an equitable way among all Members, having regard to non-trade concerns, including food security and the need to protect the environment; having regard to the agreement that special and differential treatment to developing countries is an integral element of the negotiations, and taking into account the possible negative effects of the implementation of the reform programme on least-developed[2] and net food-importing developing countries.

Agreement on the application of sanitary and phytosanitary measures (SPS)

Sanitary measures are those that relate to the safety of food for human and animal consumption. Phytosanitary measures relate to protecting plant health. The SPS

---

[1] There are no WTO definitions of 'developed' and 'developing' countries. 'Developing countries' in the WTO are designated on the basis of self-selection although this is not necessarily automatically accepted in all WTO bodies.

[2] The WTO recognizes as 'least-developed countries' those countries which have been designated as such by the United Nations. Over three-quarters of the WTO members are developing or least-developed countries.

Agreement is concerned with minimizing the potential use of SPS measures as unreasonable or inappropriate barriers to trade (26). The SPS Agreement contains specific rules for countries wanting to restrict trade to ensure food safety and the protection of human life from plant- or animal-carried diseases. While recognizing the sovereign right of Members to decide upon the level of health protection they deem appropriate, the main purpose of the SPS Agreement is to restrict the use of technical regulations and conformance procedures as disguised trade barriers.

Agreement on technical barriers to trade (TBT)

The TBT Agreement applies to all products, including industrial and agricultural products, but excluding sanitary and phytosanitary measures as defined in the SPS Agreement. Technical barriers to trade are those official national requirements with which products entering a country must comply. In the food trade the sources of technical barriers include regulations and standards as to food safety, quality, or other attributes, including labeling, and conformity assessment procedures. The TBT Agreement (26):

> tries to ensure that regulations, standards, testing and certification procedures do not create unnecessary obstacles. The agreement recognizes countries' rights to adopt the standards they consider appropriate – for example, for human, animal or plant life or health.

Countries that are not WTO members

Many developing countries are not Members of WTO and hence are not bound by the rules and provisions in its agreements. In the absence of such obligations, non-members of the WTO have greater flexibility in pursuing regulatory approaches that influence their food and nutrition systems. However, trade-restrictive behaviors that appear to be outside the terms of the relevant WTO agreements may expose nations to retaliatory measures with respect to access to development aid, harm international relationships, and diminish participation in other political agendas. Also, observer governments[3] to the WTO that do not abide by the rules and provisions of its agreements may influence detrimentally their prospects for future WTO membership.

Assessment of regulatory approaches to prevent obesity

When the original multilateral trade agreement, that is the General Agreement on Tariffs and Trade (GATT), was prepared it made special reference to the importance of taking into account national public health policy objectives in the decision-making process of trade negotiations. Specifically, Article XX (26):

> … allows governments to act on trade in order to protect human, animal or plant life or health, provided they do not discriminate or use this as disguised protectionism.

---

[3] An observer government is one that is in the process of acceding to WTO membership.

However, some commentators assert that the rules and provisions prescribed in the WTO agreements serve to promote food trade practices contrary to public health interests and obstruct the development of potential food regulatory approaches that might otherwise help to tackle obesity. In response to these public health concerns, a joint study that had examined the WTO agreements and public health was published by the WHO and WTO Secretariat in 2002. The joint study affirms that the health protection principle espoused in the GATT is relevant in the context of the current WTO agreements when it states that (27):

> ... the rules and provisions of the WTO agreements most relevant to health generally permit countries to manage trade in goods and services in order to achieve their national health objectives, as long as health measures respect basic trade principles such as non-discrimination. Even these provisions may be waived under exceptions for public health.

The joint study states that WTO and WHO are seeking to move towards health and trade "policy coherence". Policy coherence is described as being efforts to seek synergies between policies in different areas in support of the common WTO and WHO goals of poverty reduction, human development, and economic growth. The potential to use food regulation as a policy instrument to help prevent obesity presents a test for demonstrating commitment towards health and trade policy coherence. The demonstration of this commitment will depend on two factors. Firstly, the acceptance of food regulatory approaches as legitimate policy instruments to proactively protect public health and safety. Secondly, how the 'protection of public health and safety' is interpreted in the application of the rules and provisions of the WTO agreements.

The WHO/WTO joint study does not appear to identify food regulation as a policy instrument for proactively protecting public health and safety. Also, it defines the protection of public health in terms of relatively acute food safety issues and therefore advises that the legitimacy of approaches to protect public health needs to be assessed within the parameters of the SPS agreement. In the present analysis, it is argued that obesity prevention needs to be framed as a legitimate public health concern for developing countries. The acceptance of this framing broadens the meaning ascribed to protecting public health and safety within the WTO agreements. Also, it is argued that regulatory approaches need to be permitted so as to be able to proactively protect public health and safety. This reframing of the interpretation of public health and safety protection, and the proactive pursuit of this policy objective, serve to provide the opportunity to use food regulatory approaches as policy instruments for obesity prevention.

Therefore, in contrast to the assessment provided in the WHO/WTO joint study, it would appear that the use of food regulation to help prevent obesity would come within the terms of the Agreement on Agriculture and the TBT Agreement. Because the focus of the SPS Agreement is on food safety and the protection of humans from plant- or animal-carried diseases and not broader nutrition concerns such as obesity prevention, it will not be discussed further in this chapter.

In this section, the three groupings of regulatory approaches described above (restrictions on the supply of fatty foods, pricing controls on fatty foods, and labeling requirements for foods) are assessed for their feasibility in relation to the requirements of the relevant WTO agreement. It is not possible to offer definitive assessments on the feasibility of a regulatory approach without placing the circumstances associated with the proposed regulatory approach into perspective. The assessment that is presented in this section provides an interpretation of the WTO agreement relevant to each regulatory approach, the requirements that need to be fulfilled, and clues on constructing a case within which these requirements might best be met. Additional technical information is available in a WHO publication on this topic (28).

Restrictions on the supply of fatty foods

There are three main forms of regulatory approach that can effect restrictions on the supply of fatty foods. These regulatory approaches are: bans on the import of fatty foods; prohibitions on domestic sale of fatty foods; and composition standards controlling the fat content of specific foods.

Import bans, prohibitions on domestic sales, and composition standards are technical regulations and as such fall under the TBT Agreement. The favorable assessment of these regulatory approaches depends on their adherence with requirements set down in the rules and provisions of the TBT Agreement. These requirements are included in Article 2 of the TBT Agreement. The key requirements are that the:

- technical regulation is contributing to the fulfillment of a legitimate objective;
- regulation is not more trade restrictive than necessary to fulfill the objective, taking account of the risks non-fulfillment would create;
- legitimate objective cannot be addressed in a less trade-restrictive manner.

The legitimate objective being addressed by regulatory approaches restricting the supply of fatty foods would be obesity prevention. The regulatory approaches may be trade restrictive and it would need to be demonstrated that they are necessary to achieve the legitimate objective, taking into account the risks non-fulfillment would create. A risk assessment process would need to demonstrate that the risks of not implementing these regulatory approaches, including the health, social, and economic costs associated with obesity, outweigh any trade-restrictive effect. The justification for each of the regulatory approaches restricting the supply of fatty foods would need to be supported with scientific evidence. For example scientific evidence would be required to show that a food affected by a regulatory approach has not been selected arbitrarily but instead contributes to excessive dietary fat intake among the population.

It would need to be demonstrated that the prevention and control of obesity could not be addressed in a less trade-restrictive manner than these regulatory approaches. For example nutrition education may be an alternative and less trade-restrictive approach for addressing obesity, but generally education is a more long-term approach for achieving food and nutrition policy objectives and is more effective when implemented in combination with regulatory approaches (29). Regulatory approaches can have a relatively immediate and targeted effect in influencing the supply of foods and thereby creating an environment that will make it easier to put the nutrition education initiatives into place.

Imposing an import ban on a product is one of the more trade-restrictive measures available and it would be discriminatory in relation to national treatment if there were like products in the marketplace. Prohibiting the domestic sale of specific foods is non-discriminatory in terms of national treatment as it applies to both imported and local foods. The example of the Fijian order prohibiting the sale of lamb flaps described earlier is relevant here. The order was targeted at a specific fatty food, lamb flaps, and the order applies to all lamb flaps irrespective of whether they are derived from a local or an international source. Since Fiji does not have a local source of lamb flaps the prohibition on the domestic sale of these foods effectively is equivalent to banning their import. The setting of composition standards for the fat content of specific foods would be discriminatory if applied arbitrarily with respect to the foods that are selected and the fat content levels that are specified.

Pricing controls on fatty foods

Governments have three main regulatory approaches at their disposal within the broad grouping of pricing controls on fatty foods. These regulatory approaches are: tariffs or custom duties; domestic subsidies or other concessions; and taxes (wholesale or retail sales tax).

Tariffs and domestic subsidies are trade-related agricultural areas that address market access and domestic support and as such fall under the Agreement on Agriculture. The use of tariffs and domestic subsidies by WTO Members will depend on commitments made when signing on to the WTO agreements. Those developing countries that are observers of the WTO need to determine whether they want to introduce tariffs and domestic subsidies and, if they do, they will need to establish the contexts for food security considerations and/or special and differential treatment to justify the introduction of the pricing controls. Developing countries are allowed to use some types of investment and input subsidies under certain conditions. For example developmental measures of assistance, whether direct or indirect, designed to encourage agricultural and rural development. These domestic support schemes can help support the production, processing, and sale of local foods. Domestic taxes are not generally affected by the Agreement on Agriculture and are unlikely to fall under the rules and provisions of the WTO agreements.

Those developing countries that are WTO Members and introduce tariffs and domestic subsidies may be in contravention of the rules of the Agreement on Agriculture in relation to both market access and domestic support. Members of the

WTO make commitments towards reductions in tariffs and domestic subsidy, and the timeline for these reductions, when signing on to the WTO agreements. The viability of introducing pricing controls by WTO Members will depend on existing commitments to the Agreement on Agriculture. Least developed countries are not required to make commitments to tariff and domestic subsidy reduction.

It is noted in the Agreement on Agriculture that special and differential treatment for developing countries is an integral element of negotiations. National health plans are legitimate concerns of developing countries and need to be considered in negotiations associated with setting commitments on tariffs and domestic subsidies. Tariffs would need to be shown to be essential components of the policy framework for obesity prevention.

The justification for setting tariff levels for fatty foods would need to be supported by a rational basis, demonstrating how it is relevant to food security and/or the legitimate concerns of a country. For example the introduction of a differential tariff or tax scheme based on the fat content of food products would need to have established that the criteria have not been set arbitrarily but instead relate to those foods that contribute to excessive dietary fat intake among the population.

Labeling requirements

There are three main forms of regulatory approach within the broad grouping of labeling requirements for fatty foods. These regulatory approaches are: nutrition claims; warning statements; and nutrition information panels.

Nutrition claims, warning statements, and nutrition information panels are technical regulations and as such fall under the TBT Agreement. The use of labeling requirements is relatively straightforward in relation to nutrition claims and a nutrition information panel as there are widely accepted guidelines and standards available that developing countries can incorporate into their food regulatory systems. The case to support the use of warning statements on fatty foods is similar to that constructed for regulatory approaches restricting the supply of fatty foods. In particular, the case for warning statements is strengthened by demonstrating the integral role of these regulatory approaches in a broad policy framework for obesity prevention.

Tonga as a case study of the potential for food regulation as a policy instrument for obesity prevention

Why consider food regulation to help prevent obesity in Tonga?

In Tonga, the prevalence of obesity and NCDs has reached epidemic proportions. The obesity prevalence is over 60 per cent (Palu, TT. 2003, Prevalence of diabetes, IGT and risk factors survey 1998, Presentation at the Tonga National Strategy for the Prevention and Control of NCDs workshop October 2003, unpublished). Cardiovascular diseases (including circulatory disease) are the number one cause of death in Tonga (29 per cent of all deaths). Diabetes prevalence is very high at about

15 per cent, with a further 11 per cent at high risk of diabetes. Tonga ranks amongst the highest prevalence of diabetes and impaired glucose tolerance in the Pacific region, and in the world.

The food consumption patterns of Tongans are being influenced by a complex interplay of cultural, social, economic, and political factors that are shaping the dynamics of the food production, processing, marketing, and distribution systems in the kingdom. In broad terms, the phenomenon of 'globalization' in recent decades has contributed to significant increases in the flow of goods, such as increasing reliance on imported foods (30). In particular, there has been a significant transition from traditional diets (comprising fresh fish, root crops, and fruits and vegetables) to increasing reliance on imported and highly processed foods including: imported fatty meats, tinned fish, cakes, ice cream, canned drinks, and alcohol (31, 32).

Which food regulatory approach is best for Tonga?

In recent years, regional Pacific meetings have prepared many policy recommendations aimed at preventing the obesity and NCD epidemic (33–34). At the Tonga National Strategy for the Prevention and Control of NCDs Workshop held in Nuku'alofa from 27–30 October 2003, delegates explored and assessed a range of policies for controlling obesity and NCDs in Tonga. The delegates recommended that the best regulatory option to help prevent NCDs in Tonga would be a quota system that limits the import of fatty meats for the domestic market. This recommendation was based on the following two factors.

1. **Addresses the nature of the problem:** Obesity and NCDs in Tonga are linked to excessive consumption, and in particular excessive consumption of fatty meats. Delegates commented, "If food is available it will be eaten". The best regulatory option is one that limits the availability of fatty meats. Taxes and subsidies were discussed, but it was considered that although these options might affect price, they might not significantly affect availability.

2. **Most consistent with the WTO principle of non-discrimination while contributing to a legitimate objective:** The basic WTO principle is non-discrimination. WTO members cannot discriminate between trading partners, nor between imported and locally produced foods. However, countries are permitted to negotiate this principle where a legitimate objective exists. Countries are then required to demonstrate that the regulatory option is not more trade restrictive than necessary to fulfill the legitimate objective; for example a quota system is less trade restrictive than import bans.

How might the case for the food regulatory approach be constructed?

A case for developing and implementing an import quota system will need to be constructed to demonstrate how it will protect the health of Tongans and that in acting in this way it is not discriminatory or disguised protectionism. The rules against which the case needs to be constructed are set out in the *Agreement on Technical Barriers to Trade* (TBT). The TBT Agreement itself supports the argument that an import quota system comes under the TBT Agreement where it defines a technical regulation as a "Document which lays down product characteristics … including the applicable administrative provisions, with which compliance is mandatory" (35). The import quota system might lay down 'product characteristics' in terms of basing the quota system on the quantity and quality of fat in a meat product.

The TBT Agreement permits variation to the rules of the *Agreement on Agriculture* where the case for a legitimate objective can be successfully argued with a form of evidence-based risk assessment. The legitimate objective that would be addressed by the proposed quota system is the prevention of obesity and NCDs. Although from the WTO perspective the proposed quota system would represent a restriction in trade, a powerful case can be constructed to argue for its implementation based on the following three inter-related arguments: the risk assessment process to support the legitimate objective; the evidence linking imported fatty meats to obesity and NCDs; and the quota system as an integral component of a policy framework.

Risk assessment process to support the legitimate objective

The risks of non-fulfillment of the legitimate objective from not implementing the legislation can be measured in terms of health, social, and economic costs and it needs to be demonstrated that these costs outweigh any trade-restrictive effect of the proposed quota system. From a health and social perspective, the prevalence of obesity and NCDs in Tonga is huge and increasing. From an economic perspective, NCDs are placing a significant cost burden on Tonga's health system. In 2000, doctors in Tonga estimated health-care activity due to diet-related NCDs at 50 per cent of hospital admissions, and estimated that these accounted for over 50 per cent of total hospital resources used (36). Conversely, the trade-restrictive effect of the proposed quota system can be measured in terms of the import duty and tax revenue foregone from restricting the amount of fatty meats imported into Tonga. Based on the most recently available complete food import statistical data from 1999, the total economic cost of a quota system that limits the imports of the four main sources of fatty meats by 50 per cent is estimated to be about T$ 1.4m per year.

Evidence linking imported fatty meats to obesity

The scientific evidence that links imported fatty meats to the obesity and NCD epidemics is very important for making the case for introducing the proposed quota system and this is outlined below.

The increased availability of imported fatty meats has significantly displaced traditional, healthier indigenous foods, especially fish. The main imported fatty meats are mutton flaps, turkey tails, tinned corned beef, and sausages. The trends for the four

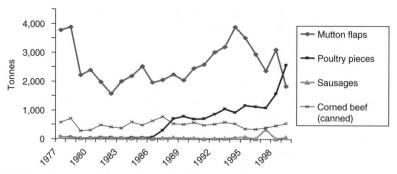

Fig. 13.3 Tonga imports of fatty meat.

main fatty meat imports (1976–1999) are shown in Figure 13.3 below. Turkey tails are not separately identified and will be one component of the general category 'poultry pieces'. The 1999 data (the last year with complete data) show that the four meat imports were over 5000 tonnes and had a value of about T\$ 9.5m. The main traditional food that these fatty meats displace appears to be fish, with fatty meat imports exceeding the availability of fish on the local market[4]. The conclusion of a 2001 study reported that economic factors are the primary reason why there has been a shift in the consumption of many local foods to an increasing reliance on imported fatty foods (30).

The increased availability of these imported fatty meats has transformed the dietary intake pattern of Tongans. Food composition data show that the four main fatty meats identified are high in total fat (over 50 per cent of energy) and saturated fat. Food supply data show that availability of mutton flaps is about 400 g/week per capita (see Figure 13.3). Of the four identified fatty meats, the mutton flaps category is of the highest priority because of its large volume and it can be specifically identified.

This dietary intake pattern is a contributing factor to the Tongan obesity and NCD epidemic. From the perspective of NCDs, saturated fat is the most important dietary factor for cardiovascular diseases (37). A high saturated fat intake from animal sources increases blood cholesterol and risk of heart rhythm disturbances (cardiac arrest and sudden death). Animal fat, such as that found in imported fatty meats, is the most import source of saturated fat. From the perspective of obesity, total energy intake is determined by serving sizes and energy density. Because fat is the most energy dense macronutrient, fatty foods promote weight gain more than other foods.

Assessed in total, the data provide strong evidence that the availability of imported fatty meats has increased and there has been a transition in the food consumption patterns

[4] In 2002, 600 tonnes of snapper, grouper and tuna and an estimated 600 tonnes of other local fish were available on the domestic market (personal communication, Ministry of Fisheries, November 2004).

of Tongans away from diets based on traditional, indigenous foods towards diets comprising increasing amounts of imported fatty meats. This has coincided with, and contributed to, the increasing obesity and NCD prevalence (36).

The quota system as an integral component of a policy framework

The food supply component of the overall plan for the prevention and control of obesity and NCDs cannot effectively be addressed in a less trade-restrictive manner than the quota system. For example, at the 2003 Tonga Prevention and Control of NCDs Meeting, delegates explained that nutrition education campaigns aimed at influencing demand for fatty food have been implemented in recent years and have achieved moderate success only in raising awareness of the problem. Moreover, given the significant and rising prevalence of obesity and NCDs, a strong response is required to tackle the serious and urgent nature of the epidemic.

Legislative and regulatory approaches can have a relatively immediate and targeted effect in influencing the supply of foods and thereby rapidly creating an environment that will make it easier to put nutrition education initiatives into place. A broad and coherent policy framework based on national health plans for obesity and NCD prevention, and involving both regulatory approaches and nutrition education as complementary and integral components, is required to fulfill the legitimate objective. The quota system has the added advantage of being an intervention that provides equitable opportunity across the population. Restrictions on food availability do not require the ability to read food labels and then motivate behavior change. The quota system is not more trade restrictive than necessary to help fulfill the legitimate objective and certainly less trade restrictive than other legislative and regulatory approaches such as import bans.

When Tonga completes it accession process and finalizes its WTO negotiations it will become the smallest member of the WTO. It will be important to raise the Kingdom's public health concerns in all health forums and trade negotiations to put some obligations on the countries that export fatty meats to the Pacific to limit such trade.

What is needed to support the development and implementation of food regulation in developing countries?

In principle, the potential of food regulation as a policy instrument to prevent obesity is especially promising in developing countries because of the special and differential treatment provisions contained in the WTO agreements that are afforded to such countries. In practice, a developing country must have the capacity to take advantage of the relevant provisions to realize the opportunities available to protect its national health needs. Generally, there are infrastructure, resource, and technical expertise constraints limiting the development and implementation of potential food regulatory approaches in most developing countries.

According to Lupien, food laws in many developing countries are copies of laws of colonial powers and date back to the early 1900s (38). There are two particular challenges facing developing countries that may wish to extend existing food laws and introduce innovative food regulatory approaches. Firstly, the limited capacity to collect, analyze, and interpret scientific evidence to construct cases for food regulatory approaches. Secondly, the technical and financial demands placed on the regulatory system then to administer, analyze compliance, enforce, and monitor and evaluate the regulatory approaches.

In looking to the future, to advance the case for incorporating food regulatory approaches as integral components within the obesity prevention programs of developing countries, a number of strategic processes will be required. Those developing countries that are WTO Members and observers should raise their public health concerns about fatty food imports and discuss any plans for introducing tariffs, quotas, taxes, and subsidies with the WTO secretariat. At relevant trade negotiations meetings the developing countries need to place their requests for regulatory approaches onto the agenda and seek the committees' support to do something about addressing these special needs and to put some obligation on the relevant countries not to allow the export of fatty foods.

Many developing countries lack the capacity and technical expertise to fully participate in the Codex standard-setting process and other fora relevant to food safety and quality issues. The WHO and FAO do provide technical assistance for developing countries. In some developing countries the Food and Agriculture Organization (FAO) has provided assistance in creating a Codex-based national food law and regulations and provided training to government and industry personnel. In 2000, the World Health Assembly passed a resolution (WHA 53.15) that has seen WHO increase efforts to support capacity building in developing countries for critical food safety activities. In the future, developing countries should consider claiming assistance and preferential treatment to build capacity for food quality issues in terms of developing and implementing food regulatory approaches to help prevent obesity.

Conclusion

Food regulation has significant potential as a policy instrument for obesity prevention in developing countries. The rationale for investing in food regulatory approaches in developing countries is two-fold. Firstly, the prevalence and serious implications of obesity in terms of the personal, social, and economic impact of consequent NCDs in many developing countries demands a powerful policy response that can create a relatively immediate structural change across the food and nutrition system. Secondly, food regulatory approaches are able to directly tackle a major causal factor, that is they can be targeted to moderate the potential detrimental impacts of trade liberalization on domestic food and nutrition environments.

When developing and implementing food regulatory approaches, policy-makers need to be aware of any commitments they have made within the context of international trade agreements. The primary purpose of the WTO agreements is to facilitate trade liberalization and not to actively promote public health interests as such. However, there are opportunities to work within the rules and provisions of the WTO agreements. The assessment of whether or not a food regulatory approach to help prevent obesity is justified depends on its adherence to the rules and procedural requirements set down in the relevant WTO agreement. Although developing countries face particular challenges in constructing a case to justify food regulatory approaches, they can seek assistance through the WTO secretariat and take advantage of special provisions with the WTO agreements to support their health objectives.

Expectations for food regulation need to be placed into perspective. In constructing the case for the regulatory approaches it needs to be argued that tackling the extreme nature of obesity prevalence requires a strong response that is part of a broader policy framework for obesity prevention. The policy framework would need to involve both regulatory approaches and nutrition education as complementary and integral components in fulfilling the legitimate objective. Whereas nutrition education will help motivate people about the need for behavior change and inform them about how to make such a change, it is the regulatory approaches that will create significant and sustainable structural changes that will then help make the healthier choices easier.

References

1. **Monteiro CA, Conde WL, Popkin BM** (2004). The burden of disease from undernutrition and overnutrition in countries undergoing rapid nutrition transition: a view from Brazil. *Am J Public Health* **94**, 433–4.

2. **Vio F, Albala C** (2000). Nutrition policy in the Chilean transition. *Public Health Nutr* **3**, 49–55.

3. **Filozof C, Gonzalez C, Sereday M, Mazza C, Braguinsky J** (2001). Obesity prevalence and trends in Latin-American countries. *Obes Rev* **2**, 99–106.

4. **Du S, Lu B, Zhai F, Popkin BM** (2002). A new stage of the nutrition transition in China. *Public Health Nutr* **5**, 169–74.

5. **Shetty PS** (2002). Nutrition transition in India. *Public Health Nutr* **5**, 175–82.

6. **Ghassemi H, Harrison G, Mohammad K** (2002). An accelerated nutrition transition in Iran. *Public Health Nutr* **5**, 149–55.

7. **Mokhtar N, Elati J, Chabir R, et al.** (2001). Diet culture and obesity in Northern Africa. *J Nutr* **131**, 887S–92S.

8. **Popkin BM, Doak CM** (1998). The obesity epidemic is a worldwide phenomenon. *Nutr Rev* **56**, 106–14.

9. **Sen K, Bonita R** (2000). Global health status: two steps forward, one step back. *Lancet* **356**, 577–82.

10. **Popkin BM** (1994). The nutrition transition in low-income countries: an emerging crisis. *Nutr Rev* **52**, 285–98.

11. **Chopra M, Galbraith S, Darnton-Hill I** (2002). A global response to a global problem: the epidemic of overnutrition. *Bull WHO* **80**, 952.

12. **Milio N** (1990). *Nutrition policy for food-rich countries: a strategic analysis.* The Johns Hopkins University Press, Baltimore.

13. **World Health Organization** (2004). *Global strategy on diet, physical activity and health.* World Health Organization, Geneva.

14. **Hughes R, Lawrence M** (in press). Globalisation, food and health in Pacific Island countries. *Asia Pacific J Clin Nutr.*

15. **Commonwealth Foundation** (2002). *South Pacific Consultation on the 2002 Commonwealth Finance Ministers' Meeting Suva, Republic of the Fiji Islands, 13–14 June.* Available from http://www.commonwealthfoundation.com/documents/pacific_final.pdf. Accessed on 6 July, 2004.

16. **Haddad L** (2003). *What can food policy do to redirect the diet transition?* FCND Discussion Paper No. 165. International Food Policy Research Institute, Washington, DC.

17. **Fiji House of Representatives** (2000). Legal Notice No 14 of 9th February 2000. Suva Fiji.

18. **Office of the United States Trade Representative** (2002). *Foreign trade barriers, Ghana.* Available from http://www.ustr.gov/assets/Document_Library/Reports_Publications/2002/2002_NTE_Report/asset_upload_file683_6403.pdf. Accessed on 22 March, 2005.

19. **Jacobson M, Brownell K** (2000). Small taxes on soft drinks and snack foods to promote health. *Am J Publ Health* **90**, 854–7.

20. **Royal Norwegian Ministry of Agriculture** (1975). Report no. 32 to the storting: on Norwegian nutrition and food policy.

21. **Caswell J** (1992). Towards a more comprehensive theory of food labels. *Am J Agric Econ* **460**, 463–6.

22. **Codex Alimentarius Commission** (2001). *Guidelines for use of nutrition claims.* CAC/GL 23–1997.

23. Fiji House of Representatives (2003). *Fiji Food Safety Act 2003.*

24. **Food Standards Australia New Zealand** (2004). *Australia New Zealand Food Standards Code. Food standard 1.2.8 – nutrition information requirements.* Food Standards Australia New Zealand, Canberra.

25. **World Trade Organization** (1994). *Agreement on Agriculture.* Available at http://www.wto.org/english/docs_e/legal_e/14-ag_01_e.htm. Accessed on 22 March, 2005.

26. **World Trade Organization** (2003). *Understanding the WTO*, 3rd edn. WTO, Geneva.

27. **World Health Organization and World Trade Organization** (2002). *WTO agreements and public health: a joint study by the WHO and the WTO secretariat.* World Health Organization, Geneva.

28. **World Health Organization** (2003). *Using domestic law in the fight against obesity: an introductory guide for the Pacific.* World Health Organization, Geneva.

29. **Lawrence M** (1987). Making healthier choices easier choices – the Victorian Food and Nutrition Project. *J Food Nutr* **44**, 57–9.

30. **Evans M, Sinclair RC, Fusimalohi C, Liava'a V** (2001). Globalization, diet, and health: an example from Tonga. *Bull WHO* **79**, 856–62.

31. **Engleberger L** (1997). *Information paper on mutton flaps in Tonga* (Draft). Tongan National Food and Nutrition Committee, Central Planning Department, Nuku'alofa.

32. **Evans M, Sinclair RC, Fusimalohi C, Liava'a V** (2002). Diet, health and the nutrition transition: some impacts of economic and socio-economic factors on food consumption patterns in the kingdom of Tonga. *Pacific Health Dialog* **9**, 309–15.

33. **World Health Organization Regional Office for the Western Pacific** (2002). *Report: workshop on obesity prevention and control strategies in the Pacific, Apia, Samoa, 26–29 September 2000.* World Health Organization, Manila.

34. **World Health Organization Regional Office for the Western Pacific** (2003). *Report: FAO/SPC/ WHO Pacific Islands food safety and quality consultation, Nadi, Fiji, 11-15 November 2002.* World Health Organization, Manilla.

35. **World Trade Organization** (1994). *Agreement on technical barriers to trade.* Available at http://www.wto.org/english/docs_e/legal_e/17-tbt_e.htm. Accessed on 22 March 2005.

36. **Evans M, Sinclair RC, Fusimalohi C, Liava'a V, Freeman M** (2003). Consumption of traditional versus imported foods in Tonga: implications for programs designed to reduce diet-related non-communicable diseases in developing countries. *Ecol Food Nutr* **42**, 153–76.

37. **World Health Organization** (2002). *Diet, nutrition and the prevention of chronic diseases.* WHO Technical Series, Report no 916. WHO, Geneva.

38. **Lupien J** (2002). The precautionary principle and other non-tariff barriers to free and fair international food trade. *Food Sci Nutr* **42**, 403–15.

Chapter 14

The need for courageous action to prevent obesity

Marlene B. Schwartz and Kelly D. Brownell

Introduction

Experts have implored the world for years to take note that obesity, poor diet, and physical inactivity are major public health issues. The world now notices. Health authorities throughout the world now devote considerable attention to at least discussing obesity. Attention from the press and the public has grown as well. There were 4767 obesity-related stories in the media for the 12-month period ending September 2003, a ten-fold increase from the same period ending September 2000 (1).

The obesity issue is sufficiently prominent that action is inevitable. The form that action takes is being determined now, with key strategic decisions being made that may set the course for decades to come. Decisions must be made on whether to emphasize diet, activity, or both, the degree to which children or adults should be the focus, whether the food industry can be trusted and hence help establish policy, how countries might interact to create global policies, and more.

Science does not yet provide all the answers for how to proceed. It is important, therefore, to make "best guess" estimates of how and where to begin. More important for the long term will be to establish a template for how to acquire the necessary science, create a sizable funding base for both research and program implementation, and set a framework on the central questions to be addressed. Otherwise, politics, influence from industry, and lack of sustained attention to the problem will offer the illusion of progress but in fact support the status quo.

That this volume, appearing in 2005, is the first of its kind is startling testimony to how public policy and the prevention of obesity have been ignored. This happens to be the same year that the US Centers for Disease Control and Prevention estimates that the death and disability attributable to poor diet, inactivity, and obesity would surpass those from smoking.

It is tempting to declare that a golden era of progress on obesity is beginning. More press attention to the problem, increased government funding, and global calls for action are better than the silence that reigned for decades. But consider a few facts:

1. At its peak, the main US government nutrition education program (Five-a-Day) was given $3 million for promotion. The food industry spends one hundred times that, $3 billion, just to advertise fast foods, just to children.

2. Child marketers have declared the next horizon to be the cell phone. Knowing that tens of millions of children turn on a cell phone as the school day ends, marketers will be able to detect a child's precise location and beam advertisements, directions to nearby eating establishments, and coupons to the child's phone.

3. The US Food Guide Pyramid, developed by the Department of Agriculture, recommends that 14 per cent of the diet be comprised of meat, poultry, fish, and eggs, but 52 per cent of USDA food promotion resources go to these foods. In contrast, fruits and vegetables are to comprise 33 per cent of the diet, yet only 5 per cent of the USDA budget for food promotion focuses on these foods.

Consider also that the factors most influential in food intake lean strongly in favor of unhealthy eating (Table 14.1). If one were designing a society from scratch with the purpose of maximizing obesity, current conditions might well be optimal. Reversing the obesity crisis will be a daunting task and will thwart any single approach. Doubling, tripling or even quadrupling government budgets for obesity-related research and prevention programs (which is unlikely) could not compete with what is spent (some by governments themselves) to encourage unhealthy eating and physical inactivity. Many things must be done by many people, many institutions must be involved, and many aspects of the environment must be addressed.

In this chapter, we draw on examples from the US, because the epidemic is so well established in that country. However, the issues we address are not unique to the US and are common to most developed countries. This chapter focuses on three key issues: (a) the necessity of a shared vision; (b) whether or not to trust the food industry; and (c) what we should do next. In order to move forward, we need a shared vision of the causes of obesity and a philosophy of prevention. The strategy of trying to increase personal responsibility has not worked. Instead, we must shift our focus to changing our environment into one that facilitates healthy eating behaviors and physical activity. We also need to determine

Table 14.1 A ledger of human eating

Unhealthy foods	Healthy foods
Highly accessible	Less accessible
Convenient	Less convenient
Promoted heavily	Barely promoted
Good tasting	Less tasty
Cheap	More expensive

if the food industry can be trusted. In watching the behavior of the food industry in recent years, their strategies have become apparent. We describe elements of the food industry "playbook" and question the influence of the industry on the government. Finally, we recommend a number of targeted actions. Among these are making policy changes to protect children from commercialism, and creating coalitions with groups concerned about the environment and sustainability. We describe a more productive role for the food industry, and end with example innovations that have succeeded at the local level.

The necessity of a shared vision

There is considerable risk that efforts to address obesity will be ineffective due to inadequate and non-sustained funding and lack of agreement on how to proceed. At its most basic level, there are disagreements on the causes of obesity and whether diet or physical activity should be the primary focus. Beyond this are disputes over strategy. An example would pit scientists' recommendations to limit children's food advertising against industry claims that advertising has no impact on children's diets. To prevent this risk from becoming reality, agreement should be reached on several key issues.

Causes of obesity

Experts agree that obesity has multiple causes: genetic and biological vulnerability, social and psychological issues, and an environment that promotes poor eating and sedentary behavior are cited. This explanation includes the key inputs that affect body weight in an individual, but is distracting when one looks for population causes. We need to know why countries around the world have more obesity this year than last, why some nations are heavier than others, and why the population gains weight year after year. Genetics, psychological weakness, or eroding personal responsibility cannot explain these changes. What can is a toxic environment.

Toxic is a strong word. It implies that an exposed population will become sick. Returning to the factors that affect eating (Table 14.1) we see conditions ripe for producing overconsumption. Conditions strongly favor inactivity as well, hence energy imbalance is a virtual certainty. These environmental causes take place against a genetic background that permits obesity to occur, but in the final analysis, the environment is causing prevalence to increase.

The specifics of the toxic environment have been discussed in detail elsewhere (2–4). The environment grows worse with time and has spread from the US and other industrialized nations to the rest of the world. Part of the shared vision must be agreement that the environment is the causal agent and the resolve to change the environment, even in the face of powerful interests. Otherwise, the future will bring calls for more education (intervention only at the individual level), supported by inadequate resources, and the problem will continue.

The role of personal responsibility

A major barrier to attacking obesity is the belief that personal irresponsibility is its primary cause, a position voiced strenuously by the food industry and its allies in government. A 2004 poll by ABC News and Time Magazine found that Americans feel that people are primarily responsible for their own weight loss (5). The same people, however, favor structural changes to address obesity (changing advertising, improving foods in schools, etc.).

This personal responsibility attribution is woven throughout programs sponsored by the US government, exemplified by the Department of Health and Human Services campaign called "Small Steps" (www.smallsteps.gov). It focuses on behaviors individuals might change and does not address the social conditions that make it difficult for people to make healthy choices.

It is not surprising that the personal responsibility attribution is central to the food industry's playbook (discussed below). Precisely as big tobacco did, the food industry asks over and over why people cannot be more responsible, presumably to maneuver blame from corporate to individual behavior. Personal responsibility is central to American thinking. Driven by Puritan philosophy, the Protestant work ethic, and the tenets of capitalism, success is attributed to motivation and hard work and lack of success to personal failing. It follows, therefore, that obesity results from personal misbehavior and that educating people about nutrition and physical activity is the key to victory.

The personal responsibility/education approach was worth a try, but it is an experiment in shambles; those believing in this approach have had their chance and have failed. Allowing the environment to worsen while blaming personal responsibility has led to increasing obesity and epidemic diseases like diabetes, now even in children. Even our smallest citizens understand the importance of a healthy diet; kindergarten children know that foods with excess sugar, salt, and fat are unhealthful, yet they still prefer to eat those foods (6). Knowledge will not get the job done.

Research documenting the addictive nature of certain substances, such as alcohol and nicotine, has moved society away from blaming individuals to a more empathic stance. The idea that food can be addictive is found in the popular press and self-help groups such as Overeaters Anonymous. Critics of the food addiction concept in the scientific community (7) were justified to this point because there was little research on the topic. Just recently, however, research has begun to suggest a possible physiological process with some foods, particularly sugar, that is similar to that seen in classic addictive substances such as morphine and nicotine (8–9). As this research matures, it will potentially have very important implications for issues such as marketing certain foods to children, having these foods in schools, etc.

Brownell and Nestle have summed up the deficiencies in the personal responsibility approach:

> First, it's wrong. Year after year the prevalence of obesity has increased. Were people less respon-
> sible in 2002 than in 2001? Obesity is a global problem; a global epidemic of irresponsibility?

Second, it ignores biology. Situated deep in human genes is a desire for foods high in sugar and fat, foods with sufficient energy to help a person survive famine.

Third, the argument does not lead to constructive action. Intensified imploring of people to eat better and exercise, the US administration's main approach, has been the default for years, with little evidence of success. How high must obesity rates rise before we declare this a failed experiment?

Fourth, the personal responsibility argument is a trap. Its rhetoric is startlingly similar to tobacco industry arguments designed to stave off legislative and regulatory attempts to protect public health. The nation tolerated these arguments for decades, with disastrous results (10).

The most important question is what has undermined personal responsibility to such a degree and what might be done to help people eat better and be more active.

Protecting children, helping parents

The most disturbing trends in obesity involve its rising rates in children and the accompanying risk for diseases such as diabetes. It is intolerable that generations of children will have serious diseases associated with poor diet and inactivity, when exposure to a healthy food and activity environment should be a basic right. Children should live better lives than their parents, but under modern conditions, the opposite may be true.

While public health actions for adults are sometimes blocked based on the personal freedom argument, society steps in much more readily to defend children. It is illegal to sell addictive substances to children, efforts are made to protect children from exposure to images or messages that may be disturbing, and, above all, we protect the rights of parents to raise their children according to their own family's ideals and values (the right to teach children about religion, for instance).

Parents' rights to raise children free of commercial exploitation, particularly in the area of food, has been usurped. Parents may wish to protect children from food advertisements and not allow children to watch commercial television, but cannot avoid product placements in movies and video games. When a child goes to school there are advertisements on soft drink machines, scoreboards, and perhaps the school bus itself. Frustrated by the constant struggle with a child who wishes to eat what is advertised, even the most intrepid parent is subverted by the environment. As much as children need to be protected, parents do as well.

Biological preferences for sweet and high fat foods combine with heavy promotion of these foods in ways that conflict with parent desires to raise healthy children. Debate is often framed in ways that portray adults as ineffective parents. This is superficial, misleading, and unfair. The challenge is to change conditions so parents are helped rather than hindered in encouraging children to make healthy choices.

Certainly it is important to develop methods for parents to feed children more reasonably. A number of research questions arise in this context (11). One is whether parents should restrict children's access to unhealthy foods, and if so, how. Others are how parents can encourage children to eat healthier foods, buffer children from pervasive marketing, or change things like television viewing patterns (12).

The sad fact is, however, that vast amounts of education and efforts to scold parents into behaving better may have little effect when the toxic environment is exerting such a profound impact. Parents deserve conditions that help them become better parents, not ones that undermine their actions in such powerful ways. This is a key social value that when shared and organized could unite people in efforts to change environmental conditions such as foods offered in schools, advertising practices, and more.

Quality vs. quantity of food, health vs. convenience

One helpful shift would be to decrease emphasis on quantity and instead value quality. A philosophy of quality could mean smaller portions of better tasting food (food to be savored rather than gobbled) and of course could include health as a key feature of the food. Rozin and colleagues believe that such philosophical difference in countries like the US vs. France help explain differences in obesity rates (13). People in France value family meals, linger over meals (even at fast food restaurants), are less accustomed than people in the US to buffets, have smaller servings in cookbooks, and eat less.

In cultures like the US, "value" (more product per unit price) is typically achieved by offering more food for what seems a small price increase ("supersize" is a household word), where in other countries it is more likely that size remains constant and price decreases. As an aside, profits improve greatly from the American approach. The incremental cost to a company for offering larger drinks and French fries at a fast food restaurant, once the consumer is there and the restaurant has the food, is minimal and is far less than the consumer is willing to pay.

The concept of more product for less money is not inherently bad, we suppose, but in the case of food this strategy is applied disproportionately to unhealthy choices. Large sizing at fast food restaurants is well known, but the concept is used in other settings as well (e.g. movie theatres urge customers to buy large containers of popcorn and soft drinks). When one buys broccoli, oranges, or whole grains, the unit price does not decrease as one purchases more. There are heavy incentives to buy more of foods that hurt us and not for foods that help. Consumer research shows that people believe that larger packages are a better value, but also use more of a product when it comes in a larger package (14). This has been shown with eating behavior (i.e. people eat more when given larger portions) and use of non-food products such as laundry detergent (i.e. people use more detergent per wash when it comes from a larger container) (14, 15).

Another key driver of consumption can be convenience. Modern life often involves "multitasking", so eating while otherwise engaged is common. This places a premium on food that is fast, easy, fits in a cup holder, etc. The most convenient foods, such as those available in drive-through windows and vending machines, tend also to be the least healthy.

Ranking health above price and convenience, encouraging slower eating of better foods, and promoting pricing incentives that direct consumers to healthier foods, might help curb rates of obesity, but implementation might require new skill sets for some consumers. Family consumer science (formerly known as home economics), in the past a required course in most schools, has become an elective with a tarnished reputation. Feminism and young women learning there were career choices beyond the home, made something like home economics unnecessary (working parents would have little time to prepare traditional family meals) and even undesirable. Many people are not capable of preparing meals. This is relevant because the most healthful meals are often the ones made at home with fresh ingredients, rather than ones concocted from processed and prepackaged foods.

Changing such ingrained social values will not be a simple task. It will take an effort of government, educational institutions, the food industry and more, and children will have to begin learning new values regarding food at an early age. Some of the programs mentioned below (notably the Edible Schoolyard Project) are likely to be shining stars in this regard.

Reconciling eating disorder and obesity concerns

Public health issues around obesity occur alongside concerns about eating disorders. One worry is that large scale efforts to help children eat less may inadvertently increase risk for eating disorders, and as a consequence the obesity and eating disorders fields are sometimes at odds. The most obvious source of conflict is over dieting itself, where one field sees dieting as a solution and for the other it is central to the pathology. We believe this conflict is not necessary and in fact the two fields might share common strategies.

Media attention to eating disorders gives the impression that they are more common than they are. Among young women the prevalence of anorexia nervosa is 0.28 per cent and of bulimia nervosa is 1 per cent (compared to rates of 25 per cent or more for obesity) (16). Despite research on etiology, few specific risk factors have been identified. In one of the best controlled studies of risk factors for bulimia nervosa only two factors were significant specific predictors, childhood overweight and parental criticism of weight and shape (17), suggesting that one key to preventing eating disorders may be healthier messages given to children about eating and weight.

Messages might be quite similar for the prevention of both eating disorders and obesity. Examples would be to eat in the service of health and vitality (and not appearance), to attend to the body's hunger signals, to nurture the body with healthy foods, and to be active in reasonable amounts. Even an issue such as preventing the stigma of overweight (18) could be helpful to both fields, as the dread of gaining weight often precipitates harmful dieting.

One symptom of eating disorders is preoccupation with eating, shape, and weight. It is likely that people with valid reasons to lose weight will become somewhat preoccupied with eating and weight. There is a grey area between pathological preoccupation and appropriate concern. It is appropriate for people with food allergies to be vigilant in knowing food ingredients and for diabetics to be preoccupied with tracking carbohydrate intake and blood sugar level. Obesity can be viewed as another metabolic disease requiring significant attention, sometimes bordering on preoccupation. An environment making it easy to eat well and difficult to eat poorly would not demand such vigilance, but such is not our fortune.

An increase in concern about eating and weight is probably part of addressing the obesity epidemic, but at the same time the overvaluation of shape and weight in one's self appraisal must be prevented. A fattening environment, part of which is constant messages to eat unhealthy foods in large amounts, is damaging to those at risk for both eating disorders and obesity. The two fields joining forces to create a healthier food environment could be beneficial in both cases.

Can the food industry be trusted?

The food industry has a heavy stake in the obesity crisis. Most fundamentally it confronts a basic fact; if the population is to weigh less, it must eat less food (4). Industry spokespeople often say that people must eat and that a switch to healthier foods would simply mean the industry sells different products. This is true to an extent, but the flaw in this statement is that a switch to healthier foods means lower sales of high-profit-margin products (the most processed, energy dense foods), and again, less food must be eaten overall. When public health and industry profits are in conflict, one can look to examples like tobacco to get clues as to how an industry will behave.

There are striking similarities in the way the food industry is responding to the obesity issue and how big tobacco reacted when health officials questioned its practices (19). It may be informative to compare the scripts or "playbooks" of the two industries.

In his book *A Question of Intent*, former Commissioner of the US Food and Drug Administration David Kessler wrote:

> Devised in the 1950s and 60s, the tobacco industry's strategy was embodied in a script written by the lawyers. Every tobacco company executive in the public eye was told to learn the script backwards and forwards, no deviation was allowed. The basic premise was simple – smoking had not been proved to cause cancer. Not proven, not proven, not proven – this would be stated insistently and repeatedly. Inject a thin wedge of doubt, create controversy, never deviate from the prepared line. It was a simple plan and it worked (20).

This script was followed by all in the employ and orbit of influence of the industry, lobbyists, public relations firms, scientists, members of congress, the Tobacco Institute (the main industry trade association), and company executives.

Is there a similar script for the food industry? For the answer, one can examine speeches, editorials, and articles written by food industry trade associations, scientists

Box 14.1: Food industry playbook (Brownell and Warner, 2004 (19))

- Introduce products perceived to be healthier.
- Publicize corporate social responsibility.
- Fund programs focusing on physical activity.
- Claim that lack of personal responsibility is at the heart of the nation's unhealthy diet.
- Plead that personal freedom is at stake, hence government should not contemplate regulation or legislation.
- Vilify critics with totalitarian language, characterizing them as the food police, leaders of a nanny state, and even "food fascists," and accuse them of desires to strip people of civil liberties.
- Emphasize physical activity over diet.
- State there are no good or bad foods, hence no food or food type (soft drinks, fast foods, etc.) should be targeted for change.
- Dispute the science to plant doubt.

funded by the industry, public relations and advertising agencies (some of the same ones formerly employed by the tobacco industry), and executives from specific companies. The key elements of the food industry playbook are outlined in Box 14.1.

The first three playbook entries could be beneficial. Introducing healthier products (as long as they are truly healthier) is an advance, but cannot excuse the heavy promotion of unhealthy choices. Social corporate responsibility is charitable activity undertaken by industry such as the Ronald McDonald House. What industries are buying for this money needs to be evaluated. In 2000, Philip Morris spent $115 million on social causes such as the arts, helping flood victims, and supporting shelters for abuse victims, and spent $150 million publicizing these acts. The remaining playbook entries are likely to be damaging.

The personal freedom card is played often and is used repeatedly when public health actions that might affect food sales are suggested. Laws mandating seatbelts, setting speed limits, and creating blood alcohol limits all faced the personal freedom argument. The freedom argument strikes a resonant chord with the public, but its power fades when a health crisis exists. Perhaps we approach this point with obesity.

The food industry funds trade organizations and front groups who attack public health advocates by labeling them "food police," "nannies," and "food fascists." Totalitarian language frightens people, so this is probably a useful strategy for the industry.

It is important to make clear to the public that there really are "food police" who tell people what to eat and have billions of dollars to do so. It is an industry that seeks the hearts and minds of children at the earliest ages, seduces school systems into sharing profits from the sale of unhealthy foods, and much more.

Shifting the focus to physical activity is a key industry strategy. No one can dispute the importance of increasing physical activity. Theoretically, one could exercise more, eat the same amount, and lose weight, but there is little hope of addressing obesity without changing food intake. It would be a tragic mistake to do as the industry wishes and focus solely on activity and hope that food practices will be overlooked.

The idea that any food can fit into a healthy diet (i.e. "there are no bad foods"), has been embraced in a collusive way by the food industry and the American Dietetic Association. This message was designed originally to combat rigid rules about what foods are good or bad and to encourage people to eat reasonably, but now has become perverted to say that no food (like soft drinks or fast foods) should be targeted in the fight against obesity. To eat a balanced and nutritious diet, variety is important; however, the range of foods that are included in this "variety" is skewed in the direction of highly processed, high fat, and high sugar foods.

The no bad food argument diverts attention from the central truth that people eat too much of some foods and too little of others; too many hot dogs and too little broccoli, too much fast food and too few vegetables, too many soft drinks and too few servings of fruit. The food industry would like nothing better than to have every product it makes exempted from criticism because no food can be considered "bad."

Another classic strategy is to undermine the impact of science on public opinion and policy. Tobacco companies were notorious for claiming that smoking does not cause cancer, second hand smoke is not dangerous, and nicotine is not addictive, even when their own internal science proved otherwise. The food industry often uses science in self-serving ways, in some cases stating the opposite of what science has proven to be true.

One tactic is to take the complicated world of dietary advice and turn it into a sea of marketing opportunities. People know that sugar, fat, and carbohydrates are all potential culprits in the cause of obesity, so companies reduce one ingredient (perhaps fat), sometimes simultaneously increasing another (like sugar), and lay claim to selling healthy foods. For example one could eat an American Heart Association approved breakfast cereal, an "Atkins approved" lunch, and an American Diabetes Association approved dinner and still consume too much energy and miss out on major nutrients. It is possible that the new generation of snack foods "approved" by health experts or organizations will harm rather than hurt the national diet.

A key example of industry distorting science is its denial of the impact of children's food advertising. Marketing to children is big business. For example American children under age 12 spend $35 billion a year on their own, and influence another $200 billion of household spending (21). A number of authoritative organizations and scientists have examined the available research and have reached quite consistent conclusions:

World Health Organization (22):

> …marketing affects food choice and influences dietary habits, with subsequent implications for weight gain and obesity.

American Psychological Association (23):

> Such advertising efforts, in our view, are fundamentally unfair because of young children's limited comprehension of the nature and purpose of television advertising, and therefore warrant government action to protect young children from commercial exploitation.

American Academy of Pediatrics position statement (24):

> Advertising and promotion of energy-dense, nutrient-poor food products to children may need to be regulated or curtailed.

Kaiser Family Foundation (25):

> … it appears likely that the main mechanism by which media use contributes to childhood obesity may well be through children's exposure to billions of dollars of food advertising and cross-promotional marketing year after year, starting at the youngest ages, with children's favorite media characters often enlisted in the sales pitch.

Review paper by Mary Story and Simone French (26):

> The research evidence is strong showing that preschoolers and grade school children's food preferences and food purchase requests for high sugar and high fat foods are influenced by television exposure to food advertising…. The heavy marketing of high fat, high sugar foods to this age group [< age 8] can be viewed as exploitative because young children do not under-stand that commercials are designed to sell products.

Contrast these conclusions to the industry's position:

Statement of William McLeod, representative of the Grocery Manufacturers of America (the world's largest food industry lobbying group), in response to questions about the damaging effects of advertising in children at the release of the Kaiser Family Foundation Report (27):

> There is very little evidence that we have seen. As a matter of fact, I think the conclusions in the report we've heard today indicate that the jury is still out…. The evidence that is not in these studies and the evidence that I don't think we are ever going to see is that advertising is telling kids or encouraging kids to eat too much or exercise too little.

Shelley Rosen, spokesperson for McDonald's when asked, "What, if any, is the relation-ship between marketing and obesity?" replied (28):

> There is no connection…. When you ask if obesity is a marketing and communications issue, the answer is no.

This process has also occurred with studies on the association of soft drink consumption and body weight. A considerable literature ranging from laboratory studies with animals to large-scale human epidemiology studies has led to the following conclusions from scientists:

Research paper by David Ludwig (29) and colleagues on soft drinks and childhood obesity:

> Consumption of sugar-sweetened drinks is associated with obesity in children

Research paper by George Bray, Samara Nielson, and Barry Popkin on obesity and high fructose corn syrup (HFCS) in beverages (30):

> It is becoming increasingly clear that soft drink consumption may be an important contributor to the epidemic of obesity, in part through the larger portion sizes of those beverages and from the increased intake of fructose from HFCS and sucrose.

Research paper by Samara Nielsen and Barry Popkin on changes in beverage consumption (31):

> ...soft drink consumption is rising and is a significant contributor to total caloric intake for many individuals, especially children and adolescents.... This would seem to be one of the simpler ways to reduce obesity in the United States.

The soft drink industry position, as stated by the industry's trade association, bears further on the question of whether the industry can be trusted:

Statement of the National Soft Drink Association (32):

> ...soft drink consumption by children is not linked to pediatric obesity, poor diet quality, or a lack of exercise.

Reaction of National Soft Drink Association spokesperson Sean McBride (33) in response to schools eliminating soft drinks from machines, using the oft-employed industry strategy to divert attention to physical activity, stating that obesity:

> is about the couch and not the can.

Whether to declare the industry trustworthy is an issue of enormous consequence. Should industry executives help establish national nutrition policy, can nutrition policy remain in the hands of the USDA (which is generally led by former food industry people), might the press trust what industry people say, should industry-produced education materials be permitted in schools? These are just a few of the relevant questions. We believe that they are many instances of industry behaving in untrustworthy ways and that the tobacco history should serve as a warning of the tragic consequences visited on public health by not confronting industry early enough and in sufficiently aggressive ways. Stated another way, the default position of trusting the industry is simply too dangerous. Instead, industry should be required to meet a series of benchmarks before earning the right to be included and heard.

Can politicians resist industry influence?
Top down vs. bottom up change

Much depends on how government leaders react to industry pressure. It is expected that companies will do whatever is required to increase profits, but in cases where this competes with public health, the public expects government to step in and offer protection. If central government does this in a capable manner, the public is well-served, but when government leans far in the direction of protecting big business, an alternative is available – change from the bottom up.

How do social movements grow? Some changes occur from the top down when a federal government issues mandates, such as nutrition requirements for WIC (Women Infants and Children) and the National School Lunch Program in the US. Legislation and regulation can be used to address most issues, if there is a will. For example the US Department of Education could work with the USDA to change the food environment in schools. The Federal Trade Commission could be given the authority by Congress to regulate food advertising directed at children. Legislation could require chain restaurants to post calorie information on menu boards. Countless other examples exist where central government action could dramatically influence the food and physical activity landscape.

Given the influence of the food industry on the US federal government, it is proving more likely for progress to come from state and local levels (and perhaps from litigation). The opposite may be true in other countries, but if the US tobacco experience in any guide, change will occur from grass roots and state levels and finally reach a crescendo where federal legislators can no longer side with the industry.

Two examples of state governments in the US taking innovation action come from Maine and Texas. In Maine, a state legislator, named Sean Faircloth, and colleagues have mobilized state health organizations around the theme of increasing freedoms; freedom to have transportation alternatives like biking and walking, freedom to know the energy content of foods at restaurants, and the freedom to send children to commercial free schools. Legislation is pending, and is a serious enough threat for the industry to send in national lobbyists.

Texas Agriculture Commissioner Susan Combs is an example of a state official taking innovative action despite some opposition. In an unusual move, she asked the federal government to give her power to make new laws about the foods sold in Texas schools, which they granted with record breaking speed. She then banned all soft drink and snack machines from the schools and prohibited the use of food as a fundraiser and reward in the classroom. At a conference in the spring of 2004 when asked about her hard hitting tactics she replied, "I tried the carrot, but the stick worked better for me" (34).

There might be exciting possibilities for citizens to band together, as has occurred with other advocacy issues. Mothers Against Drunk Driving (MADD) offers an example of how the personal experience of one or two people can change how society responds to a problem. MADD was formed by two mothers – Cindi Lamb, whose 5 1/2-month-old daughter became a quadriplegic when they were hit by a drunk driver in 1979 in Maryland, and Candace Lightner, whose 13-year old-daughter was killed by a drunk driver less than a year later in California. These two women began by fighting drunk driving in their home states and then joined forces. In 1981, there were 11 MADD chapters in four states; by 2001 MADD had more than 600 chapters and Community Action Teams in all 50 states (35).

Federal action sometimes occurs in response to pressure from grassroots efforts. MADD increased public awareness of the problem of drunk driving, provided victim assistance, conducted youth programs, and affected public policy. Their activism assisted the passage of numerous federal and state anti-drunk driving laws, including a 1984 federal law mandating the increase of the legal drinking age to 21 in order to retain highway funding.

There are not yet parallel advocacy movements related to nutrition, but it is not far fetched to expect something soon. An example might come from parents working hard to rid schools of commercial food interests. One can imagine such individuals banding together, perhaps with help from state groups like the PTA (Parent Teachers Association), to form regional, then state, and then national advocacy groups to protect children from unhealthy food influences. It may not be overstatement to say that a single parent or school official might have more ultimate impact on the obesity problem than someone like the US Surgeon General, when one considers that central government collusion with the food industry prevents innovative central action and that local victories can become contagious and spread in ways that change public opinion.

What to do?

Based on what is known, a number of actions have been suggested to reduce the prevalence of obesity. Box 14.2 presents a summary of such actions.

For innovative action to occur, it is imperative that we move beyond the superficial knowledge that people are making bad choices and turn instead to environmental changes that permit and encourage healthy choices to occur. Modern food conditions undermine personal responsibility. Examining Box 14.2 shows that many, many approaches are possible. Time and more science will determine which will have the greatest impact and what might be the logical priorities for beginning. Here we would like to discuss several topics we feel are especially important.

Demand more from industry

Earlier we discussed the food industry playbook. While it has some positive features, it contains components made to protect "business as usual" at the expense of improving nutrition. The industry should develop a new playbook, one that acknowledges that its role must change if diet and health are to improve (Box 14.3).

Box 14.2: Summary of actions recommended by Brownell and Horgen (2)

Social attitude change

◆ Focus on environmental change and recognize that personal resources (responsibility) can be overwhelmed when the environment is toxic.

◆ Replace the "no good foods or bad foods" stance with a public health focus on what foods must be consumed more or less overall.

◆ Recognize that treating obesity is very difficult and can be costly, thus making prevention the priority and children the group needing attention.

◆ See obesity as a matter of social justice: With the prevalence of obesity being highest in low income groups, social justice and race issues are linked with diet, inactivity, and obesity. Social conditions are central to this disparity, thus making the correction of such disparities one means for fighting obesity. Civil rights, antipoverty, community organizing, and antihunger groups might be allies for public health experts working on obesity.

Global priorities

◆ Learn from successes in countries such as Finland and Mauritius about large-scale efforts to change diet and activity.

◆ Support research to understand transitions in nutrition and activity.

◆ Emphasize disparity issues and the impact of obesity on developing countries.

◆ Work with the WHO as the prime organizing unit.

◆ Establish a world culture where promoting unhealthy food is unacceptable.

Physical activity

◆ Develop national strategic plans to increase physical activity.

◆ Earmark transportation funding for non-motorized transport.

◆ Design activity-friendly communities and offer incentives for activity.

◆ Build and promote exercise opportunities in communities, schools, worksites, and physician practices. Promote walking and biking to school.

Commercialization of childhood

◆ Prevent exploitation of children as market objects.

◆ Protest the use of cartoon characters by companies like Disney and Nickelodeon and celebrity endorsements to promote unhealthy foods.

◆ Discourage product placements in movies, TV shows, videogames, and food company websites with games for children.

Continued

Box 14.2: Summary of actions recommended by Brownell and Horgen (2) *(continued)*

- Encourage legislators to prohibit marketing of products to children or at least to create equal time for pro-nutrition messages.
- Create a nutrition "superfund" to promote healthy eating, perhaps from fees placed on food advertisements or small taxes on the sale of unhealthy foods.
- Promote media literacy (advertising inoculation) among children.

Food and soft drinks in schools

- Identify how eating and activity affect academic performance. Education and public health officials should be allies in this effort. Soft drinks and snack foods will be banished from schools the instant schools officials learn that poor diet is affecting standardized test scores.
- Prohibit TV programming with food promotion, rid schools of food company logos and references to unhealthy foods in educational materials, have only non-food fundraisers, and use only healthy foods as academic incentives.
- Improve school lunch programs and use the cafeteria as a learning laboratory
- Find alternatives to snack foods, soft drinks, and fast foods.
- Improve nutrition and activity instruction.
- Use zoning laws to prohibit food establishments from operating near schools.
- Have only healthy foods/beverages in vending machines.

Portion sizing

- Raise awareness that larger portions lead to greater eating, encourage companies to sell and advertise reasonable portions, and educate people on serving sizes.
- Require food labeling at restaurants and food companies to list the number of USDA servings on the front of containers.

Economic issues

- Increase awareness of the fundamental imbalance of incentives to eat well vs. poorly, and highlight the connections of poverty with obesity.
- Engage the National School Lunch Program, Food Stamp Program, Head Start, and WIC to fight poor diet.
- Change the price structure of food, first by lowering costs of healthy foods and perhaps by increasing the costs of unhealthy foods.
- Think of food taxes not as punitive measures but as a means to support nutrition programs.

Continued

Box 14.2: Summary of actions recommended by Brownell and Horgen (2) *(continued)*

Interacting with the food industry and government

- Support positive industry changes, but also increase awareness of industry tactics to influence policy and promote unhealthy eating.
- Challenge the industry for hidden funding of political and nutrition front groups.
- Encourage bold action free of industry influence among political leaders.
- Curb food commercialism in public institutions (museums, hospitals, ads on police cars, etc.).
- Promote activities known to help with body weight (e.g. breast feeding, decreased television watching).
- Mobilize parents to demand a healthy environment for their children.

Explore innovative coalitions

- Making coalitions of concerned groups increases the power of social movements. In the case of diet and obesity, there are coalitions to be made with education groups because improved diet should boost academic performance, and with fields in traditional medicine, but there are also other creative avenues to explore. One would be connection with environmental groups and groups focused on sustainability (36–39). Improving dietary habits would benefit the aims of these groups as well as public health.

Changing government structures

Structural problems in government can sometimes create problems for public health. An example occurs in the US where the agency empowered to set nutrition policy is the USDA. The agency's main priority is to promote agriculture and its leaders commonly come from food and agriculture industries. Obvious conflicts of interest exist, and it is no surprise that serious concerns are often voiced about nutrition guidelines the agency issues. One solution would be to remove nutrition policy from the USDA and instead place it with an agency focused on public health, in particular the Centers for Disease Control and Prevention. There are other examples, such as whether the Federal Trade Commission has the power to regulate food advertising to children.

Changing the structure of government might seem a pipe dream, and in fact may never occur, but it is important at least that the debate occur. If the obesity problem continues to grow, there may be no choice but to take bold action and to remove some

---

Box 14.3: Proposal for a more constructive food industry playbook (adapted from Brownell and Warner (19))

- Introduce products that are truly healthier.
- Be truly responsible with corporate social responsibility, spending more on programs and less on boasting of them.
- Promote only healthy foods to children, and ultimately, minimize promotion of unhealthy foods to adults.
- Cease sales and promotion of unhealthy foods in schools.
- Change marketing, pricing, and promotion strategies that encourage overeating and the consumption of unhealthy foods.
- Alter the industry focus from personal responsibility to environmental changes that encourage and enable people to make healthy decisions.
- Place approximately equal emphasis on diet and physical activity.
- Permit objective parties to interpret science and avoid manipulating science as a marketing and public relations tool.
- Acknowledge that personal freedom is enhanced as the environment becomes healthier.

---

of the barriers to change. Government structures might then be created to support, rather than undermine, public health.

Schools

As mentioned earlier, children are the logical group to target first in efforts to change eating practices. In most schools, unhealthy foods are available and even promoted, and healthy options are not featured or prepared in attractive ways. Many schools have "pouring rights" contracts with soft drink companies, multiple snack food machines with high-energy products, food company logos on scoreboards, abundant food advertising on "free" news channels, and homework programs rewarding children with free food from companies like Dunkin Donuts and Pizza Hut.

These arrangements might seem reasonable because they fund important educational programs. The soft drink industry exploits this perception and lays claim to helping education. However, it is the children who put money into the machines. They and their parents are therefore paying for the band uniforms or school trips, after the industry takes its share of the money. In addition, the industry achieves mass advertising exposure by putting logos machines, scoreboards, and more.

Clearly, schools are caught between needing revenue and concerns with the health of children. At its worst, this battle deteriorates to finger pointing with schools blaming parents for not feeding their children well at home (the industry position), and parents blaming the schools for facilitating poor nutrition. At its best, school districts are making positive changes and are encountering an unexpected result, the fear that schools will not be able to recoup the losses from selling healthier foods is not proving to be the case. Preliminary data from schools in California, Kentucky, Maine, Massachusetts, Minnesota, Mississippi, Montana, and Pennsylvania suggest that it is possible to replace unhealthy vending and cafeteria foods with healthier options and maintain profits (40). One key component of these programs appears to be involving the students and having them taste test new options.

Vending machine and a la carte items have typically been used to compensate for low lunch sales. Another possible strategy is to decrease the reliance on snack foods, and improve the school lunch options to encourage higher participation. Increasing lunch sales (with healthy choices) might create less dependence on the income from other foods. Research is desperately needed to guide schools on the best way to sell healthy foods and keep their food service program solvent.

Another problem in schools is declining physical activity due to cuts in physical education and extracurricular athletic activities, prompted by budget shortfalls. The concern that putting physical education back into the schedule would adversely affect academic performance (because it crowds out class time) is not supported by available research (41).

Education and public health officials could be allies with the shared goal of protecting the physical health of the students, the financial health of schools, and the academic development of students. Schools are becoming more aware that childhood obesity is affecting the well-being of their pupils and of the possibility that poor eating and inactivity are affecting the academic performance of their pupils. If school officials learn that poor diet affects standardized test scores, there will be a rush to improving nutrition, hence the need for research on this topic.

Develop new coalitions

Concerned groups can join forces and increase the power of social movements. Obvious coalitions would be between professional fields interested in obesity, such as public health, nutrition, exercise science, psychology, communications, and traditional fields of medicine. But there are some non-traditional coalitions built around themes that might be especially fruitful.

Social justice

The prevalence of obesity is highest in low income groups. This suggests a link among social justice, race, diet, inactivity, and obesity issues. There are a number of factors that might explain the increased risk experienced by poorer individuals, including stress, less leisure time to be physically active, unsafe neighborhoods, access primarily

Table 14.2 Percentage of US environmental impact attributable to food production (38)

Climate change (%) Greenhouse gases	Air pollution (%)		Water pollution (%)		Habitat alteration (%)	
	Common	Toxic	Common	Toxic	Water	Land
12	17	9	38	22	73	45

to processed and fast foods, higher costs for healthy foods, and more. Coalitions might be formed between those expert in public health, civil rights, antipoverty efforts, community organizing, city planning, and antihunger campaigns.

Protecting the environment

Today's eating patterns come with an environmental cost, an issue rarely mentioned in the obesity field. Overconsumption is made possible by abundant food, itself made possible by modern agriculture. Highly processed food and many meats are resource intensive, raising serious questions about sustainability. Mass produced cows, for instance, are raised on corn and other grains grown with petroleum-based pesticides and fertilizers. The cows are administered hormones to maximize growth, requiring energy to produce. Beef and other foods are often shipped long distances, requiring energy for trucking. In addition to damaging the environment and possibly affecting the health of people who eat the food, much more energy is used to produce some foods (more than 870 litres of petroleum to raise a 567 kg steer, for example) than the food provides in return. This depletion of natural resources is an issue that could cerate interesting coalitions.

Some foods require energy to produce and provide no energy in return (e.g. 2200 kcal of energy are needed to produce a 1 kcal can of Diet Coke). Public outcry and even the denial of water licenses to Coca Cola and Pepsi have occurred in India for depleting ground water resources to the point of creating shortages for local residents. Table 14.2 shows estimates of the environmental impact of food production.

Unexplored coalitions might be developed between people involved in the environmental and sustainability movements and those working toward healthy eating and obesity prevention. The first step in creating such a coalition would be education of each field of the importance of the others.

Existing innovations

There is growing hope that significant progress on the obesity issue will be made by efforts at the local level. Some of the innovations we have learned about are outlined below.

The edible schoolyard

Well-known US chef and author, and owner of Chez Panisse restaurant in Berkeley, California, Alice Waters, has taken her passion for organic farming and created the Edible Schoolyard (www.edibleschoolyard.org). Located at the Martin Luther King, Jr.

Middle School in Berkeley, California, the garden is a means for teaching children where food comes from and how to prepare healthy meals. Teachers integrate the garden into the curriculum in creative and surprising ways; there are science lessons on worms, math lessons that use the weights of pumpkins to learn about the mean, median, and mode, and English lessons that teach children to experience a piece of fruit with all of their senses in order to write a poem. It is impressive how this garden has been integrated into the lives of the children and teachers.

Sustainable South Bronx

In 2001, Majora Carter founded Sustainable South Bronx (www.ssbx.org), a community organization whose mission is to "implement sustainable development projects for the South Bronx that are informed by the needs of the community and the values of Environmental Justice". This organization implements policy and planning for land use, energy, transportation, water, waste, and sustainable development. One project to increase access to physical activity is the South Bronx Greenway, which consists of bike and running paths and parks on the edge of the Bronx River. Another project, the Hunts Point Market, is designed to increase access to fresh produce.

Ruby Tuesdays Restaurants

While the restaurant industry as a group lobbies strenuously against required energy content labeling on menus and menu boards, Ruby Tuesdays decided to take action on its own (www.rubytuesday.com). Seeing an opportunity to lead the industry, the company took the risk of printing nutrition information on its menu. The chain created a line of "smart eating" choices, and became the first chain to our knowledge to create a healthy children's menu that include broccoli and mashed potatoes as the side dishes instead of French fries. The chain later retreated on its promise and removed nutrition labeling from the menus and placed it in a table display. The stated reason was that recipes kept changing and it was too expensive to amend menus. Another explanation may be that sales of certain items were affected adversely, but we can only speculate. What is promising is that the labeling was possible and earned the chain considerable visibility. We hope more restaurants follow suit.

Soft drinks and snacks in schools

Important changes have occurred in some US schools. Led by Marlene Canter, a particularly effective and inspired member of the school board, Los Angeles removed soft drinks from the entire school district (more than 600 000 children). Philadelphia, Los Angeles, New York, Chicago, and the state of Texas have now created policies to remove soft drinks from the public schools. Some policies also include the removal of candy, donuts, and other high-calorie snacks from vending machines.

These are but a few example of innovative work occurring at local levels. Other are farmer's markets in inner cities, schools with classes on food and agriculture, restaurants committed to buying local and organic produce, and courses on media literacy. Right now these programs have not been organized and for the most part, have not been evaluated. We cannot say whether they are effective, but it can be said that they are possible. Encouraging local creativity, evaluating such programs, and spreading the word to other communities is one task public health researchers might profitably undertake.

Conclusions

Obesity, poor diet, and inactivity are severe global problems, a consequence of the current environment. To make progress, the environment must change. This will require close attention to both food and physical activity environments, courageous action on the part of national leaders (including separation from food company interests), support of inventiveness at the community level, increased funding, and perseverance despite deeply rooted systemic problems.

The default strategy of the food industry, and the people in government who support it, has been to pound the table with exhortations for more personal responsibility. This approach is flawed, protects the interests of the food industry, and does little to advance public health. Blaming obese individuals has not led to behavior change. The most logical (and humane) approach will be to change conditions so that people are supported in efforts to be healthy. This will require fundamental changes in the economics of food, the way the food industry does business, and the activity environment.

There are positive signs. People are aware of the problem, the media is discussing obesity as a public health issue (not just reporting on diets), and some government leaders are resisting pressure from the industry. There have been grass roots victories. The field should seek ways to make these contagious. We believe that supporting local movements, helping people organize into larger coalitions, and working to foster effective changes through legislation, regulation, and (if needed) litigation, offers the greatest hope of progress.

References

1. International Food Information Council (2003). *Trends in obesity-related media coverage.* Available at www.ific.org/research/obesitytrends.cfm Accessed 21 June 2004.
2. **Brownell KD, Horgen KB** (2003). *Food fight: the inside story of the food industry, America's obesity crisis, and what we can do about it.* McGraw-Hill, New York.
3. **Critser G** (2003). *Fat land: how Americans became the fattest people in the world.* Houghton Mifflin, Boston.
4. **Nestle M** (2002). *Food politics : how the food industry influences nutrition and health.* University of California Press, Berkeley.

This chapter was written concurrently with a chapter written by K. Brownell to be published in Heintzman A, Solomon E, eds. *Feeding the Future* (in press). Anasi, Toronto. Some overlap in content will occur.

5. Lemonick M, Bjerklie D (2004). Poll on American's views of obesity. *TIME* **163**, 58.

6. Murphy AS, Youatt JP, Hoerr SL, Sawyer CA, Andrews SL (1995). Kindergartener student's food preferences are not consistent with their knowledge of the Dietary Guidelines. *J Am Diet Assoc* **95**, 219–23.

7. Wilson GT (1999). Eating disorders and addiction. *Drugs Soc* **15**, 87–101.

8. Spangler R, Wittkowski KM, Goddard NL, Avena NM, Hoebel BG, Leibowitz SF (2004). Opiate-like effects of sugar on gene expression in reward areas of the rat brain. *Mol Brain Res* **124**, 134–42.

9. James GA, Gold MS, Liu Y (2004). Interaction of satiety and reward response to food stimulation. *J Additive Diseases* **23**, 23–37.

10. Brownell KD, Nestle M (2004). Are you responsible for your own weight? *TIME* **163**, 113.

11. Schwartz MB, Puhl RM (2001). Childhood obesity: a societal problem to solve. *Obes Rev* **4**, 57–71.

12. Robinson T (1999). Reducing children's television viewing to prevent obesity: a randomized controlled trial. *JAMA* **282**, 1561–7.

13. Rozin P, Kabnick K, Pete E, Fischler C, Shields C (2003). The ecology of eating: smaller portion sizes in France than in the United States help explain the French paradox. *Psychol Sci* **14**, 450–4.

14. Wansink B (1996). Can package size accelerate usage volume? *J Mark* **60**, 1–14.

15. Wansink B (2004). Environmental factors that increase the food intake and consumption volume of unknowing consumers. *Ann Rev Nutri* **24**, 455–79.

16. Hoek HW (2002). Distribution of eating disorders. In: Fairburn, CG, Brownell KD, eds. *Eating disorders and obesity: a comprehensive handbook,* 2nd edn, pp. 233–7. Guilford, New York.

17. Fairburn CG, Welch SL, Doll HA, Davies BA, O'Connor ME (1997). Risk factors for bulimia nervosa: a community-based control study. *Arch Gen Psy* **54**, 509–7.

18. Puhl R, Brownell KD (2001). Bias, discrimination, and obesity. *Obes Res* **9**, 788–805.

19. Brownell KD, Warner KE (2004). *The perils of ignoring history: Big Tobacco played dirty and millions died; how similar is Big Food?* Unpublished manuscript.

20. Kessler DA (2002). *A question of intent: a great American battle with a deadly industry.* Public Affairs, New York.

21. Kane C (2003). TV and movie characters sell children snacks. *New York Times* 8 December, Section C, p. 7.

22. World Health Organization (2004). *Marketing food to children: the global regulatory environment.* Available at http://www.who.int/dietphysicalactivity/publications/en/. Accessed 14 July 2004.

23. American Psychological Association (2004). *Report of the APA task force on advertising and children: psychological issues in the increasing commercialization of childhood.* Available at: www.apa.org/releases/childrenads_summary.pdf. Accessed 14 July 2004.

24. American Academy of Pediatrics (2003). Prevention of pediatric overweight and obesity. *Pediatrics* **112**, 424–30.

25. Kaiser Family Foundation (2004). *The role of media in childhood obesity.* Available at http://www.kff.org/entmedia/entmedia022404pkg.cfm. Accessed 14 July 2004.

26. Story M, French S (2004). Food advertising and marketing directed at children and adolescents in the US. *Int J Behav Nutr Physical Activity* **1**, 3–20.

27. McLeod W (2004). *Statements at a public meeting of the Kaiser Family Foundation on food advertising directed at children.* Available at http://www.kaisernetwork.org/health_cast/uploaded_files/022404_Media_and_Obesity1.pdf. Accessed Jul 14, 2004.

28. Rosen S (2003). *Comments of McDonald's in response to a Reveries Magazine survey.* Available at http://www.reveries.com/reverb/revolver/obesitymarketing/. Accessed 14 July 2004.

29. **Ludwig DS, Peterson KE, Gortmaker SL** (2001). Relation between consumption of sugar-sweetened drinks and childhood obesity: a prospective, observational analysis. *Lancet* **357**, 505–8.

30. **Bray GA, Nielsen SJ, Popkin BM** (2004). Consumption of high fructose corn syrup in beverages may play a role in the epidemic of obesity. *Am J Clin Nutr* **79**, 537–43.

31. **Nielsen S, Popkin BM** (2004). Changes in beverage intake between 1977–2001. *Am J Prev Med* **27**, 205–10.

32. National Soft Drink Association. Available at http://www.nsda.org/softdrinks/CSDHealth/Nutrition/NutritionPR/Consumption43.html. Accessed 14 July 2004.

33. **Severson K** (2002). LA schools to stop soda sales: district takes cue from Oakland ban. *San Francisco Chronicle* 28 August, A1.

34. **Combs S** (2004). *TIME-ABC obesity summit*, 1 June. Williamsburg, VA.

35. MADD Online (2000). *Really MADD: looking back at 20 years.* Available at www.madd.org/aboutus. Accessed 23 May 2004.

36. **Lappe FM, Lappe A** (2002). *Hope's edge: the next diet for a small planet.* Tarcher/Putnam, New York.

37. David Suzuki Foundation (2003). *Nature challenge newsletter, edition 2.* Available at http://www.davidsuzuki.org/WOL/Challenge/Newsletter/Two.asp. Accessed 12 July 2004.

38. **Browner M, Leon W** (1999). *The consumer's guide to effective environmental choices: practical advice from the Union of Concerned Scientists.* Three Rivers Press, New York.

39. **Fowler C, Mooney P** (1996). *Shattering: food, politics, and the loss of genetic diversity.* University of Arizona Press, Tucson.

40. Center for Science in the Public Interest (2003). *School vending machine case studies.* Available at: http://www.cspinet.org/new/pdf/school_vending_machine_case_studies. pdf. Accessed 28 July 2004.

41. **Shepherd RJ** (1997). Curricular physical activity and academic performance. *Pediatr Exerc Sci* **9**, 113–26.

Index

ABC News 310
ABI/Inform Global 56
acceptability curve approach 188
accessibility 210, 211, 212–13
active transport approaches 137–8
'Active Winners' 136, 137
advertising 237–9
Agreement on Agriculture 292, 294, 296, 297
Agreement on the application of Sanitary and
    Phytosanitary Measures 292–3, 294
Agreement on Technical Barriers to Trade 293, 294,
    295, 297, 299
Altria 277
American Academy of Pediatrics 238, 317
    Committee on School Health 242
American Cancer Society 247
American Diabetes Association 316
American Heart Association 247, 316
American Psychological Association 317
Americans' Use of Time Study 28–30, 32
angina pectoris 17
animal source foods 84, 87
APPLES 134
Asia 4, 15, 43, 90, 277
    Pacific 15, 47
Assessing Cost-Effectiveness (ACE) 197–8
AusDiab study 14
Australasia 46
    see also Australia; New Zealand
Australia:
    cost-effectiveness of prevention 165, 173, 175,
        177, 190, 191, 192, 196, 197
    ecological approach 212
    environmental factors 60, 67
    epidemiology 3, 16, 18
    food regulation 287, 291
    and New Zealand Food Standards Code 291
    obesity prevention 156, 158–9
    physical activity 129–30, 133, 141–2
    prevalence and trends in adults 14–15
    socio-cultural factors 39
    tobacco control experience 232, 240, 244
    see also case study: estimating burden of disease
        and cost of illness

back problems 175–8, 180–1
Bahrain 14
Baltic states 10
Baltimore Longitudinal Study on Aging 26
BBC 277

behavioral change 77, 143
Behavioral Risk Factor Surveillance System 6, 27–8,
    59, 244
behavioral risk factors 40–1
Belgium 10, 16, 43
beliefs 209, 210–11, 212
body mass index 15, 16, 18, 133, 236
    cost-effectiveness of prevention 173, 174,
        192, 193
    environmental factors 55, 65, 67
    epidemiology of obesity 3–4, 5, 7
    obesity prevention 153–4, 157, 158, 159, 160
Bogalusa Heart Survey 23–4
bottom up change 319–20
bowel cancer 175–8, 180–1
Brazil 16, 90, 91, 266, 278
breast cancer 175–8, 180–1
burden of disease 167, 174, 177, 179, 181, 191–2
    see also case study: estimating burden of disease
Bureau of National Statistics (Australia) 47
Business and Industry 56

Cadbury Schweppes 276, 277
Call to Action to Prevent and Decrease Overweight
    and Obesity, The 266–7, 272
caloric sweetener 83–4, 85
Canada 7, 8, 16, 18, 173
    tobacco control experience 232, 240, 245
cancer 17, 175–8, 180–1
cardiovascular disease 4, 190, 297
Cardiovascular Risk in Young Finns 83
case study: estimating burden of disease and cost of
    illness in Australia 174–81, 191–7
    diseases identification causally related to
        overweight/obesity 175–6
    health burden and health-care expenditure
        179–81
    health gains and health cost offsets 192–3
    level of investment 194–6
    link between reduction in childhood and
        consequently adult obesity 193–4
    overview of method 191–2
    prevalence and excess relative risk 176–7
    threshold analysis 196–7
    total health burden and health-care expenditure
        177–9
causes of obesity 309
Census Bureau (United States) 31–2
Center for Science in the Public Interest, 64,
    218, 247

Centers for Disease Control and Prevention 65, 249, 269, 307, 323
 Office on Smoking and Health 245
 Public Health Law News 279
 State-Based Nutrition and Physical Activity Program to Prevent Obesity and Other Chronic Diseases 248
 Steps to a Healthier United States 248
 VERB campaign 239
Central and Eastern Europe 9, 10
Cheeseburger bill
 see Commonsense Consumptin Act; Personal Responsibility in Consumption Act
Changing Individuals' Purchase of Snacks (CHIPS) 116
Child and Adolescent Trial for Cardiovascular Health 113–15, 158, 159
child characteristics 214–15
childhood, commercialization of 321–2
childhood obesity 15–16
children: ecological approach 207–25
 advocacy and healthy environments 221
 eating behaviors 209–10
 increasing access to healthy options 220–1
 parents as role models and children as coparticipators 219
 physical activity 210–12
 practitioners and policy makers supporting efforts at healthy lifestyles 221–5
 sedentary behaviors 212–13
 supporting and encouraging healthy behaviors 221
 see also parenting, ecology of
children, protection of 311–12
China 16, 89, 90, 91
circulatory disease 297
classification 3–5
clinical intervention and management 234–6
coalitions:
 innovative 323
 new 325–6
Coca-Cola 275, 276, 277–8, 326
Codex 290–1, 302
colon cancer 17
commercialization of childhood 321–2
Committee on the Prevention of Obesity in Children and Youth 268
Commonsense Consumption Act (Cheeseburger bill) 269
Commonwealth Finance Ministers Meeting 287
communities 119–23
Community Action Teams 320
community characteristics 217–18
community interventions and programs 245–8
Community Preventive Services Task Force 245–6
community-based approaches 136–7
composition standards for fat content 289
comprehensive approaches, necessity for 232–3
comprehensive programs 244–8
Congress (United States) 241, 267, 269, 319

Continuing Survey of Food Intake in Individuals 22, 59
convenience 312–13
coronary heart disease 175–8, 180–1, 190
cost of illness 17, 166–8, 173, 174, 179, 182, 191–2
 see also case study: estimating burden of disease and cost of illness
cost-benefit analysis 188
cost-effectiveness 165–98
 analysis 188
 economic literature review 168–74
 economics discipline contribution 165–7
 from evaluation to decision-making 197–8
 interventions for prevention 183
 interventions for treatment 183–90
 prediction: future trends 182–3
 see also case study: estimating burden of disease and cost of illness in Australia; incremental cost-effectiveness ratios
cost-minimization analysis 188
cost-utility analysis 188
counter-marketing 237–9
county-wide programs 247–8
courageous action, necessity for 307–28
 causes of obesity 309
 coalitions, innovative 323
 coalitions, new 325–6
 commercialization of childhood 321–2
 eating disorder and obesity concerns 313–14
 economic issues 322
 food industry and government, interaction with 323
 food industry and trust issues 314–20
 food and soft drinks in schools 322
 global priorities 321
 government structures, changing 323–4
 innovations, existing 326–8
 personal responsibility 310–11
 physical activity 321
 portion sizing 322
 protecting children and aiding parents 311–12
 quality versus quantity of food and health versus convenience 312–13
 schools 324–5
 social attitude change 321
Crete 16, 134, 159
cultural approaches 38–9, 139–40
 see also socio-cultural
customs duties 289
Czech Republic 11, 189

Dairy and Fluid Milk Acts 64
Denmark 10, 16
Department of Agriculture see United States
Department of Education (United States) 319
Department of Health and Human Services 22, 310

developing countries *see* food regulation in developing countries
diabetes 297–8, 310
  see also Type 2 diabetes
Diageo 276
diet 42–4, 57–8
Diet, Nutrition and the Prevention of Chronic Disease 276
dietary behaviors 143, 144
Dietary Guidelines for Americans 64, 241
dietary intake pattern 300–1
dietary shifts 77–89
  higher income developed world 77–83
  lower and middle income developing world 83–9
disability adjusted life year 168, 177–8, 181, 193, 194, 198
Disease Costing Methodology used in the Disease Costs and Impact Study 178, 179
domestic taxes 289–90
domestic-related physical activities 32–3
Dunkin Donuts 324

Eastern Mediterranean 13–14
eating:
  behaviors 209–10
  location 79
  occasions 82
ecological approach *see* children: ecological approach
Ecological Systems Theory 207–8
economic appraisal terminology 188
economic approaches 242–4
economic issues 322
Economic Research Service 25
edible oil 83
Edible Schoolyard Project 313, 326–7
educational strategies 236–9
Egypt 14, 90, 91
endometrial cancer 175–8, 180–1
energy expenditure 25–33
  domestic-related physical activities 32–3
  involuntary activity 26–7
  leisure time pursuits 27–30
  occupation-related physical activities 30–1
  transportation-related physical activities 31–2
energy intake 22–5
environment protection 326
environmental factors 55–69
  diet versus exercise 57–8
  exercise exposures, temporal trends in 62–3
  food supply 60–2
  information, temporal trends in 64–6
  trends in weight-related behavior 58–60
  and weight/weight-related behaviors 66–8
epidemiology: global perspective 3–18
  childhood obesity 15–16
  classification and fat distribution 3–5
  health consequences 16–18

  see also prevalence and trends in adults
Estonia 13
ethnicity 38–9
Europe 276
  epidemiology of obesity 3, 4, 9, 15, 16, 18
  nutrition transition 90
  obesity prevention 156
  prevalence and trends in adults 8–13
  socio-cultural factors 46, 47
  tobacco control experience 232
European Commmission 241
European Prospective Investigation into Nutrition and Cancer 10
evaluation issues 104–5
exercise 57–8
  exposures, temporal trends in 62–3
  see also physical activity

Fair Trading Decree 1992 289
family:
  -based approaches 135
  demographics 214
famine 76
  receding 76–7
fat:
  content 289
  distribution 3–5
  -free mass 26
  mass 26
fatty foods 299–301
  labeling requirements 290–1
  pricing controls 289–90, 296–7
  restriction of supply 288–9, 295–6
Federal Trade Commission 319, 323
Fiji 240, 289, 296
  Food Safety Act 2003 291
Finland 9, 10, 12
  see also North Karelia Heart Health Program
Five A's 234–5
Five R's 234
Five-A-Day for Better Health campaign 110, 115
Food and Agriculture Organization 58, 302
food availability 117–18
Food Balance Sheets 34
food collection 76
food disappearance data 24–5
Food Guide Pyramid 308
food industry, interaction with 323
food industry and trust issues 314–20
Food and Nutrition Service 237
Food Politics 273
food pricing 116–17
food promotion 118
food quality versus quantity 312–13
food regulation in developing countries 285–303
  development and implementation 301–2
  fatty foods, labeling requirements of 290–1
  fatty foods, pricing controls on 289–90, 296–7
  fatty foods, restriction of supply of 288–9
  fatty foods, restriction on supply of 295–6

food regulation in developing countries
   (Continued)
   labeling requirements 297
   Tonga 297–301
   World Trade Organization agreements 292–3
food and soft drinks in schools 322, 327–8
Food Standard 1.2.8 291
food supply 60–2
Food Supply Series (United States) 24–5, 33
Framework Convention on Tobacco Control 241, 242
France 10, 16, 43, 312
Frito-Lay 266, 275
fruit drinks 79
Fruit and Vegetable Environment, Policy and
   Pricing 243–4

gall bladder disease 17, 175–8, 180–1
General Agreement on Tariffs and Trade 268, 293–4
General Foods 272
Germany 39, 47, 277
   epidemiology of obesity 9–10, 13, 16
Ghana 289
Girls Health Enrichment Multi-Site project
   (GEMS) 135, 137
global priorities 321
Global Strategy on Diet, Physical Activity and
   Health 286
GO GIRLS! 137
gout 17
government:
   interaction with 323
   structures, changing 323–4
Greece 10, 16, 47
   Food Balance Sheets 34
   see also Crete
Grocery Manufacturers of America 317
grocery stores 121–2
gross national product 83–4, 90
Guide to Community Preventive Services 243
Guidelines for Use of Nutrition Claims 291
Gulf States 13

Halting the Obesity Epidemic 266, 269, 273
Harris-Benedict equation 26
Harvard Business Review 279
health consequences 16–18
Health and Human Services Department (United
   States) 267
Health Lifestyles and Prevention (HeLP) American
   Act 2004 269
Health and Nutrition Survey (China) 87
health versus convenience 312–13
healthful eating behaviors promotion *see*
   population approaches
healthful physical activity 144
Healthier US initiative 267

heart disease *see* cardiovascular; coronary; ischemic
Hershey 277
higher income developed world 77–83
   United States 78–83
House of Representatives (United States) 269, 279
Hunts Point Market 327
hypercholesterolemia 175–8, 180–1
hypertension 17, 175–8, 180–1, 190

Iceland 10
imports:
   bans on specific foods 288
   tariff or custom duties on 289
Improved Nutrition and Activity (IMPACT) Act
   269
incremental cost-effectiveness ratios 183, 188, 197
India 244, 326
information, temporal trends in 64–6
innovations, existing 326–8
Institute of Health and Welfare (Australia) 178
Institute of Medicine 65
   Committee on the Prevention of Obesity in
      Children and Youth 268
Institute of Medicine (United States) 93
International Diabetes Institute 15
International Obesity Task Force 15, 176–7
interventions:
   for prevention 183
   surgical 189–90
   for treatment 183–90
involuntary activity 26–7
ischemic stroke 175–8, 180–1
Italy 10, 13, 16, 26, 47, 158

Japan 3, 14–15, 43, 77
Jerusalem 159
Jordan 14
JP Morgan's European Equity Research 276

Kaiser Family Foundation 317
Kazakstan 13
kidney cancer 175–8, 180–1
Know Your Body program 159
knowledge 209, 210–11, 212
Kraft Foods 266, 275, 277
Kuwait 14

labeling requirements 290–1, 297
Latin America 90
Latvia 13
legislation 269–70
leisure time pursuits 27–30

life-course issues 144
Lifelong Improvements in Food and Exercise
    (LIFE) Act 269
lifestyle interventions 190
Lithuania 13
litigation 270–80
lower and middle income developing world 83–9
    animal source foods 84, 87
    caloric sweetener 83–4, 85
    edible oil 83
    physical activity 87, 89

M-SPAN 134
McDonald's 266, 276, 317
    see also Pelman vs. McDonald's
Malta 16
mass media 237–9
    campaigns 119–21
Masterfoods 277
Mauritius 160
media influences 218–19
    see also mass media
Medicaid 273
Medline 56
Metformin 189
Mexico 90, 91
Middle East 13, 14, 15, 61
Minnesota:
    Heart Survey 23, 59, 119, 160
    Leisure Time Physical Activity Questionnaire 59
modeling 209–10, 211, 212
MONICA study 8–9
Morocco 14, 90, 91
Mothers Against Drunk Driving 319–20
multiples of resting energy expenditure 28
Muslim societies 43
myocardial infarction 17

National Association for Sport and Physical
    Education (United States) 247
National Audit Office (United Kingdom) 16–17
National Cancer Institute (United States) 114,
    119–20
National Coalition for the Promotion of Physical
    Activity 247
National Conference of State Legislatures 270
National Health Interview Survey 27
National Health and Nutrition Examination Survey
    6, 22, 23, 24, 32, 33
    1999–2000 22
    I 22
    II 22
    III 16, 22
National Health Survey for England 34
National Human Activity Pattern Survey 28, 30, 33
National Institutes of Health (United States) 4

National Physical Activity Survey (Australia) 34
National School Lunch Program (United States)
    241, 319
National Soft Drink Association 318
National Strategy for the Prevention and Control of
    Non-Communicable Disease Workshop
    (Tonga) 298, 301
Nationwide Food Consumption Survey 22, 59
Nauru 15
Near East 15
Netherlands 9, 11–12, 16, 39, 43, 122
'New Moves' 132
New Zealand 3, 14–15, 47, 232
    food regulation 287, 291
Nigeria 289
non-communicable disease 285, 297, 298, 299,
    300–1, 302
    see also nutrition-related
North Africa 14, 90
North America 3, 6–8, 46, 250
    see also Canada; United States
North Karelia Heart Health Program (Finland)
    119, 160
Northern Africa 13
Norway 159, 290
nutrition claims 290–1
nutrition information panels 291
Nutrition Labeling and Education Act 121
nutrition and physical activity 21–34
    energy intake 22–5
    see also energy expenditure
nutrition transition 75–94
    burden shift towards poor countries 90–2
    causes of changes 92–3
    change: obesity shifts 90
    definition 75–7
    Stage 5 93–4
    see also dietary shifts
nutrition-related non-communicable disease
    77, 83

occupation-related physical activities 30–1
Oceania 14–15
Office of National Statistics 47
Office on Smoking and Health 245
One Per cent or Less campaign 119
organizational approaches 139–40
organizational characteristics 215–17
Orlistat treatment 189
osteoarthritis 17, 175–8, 180–1
ovarian cancer 17
Overeaters Anonymous 310

Pacific Island communities 43, 240, 287, 301
Papua New Guinea 15
Parent Teachers Association 320

parenting, ecology of 213–19
    child characteristics 214–15
    community characteristics 217–18
    family demographics 214
    organizational characteristics 215–17
    policy and media influences 218–19
parents as role models 219
partnership grants 247–8
Pathways 113–15
Patient-centred Assessment and Counseling for
    Exercise plus Nutrition (PACE+) 136
Pawtucket Heart Health Program 119, 160
Pelman vs. McDonald's 274–5, 276, 277, 279
PepsiCo 276, 277, 278, 326
personal level approaches 138–9
personal responsibility 310–11
Personal Responsibility in Consumption Act
    (Cheeseburger bill) 279–80
pharmacological interventions 183, 189
Philip Morris 277, 315
Philippines 47
physical activity 42–4, 82–3, 321
    children 210–12
    domestic-related 32–3
    lower and middle income developing world
        87–9
    occupation-related 30–1
    transportation-related 31–2
    see also nutrition and physical activity;
        population approaches to physical activity
        increase
physical environment 140–2
Pizza Hut 324
Planet Health 183, 237
Poland 11, 240
policy influences 218–19
politics 319–20
population approaches to obesity prevention
    153–62
    definition of obesity 153–4
    development of obesity 154–5
    prevention in adults 160–1
    prevention in youth 156–9
population approaches to physical activity increase
    129–46
    active transport approaches 137–8
    community-based approaches 136–7
    emerging issues and directions 142–5
    family-based approaches 135
    personal level approaches 138–9
    physical environment 140–2
    primary-care approaches 135–6
    school-based approaches 132–4
    social, cultural and organizational level
        approaches 139–40
    social ecological models 130–1
population approaches to promote healthful eating
    behaviors 101–23
    communities 119–23
    environmental interventions 115–18

population approaches to promote healthful eating
    behaviors *(Continued)*
    future research directions 123
    schools 111–15
    study design and evaluation issues 104–5
    theoretical conceptualizations 101–4
    worksites 105–11
portion sizing 79, 322
population attributable factors (PAFs) 175–77,
    179, 192
Pound of Prevention study 161
prevalence and trends in adults 6–15
    Australia, New Zealand, Oceania and Japan 14–15
    Eastern Mediterranean 13–14
    Europe 8–13
    North America 6–8
Preventive Services Task Force (United States) 236
primary-care approaches 135–6
processing of local foods 290
Produce for Better Health Foundation 119
production of local foods 290
prohibitions on domestic sale of specific foods 289
province-wide programs 247–8
PsycINFO 56
Public Health Advocacy Institute's Obesity Task
    Force 272
Public Health Law News 279
Public Health Service (United States) 234

quality adjusted life year 168, 183, 189, 191, 192
quota system 301

Reducing Tobacco Use 233
regulation 266–8
regulatory efforts 239–42
Resource Guide for Nutrition and Physical Activity
    Interventions 249
restaurants 121–2
resting energy expenditure 26
risk assessment 299
Ronald McDonald House 315
Ruby Tuesdays Restaurants 327
Russia 11, 34, 159

Safe Routes to School program 138
sale of local foods 290
Samoa 15
Saudi Arabia 14
Scandinavia 46
schools 111–15, 324–5
    -based approaches 132–4
    programs 236–7
    soft drinks and snacks 322, 327–8
sedentary behaviors 143–4, 212–13
Senate (United States) 269, 280

shaping 210, 211–12, 213
Sibutramine 189
Singapore 43, 232
'Small Steps' 310
social approaches 139–40
social attitude change 321
Social Cognitive Theory 102, 113, 114, 132–3, 142
social ecological model 130–1, 142–3
social justice 325–6
social roles and relationships 38
socio-cultural factors 37–48
    behavioral risk factors 40–1
    change 46–8
    ethnicity and cultural factors 38–9
    proposed model 44–6
    social roles and relationships 38
    socio-economic status 39–40
    variations in obesity-related behaviors 41–4
socio-economic status 41–3, 48, 66, 90
soft drinks 79
    and snacks in schools 322, 327–8
South Africa 90, 91, 240
South Korea 77, 277–8
South Pacific Consultation 287
Spain 10, 11, 16, 34
SPARK 158
Stanford Five Community Study 119, 160
Stanford Three Community Study 119, 160
State-Based Nutrition and Physical Activity
    Program to Prevent Obesity and Other
    Chronic Diseases 248, 249
state-wide programs 247–8
steady-state analysis 188, 191
Steering Committee 198
Steps to a Healthier United States 248, 267
stroke 17
    see also ischemic
study design 104–5
Sub-Saharan Africa 15
subsidies 290
Surgeon General 267, 268, 320
    Call to Action to Prevent and Decrease Overweight
        and Obesity, The 266–7, 272
    Reducing Tobacco Use 233
surgical interventions 189–90
survey findings 22–4
Sustainable South Bronx 327
Sweden 10, 16, 173
'Switch-Play' 133
Switzerland 10, 16

Table of Conditions for Nutrient Contents 291
tariffs 289
Task Force on Community Preventive Services
    (United States) 138–9, 249
Tate and Lyle 276
Team Nutrition initiative 237
Thailand 90, 91, 157

theoretical conceptualizations 101–4
threshold analysis 188, 191, 196
Time Magazine 310
tobacco control experience 231–50
    clinical intervention and management 234–6
    comprehensive programs 232–3, 244–8
    economic approaches 242–4
    educational strategies 236–9
    future directions 248–50
    regulatory efforts 239–42
Tobacco Institute 314
Tonga 286, 297–301
    National Strategy for the Prevention and Control
        of Non-Communicable Disease Workshop
        298, 301
top down change 319–20
transportation-related physical activities 31–2
trends:
    in weight-related behavior 58–60
    see also prevalence and trends in adults
Trying Alternative Cafeteria Options in Schools
    (TACOS) 116
Tunisia 14
Turkey 14
Type 2 diabetes 4, 17, 143–4, 175–8, 180–1, 189,
    190, 236

UBS Warburg 278
    Global Equity Research 276
United Kingdom:
    ecological approach 217
    epidemiology of obesity 8, 10, 16
    nutrition transition 77
    obesity prevention 156
    physical activity 134, 137
    socio-cultural factors 39, 43, 46–7
    tobacco control experience 241
United Nations 58, 292n
United States 265–80, 308, 309, 310, 311–12, 316,
    319, 323, 327
    Census Bureau 31–2
    Congress 241, 267, 269, 319
    cost-effectiveness of prevention 173, 174
    Department of Agriculture 22, 23, 60, 64, 275,
        308, 318, 319, 323
    Economic Research Service 25
    Food and Nutrition Service 237
    Nationwide Food Consumption Survey 59
    Department of Education 319
    dietary shifts 78–83
    ecological approach 212–13, 215–16, 218, 224
    environmental factors 55, 57–8, 60–6
    epidemiology of obesity 3, 6, 8, 16, 18
    Food and Drug Administration: Obesity Working
        Group 268
    food regulation 289, 290
    Food Supply Series 24–5
    Health and Human Services Department 267

United States *(Continued)*
  healthful eating behaviors 105, 111–12, 117, 119–21
  House of Representatives 269, 279
  Institute of Medicine 93
  legislation 269–70
  litigation 270–80
  National Association for Sport and Physical
    Education 247
  National Cancer Institute 114
  National Institutes of Health 4
  National School Lunch Program 241
  nutrition and physical activity 21–2, 26, 27, 28,
    29–31, 32–3, 34
  nutrition transition 77, 90, 91
  obesity prevention 156, 157, 159, 160
  physical activity 130, 132, 134, 135, 136, 138,
    141, 145
  Preventive Services Task Force 236
  Public Health Service 234
  regulation 266–8
  Senate 269, 280
  socio-cultural factors 38–9, 43, 47
  Task Force on Community Preventive Services
    138–9
  tobacco control experience 232, 240, 244, 245,
    247, 249
  Youth Risk Behavior Survey 242
Uzbekistan 13

VERB campaign 239
Vietnam 47

warning statements 291
weight/weight-related behaviors 66–8
Women Infants and Children (WIC) 319
Women's Healthy Lifestyle project 161
Working Well Trial 110
worksites 105–11
World Cancer Research Fund 79
World Health Assembly 241, 302
World Health Organization 15, 276, 317
  ecological approach 225
  environmental factors 58, 59, 65, 69
  epidemiology of obesity 3–4
  food regulation 294, 295, 302
  Global Strategy on Diet, Physical Activity and
    Health 286
  MONICA study 8–9
  tobacco control experience 240–1, 242
World Trade Organization 268, 286
  Agreement on Agriculture 292, 294,
    296, 297
  Agreement on the application of Sanitary
    and Phytosanitary Measures (SPS)
    292–3, 294
  Agreement on Technical Barriers to Trade (TBT)
    293, 294, 295, 297, 299
  food regulation 295, 296–7, 298, 301, 302, 303
  Secretariat 294

youth and obesity prevention 156–9
Youth Risk Behavior Survey (United States) 242
Yugoslavia 11, 47